POLITICS AND PUBLIC HEALTH IN REVOLUTIONARY RUSSIA, 1890–1918

THE HENRY E. SIGERIST SERIES
IN THE HISTORY OF MEDICINE

Sponsored by The American Association for the History of Medicine
and The Johns Hopkins University Press

The Development of American Physiology:
Scientific Medicine in the Nineteenth Century,
by W. Bruce Fye

Save the Babies:
American Public Health Reform
and the Prevention of Infant Mortality,
1850–1929,
by Richard A. Meckel

Politics and Public Health
in Revolutionary Russia, 1890–1918,
by John F. Hutchinson

POLITICS AND PUBLIC HEALTH IN REVOLUTIONARY RUSSIA, 1890–1918

John F. Hutchinson

THE JOHNS HOPKINS UNIVERSITY PRESS
Baltimore and London

© 1990 The Johns Hopkins University Press

Printed in the United States of America

The Johns Hopkins University Press
701 West 40th Street, Baltimore, Maryland 21211
The Johns Hopkins Press Ltd., London

The paper used in this publication meets the minimum requirements of American National
Standard for Information Sciences—Permanence of Paper for Printed Library Materials,
ANSI Z39.48-1984.

Library of Congress Cataloging-in-Publication Data

Hutchinson, John F.
    Politics and public health in revolutionary Russia, 1890–1918 / John F. Hutchinson.
        p.   cm.
    Includes bibliographical references.
    ISBN 0-8018-3957-2 (alk. paper)
        1. Medical policy—Soviet Union—History—19 century.   2. Medical policy—Soviet Union—
History—20th century.   3. Public health—Soviet Union—History—19th century.   4. Public
Health—Soviet Union—History—20th century.   5. Medical care—Soviet Union—History—
19th century.   6. Medical care—Soviet Union—History—20th century.   I. Title.
RA284.H87   1990
362.1′0947′09041—dc20   89-39102
                                                                                          CIP

To the memory of a superlative under-
graduate teacher, the late Ross Macdonald.
His kindness and generosity towards students, as well as the genial persistence
with which he aroused support for Russian
studies in Canada, will be remembered by
all who knew him. This book is a heartfelt,
though belated, tribute to his memory.

CONTENTS

ACKNOWLEDGMENTS

Most of the research upon which this book is based was carried out at the National Library of Medicine in Washington, D.C., and at the Slavonic Collection of Helsinki University Library in Finland. The costs of research were borne primarily by the Social Sciences and Humanities Research Council of Canada and its antecedent, the Canada Council; the indispensable support I received from these bodies is hereby gratefully acknowledged. Additional financial support came from the President's Research Fund at Simon Fraser University. Much of the first draft of the manuscript was written during the 1983–84 academic year, when I was Hannah Visiting Professor in the History of Medicine at the Institute for the History and Philosophy of Science and Technology at the University of Toronto. At a later stage in the project, Glendon College provided both a congenial environment and a splendid secretary, Marina Sakuta. Interlibrary loan (ILL) arrangements are an enormous boon to historians in search of rare items; I am delighted to be able to acknowledge the help I have received over the years, especially from the ILL and reference staffs of the Library of the Academy of Sciences in Leningrad, the Lenin Library in Moscow, the Slavonic Collection of Helsinki University Library, the Hoover Institution, the New York Public Library, the Slavic Reference Service of the University of Illinois, and, last but by no means least, Simon Fraser University.

During my research, I was fortunate in being able to draw upon the work of several other scholars, most obviously Nancy Frieden, but also Neil Weissman, Peter Krug, and William Gleason. Naturally, none of them bears any responsibility whatever for the use that I have made of their work.

Several individuals have provided the kind of advice, encouragement, and criticism that deserves special recognition here. John Keep has maintained a friendly, if somewhat bemused, interest in my admittedly eccentric migration from Duma politics to the alcohol problem and then to medical politics; his ability to ask the arresting question at the right moment has improved a hundred projects, this one included. Richard Stites and Peter Wiesensel provided companionship and encouragement during long sojourns in Helsinki, as did many Finnish friends, particularly Goran and Larisa Lindholm. On this side of the Atlantic, Sam Ramer, Neil Weissman, Susan Solomon, Bob Joy, Pauline Mazumdar, and Bert Hansen have all shared ideas, answered questions, supplied references, and generally exemplified collegiality at its best. My own colleagues at Simon Fraser have borne with a good grace my inordinate interest in what one of them invariably dismisses as "the history of drainage"; two in particular—Douglas Cole and Hugh Johnston—were especially helpful at moments when various gremlins seemed to be conspiring to prevent me from completing this study. The final version of the manuscript benefited considerably from careful readings by Edward Ingram and Frances Wasserlein. I am, of course, solely responsible for all errors of fact and judgment that remain.

In preparing the final manuscript I have had the assistance of Marion Mitchell, an expert at the word processor, and Linda Forlifer, a splendid copyeditor. The index was prepared by Michael K. Smith.

Parts of chapters 1 and 2 appeared in article form in *Jahrbücher fur Geschichte Osteuropas* 30 (1982): 37–53; I gratefully acknowledge the permission of Franz Steiner Verlag GmbH Wiesbaden to draw upon this copyright material. Other parts of these two chapters appeared in the *Journal of the History of Medicine and Allied Sciences* 40 (1985): 420–439; the permission of the editor to draw upon this material is also gratefully acknowledged. All illustrations courtesy of the Slavonic Collection of Helsinki University Library unless noted otherwise.

NOTE
ON TRANSLITERATION
AND DATES

Transliteration follows the Library of Congress system. A few Russian words, well known to English-speaking students of Russia, have been given in Anglicized form, for example, *zemstvos*, not *zemstva; Nicholas*, not *Nikolai II.*

Dates are given Old Style, that is, according to the Julian calendar in force in Russia until the reform of 1918. Dates are thus twelve days behind western Europe in the nineteenth century and thirteen days behind in the twentieth.

A glossary of Russian terms and acronyms follows.

GLOSSARY OF
RUSSIAN TERMS
AND ACRONYMS

CMSC	Central Medical Sanitary Council
duma, municipal	Elected city government
Duma, State	Elected legislative assembly (from 1906)
feldsher, feldsheritsa	Paramedic, either trained in a special school (*shkolnyi*) or given rudimentary instruction in the army (*rotnyi*)
gorodovoi vrach	Police physician
gradonachal'nik	City prefect
guberniia	Province
GUGZ	Main Administration for State Health Protection
jurisconsult	Legal adviser
kollegia	(Collegial) board
MRC	Military Revolutionary Committee
MVD	Ministry of the Interior
nachal'nik	Head, director
narodnik, narodnichestvo	Populist, populism
NKVD	People's Commissariat of Internal Affairs
NKZ	People's Commissariat of Health Protection
oblast'	Regional administrative unit
obshchestvennost'	Public spirit, community direction
otdel	Department, section
ozdorovlenie	Making healthier, more orderly
pirogovets, pirogovtsy	Member(s) of the Pirogov Society
prikaz	Bureaucratic office
raion	Large region or group of provinces
SEC	Sanitary-Executive Commission
SMK	Council of Medical Boards

soslovie, sosloviia	Estate(s)
SPMAS	St. Petersburg Physicians' Mutual Assistance Society
tsenzovaia Rossiia	Literally, "census Russia"; a shorthand term to describe those enfranchised in zemstvo, municipal, and (after 1906) national elections
uchastok, uchastki	Bailiwick(s)
uezd	District, subdivision of a *guberniia*
uprava	Administrative board
volost'	Township, subdivision of an *uezd*
vrach	Physician
VSPOV	All-Russian Alliance of Professional Associations of Physicians
VTsIK	Central Executive Committee (of the Congress of Soviets)
zemets, zemtsy	Member(s) of a zemstvo assembly or board; by extension, a partisan of zemstvo autonomy
zvanie	Occupational title

INTRODUCTION

From the Russian word for health, familiar to all those who ever raised a glass, *Na zdorov'e*, comes *ozdorovlenie*, the meaning of which is best conveyed in English by the neologism "healthification." This book is about *ozdorovlenie Rossii*, the "healthifying" of Russia. Its principal focus is on the two decades before the Bolshevik Revolution because it was during this period that the struggle to control the nature and direction of this process of "healthification" was at its height. It is important that readers appreciate from the outset that *ozdorovlenie* has two meanings, each of which is an integral part of the theme of the book: in addition to "healthifying," or "making healthy," *ozdorovlenie* carries with it the idea of "putting things into proper order." Inevitably, therefore, *ozdorovlenie* became a political and moral as well as a medical issue. Those who joined the campaign to make Russia healthy did so not only to rid the country of cholera or to reduce child mortality, but also to make whatever changes were necessary to ensure that premature death and preventable disease would never again take such a devastating toll. The struggle to make Russia healthy was, inescapably, a political struggle, not in the narrow sense of party politics but in the larger and ultimately more important sense of a struggle to control the place that the promotion of better health would play in the political economy of Russia.

The book thus belongs to a category of historical inquiry which the Germans, who pioneered it, have called *gesundheitspolitikgeschichte*, or the history of health politics and health policy. The leading exemplar of this genre was Alfons Fischer, whose magisterial *Geschichte des Deutches Gesundheitswesens*, though published in 1933, has yet to be rivaled, let alone superceded. English-language scholarship has created no equivalent term, but there are nevertheless several authors whose work falls into this category. Jeanne Brand's *Doctors and the State* and Rosemary Stevens' *American Medicine and the Public Inter-*

est are books concerned with many of the same issues as this one, despite their (respectively) British and American subject matter. True, neither Britain nor America—at least during the first two decades of the present century—experienced a revolution comparable to that which rocked Russia in 1917. Hence, I have found it useful to bear in mind several previous instances of the interplay between medicine, politics, and revolution: Philadelphia in the 1780s, Paris in the 1790s, and Frankfort in 1848, to choose examples only from the period after 1750. Doubtless, Benjamin Rush, P.-J.-G. Cabanis, and Rudolf Virchow never heard the Russian term *ozdorovlenie,* but each of them would certainly have appreciated the connection it drew between political revolution, the reform of medicine, and the improvement of health.

With this book I aspire to add something, however modest, to both these areas of scholarly concern. Those interested in the political economy of health will find in the Russian material a debate about the moral and political obligations of physicians which is especially interesting because it was shaped both by the ethical concerns of the Russian intelligentsia and by the influential position that public physicians occupied within the prerevolutionary profession. Those interested in the question of how revolutionaries deal with issues of health policy will find that the dynamics of 1917 lent not only an exceptional urgency but also an unusually revealing clarity to debates and decisions about the goals of health care and the role of physicians in a revolutionary society. Seen from the vantage point of *gesundheitspolitikgeschichte,* several unexamined assumptions about the incapacity of the tsarist regime and the tyranny of the Bolsheviks cry out for reassessment.

Having given the reader some idea of what this book is about, I will state explicitly what will not be found in these pages. In no sense is this a comprehensive history of Russian public health, still less of Russian medicine, during the revolutionary period. Although the reader may find here passing references to both these subjects, the richness and variety of early twentieth-century Russian medicine, as well as the enormous sanitary undertakings begun before 1917 and continued during the 1920s, deserve to be treated separately elsewhere. Each of these subjects, moreover, requires an approach substantially different from that adopted here to elucidate issues of medical politics.

Two broad but related themes dominate this book: one is the question of whether Russia ought to establish a ministry of health, a matter that became a public—and ultimately a political—issue in the late 1880s and remained one until resolved by the Bolsheviks' decision to create the Commissariat of Health Protection in July 1918; the other is the question of what form of organization—professional, political, or public—best suited the needs and objectives of Russia's physicians, a question that also dates from the 1880s and was resolved—some would say overwhelmed—by the advent of the Bolsheviks. These questions were related to each other because it was literally impossible to answer one of them without at the same time dictating the limits within which the other could be answered. Not all of those who were involved with these questions appreciated this relationship from the outset, but they soon came to recognize the interdependence of the issues.

Two groups of players, both claiming to be reformers of medicine and public health, occupy center stage in this drama: (1) medical bureaucrats and academics who sought to refurbish the reputation of the tsarist regime by demonstrating a fresh, enthusiastic, and efficacious concern for the health and productivity of its subjects, and (2) public or, as they liked to call themselves, community physicians, nearly all of whom shared the conviction that the tsarist autocracy was the principal obstacle in the path of those working towards a healthy Russia. The bureaucrats and academics were almost all to be found in St. Petersburg, in the higher reaches of the Ministry of the Interior and the Imperial Military-Medical Academy; the community physicians, on the other hand, could be found in the provinces of central Russia and in the headquarters of the Pirogov Society of Russian Physicians in Moscow.

Readers unfamiliar with late Imperial Russia deserve a word or two of explanation to help orient them to what might otherwise be unknown territory. The medical bureaucrats and academics they will meet here worked within a system of state medical administration which owed a good deal to the medical police traditions of the German states in the seventeenth and eighteenth centuries. The establishment of a medical collegium during the reign of Catherine the Great was part of eighteenth-century Russia's attempt to build what Professor Marc Raeff has called "the well-ordered police state." The administrative reforms of Alexander I, including the establishment of the Ministry of the Interior in 1802, were intended to regularize and, hence, to make more effective the central administration of the empire. After Russia's defeat in the Crimean War had proven that the tsarist regime could not survive without major alterations, Alexander II's reforms during the 1860s touched virtually every aspect of Russian life, most notably in the emancipation of the serfs. For our purposes, the most significant changes were those that altered local government and encouraged higher education.

In 1864, the regime established new institutions of local government—known as zemstvos—at the provincial and district levels and transferred to them responsibility for a variety of purely local functions, including road maintenance, schools, and public health. Composed of representatives of the estates (*sosloviia*) into which Russian society was legally divided, the zemstvos soon found that performing these tasks not only demanded the hiring of professional staff such as statisticians, teachers, and physicians, but also brought them into continuous conflict with the bureaucracy in St. Petersburg and its local agents. Those employed as zemstvo, or community (*obshchestvennye*), physicians in the 1870s and 1880s tended to be idealistic young people who had studied at Russian universities (and perhaps abroad as well) during the period of relative liberalism which marked the early years of the reign of Alexander II. Most often imbued with the political and moral values of Russian populism (*narodnichestvo*), they believed that they could demonstrate their concern for and benefit to the peasantry by endeavoring to meet the medical and public health needs of rural Russia. Hence, they began to create what soon came to be known as zemstvo medicine: a system of primarily rural medical and sanitary services which was funded out of government subsidies and zemstvo taxation but which, to encourage greater utilization by a populace ignorant of scientific medicine, was made available on a no-fee basis. By the end of the nineteenth century, Russia's community physicians were justifiably proud of the greater access to medical care that community medicine had achieved, although they were only too well aware of how much more remained to be done, particularly in the cities, where a municipal counterpart to rural zemstvo medicine had been somewhat slower off the mark.

It was no easy task to be a zemstvo physician, and those who undertook the work found that they needed all the support they could get. The local aristocracy, who dominated the zemstvo assemblies, suspected—not without reason—that their professional employees were political radicals who believed that the zemstvos themselves ought to be democratized to teach the people about political participation in a future free and democratic Russia. Often hemmed in or harrassed by their employers, zemstvo physicians also faced the hostility or indifference of the local tsarist bureaucrats, as well as the ignorance and suspicion of the peasants. Understandably, zemstvo physicians bolstered their self-confidence by holding frequent conferences, by meeting each other as often as possible, and by exchanging experiences and information through regular periodical publications. During the 1890s, they began to attend and soon effectively took over the only Russian medical society that even approximated to national standing, the Pirogov Society of Russian Physicians. Founded a decade earlier largely by academic physicians from St. Petersburg and Moscow, the Pirogov Society and its regular biennial congresses and monthly journal offered the zemstvo physicians a forum in which to praise their achievements and to call for the expansion and, if necessary, protection of Russian community medicine.

All scholars interested in the medical profession in tsarist Russia—none more so than I—owe a tremendous debt to Nancy Frieden, whose pathbreaking study, *Russian Physicians in an Age of Reform and Revolution, 1856–1905*, deservedly received wide praise when it was published in 1981. Her work is, and will remain, the definitive account of the development of zemstvo medicine in Russia. Her treatment of the government's creation of zemstvo medicine, of the often tense relations between physicians and the zemstvos, and of the underlying significance of professional issues provided solid foundations for our understanding of the whole subject. No doubt readers will recall the enormous emphasis that she placed on the establishment of an independent medical profession. Indeed, she implicitly encouraged the idea that the Anglo-American model of medical professionalization was applicable to Russia because so much of her work was a search for reasons why Russian developments failed to conform to this model. To be sure, Frieden conceded that Russian physicians were different, but only because circumstances forced them to be; according to her interpretation, the tsarist regime obstinately refused to allow physicians to achieve the degree of professional autonomy that was becoming the norm elsewhere, and consequently they found themselves too weak to do anything other than seek an accord with the Bolsheviks after 1917. Her approach left intact all of the principal western assumptions about the necessity for professional autonomy and the primacy of professional over political concerns.

In the sources that I consulted for the period after 1900, however, I found neither the same emphasis on the importance of establishing an autonomous medical profession nor the same unanimity about physicians' goals and how to achieve them. To be sure, Frieden herself noted in her epilogue that the period between 1905 and 1917 was marked by considerable disunity, but she left the impression that this was simply an understandable, if regrettable, consequence of tsarist obscurantism and bureaucratic abuse. By contrast, I have been struck by the fact that, among so many physicians dedicated to the cause of making Russia healthy, few believed that achieving this goal required the creation of a Russian version of the A.M.A or the B.M.A. The increase in medical knowledge, I have found, led not to greater unanimity but to more frequent squabbles among physicians. The issue of medical reform did not invariably pit an obscurantist regime against a profession that was uniformly in the forefront of scientific advance and resolute in its defense of local autonomy. Instead, one finds pioneers of medical innovation who sought more, not less, state control over physicians and reformers who, before October 1917, had already turned a deaf ear to the evangelists of local autonomy. Thus, where Frieden discerned only a lamentable disunity during the interrevolutionary period, I found striking evidence of ferment and creativity, attributable more to the growing sophistication and complexity of medical knowledge than to the machinations of the autocracy.

Believing that the first obligation of the historian is to tell a good story, I have attempted as far as possible to organize the material in the form of a straightforward narrative. However, the reader will find that, especially in the first four chapters, I have not kept to a rigidly chronological structure wherever it made sense to adopt a more topical approach. The first chapter presents a largely descriptive overview of what might be called "medical Russia" as the twentieth century began, a necessary prelude to understanding the medical-political aspects of the 1905 Revolution, discussed in chapter 2. The next two chapters examine the quite different responses to the events of 1905 on the part of, first, the community physicians and then the bureaucrats and academics. From July 1914 onwards, strict chronology is adhered to, with separate chapters devoted to the First World War, the period of the Provisional Government, and the Bolshevik Revolution. The reader will soon find, however, that two themes find their way into almost every part of the story: the first is the bacteriological revolution and its consequences and the second is the conflict between advocates of centralized administration and defenders of local autonomy.

One final point deserves mention. The question "What impact did the Russian Revolution have on medicine?" is loaded: it assumes that the role of medicine, and indeed of physicians, was responsive and passive, rather than dynamic and active. Such a formulation does not allow for the rich and complex medical politics that existed well before 1917 and that both affected and was effected by the events of that year. For these reasons, I have tried to avoid this question and have instead asked "What role did medical reformers and medical-political issues play in Revolutionary Russia?" Whether I have been able to provide a satisfactory answer to this question is a matter for others to judge.

POLITICS AND PUBLIC HEALTH IN REVOLUTIONARY RUSSIA, 1890–1918

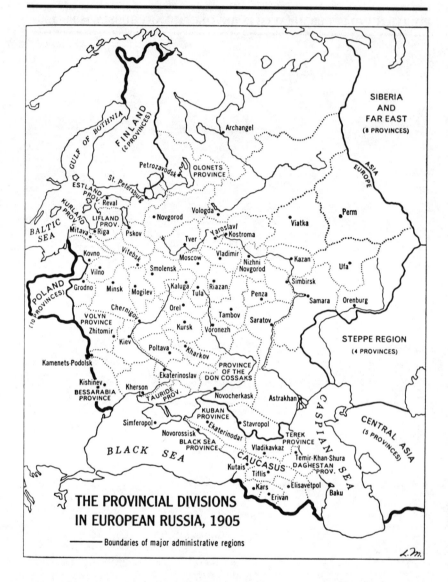

SIBERIA
AND
FAR EAST
(8 PROVINCES)

GULF OF BOTHNIA

FINLAND
(2 PROVINCES)

ASIA
EUROPE

Archangel

Petrozavodsk
OLONETS
PROVINCE

ESTLAND
PROV.
Reval
St. Petersburg

KURLAND
PROV.
LIFLAND
PROV.
Mitava
Riga
Pskov

BALTIC
SEA

Novgorod

Vologda

Viatka

Perm

Vitebsk
Tver
Yaroslavl
Kostroma

Kovno
Vilno

Moscow
Vladimir
Nizhni
Novgorod
Kazan

Ufa

POLAND
(10 PROVINCES)
Grodno
Minsk
Mogilev
Smolensk
Kaluga
Tula
Riazan
Penza
Simbirsk

Samara
Orenburg

Chernigov
Orel
Tambov
Saratov

VOLYN
PROVINCE
Zhitomir
Kiev
Kursk
Voronezh

STEPPE REGION
(4 PROVINCES)

Kamenets-Podolsk
Poltava
Kharkov

PROVINCE
OF THE
DON COSSAKS

Kishinev
Kherson
BESSARABIA
PROVINCE
TAURIDE
PROV.
Ekaterinoslav
Novocherkask
Astrakhan

CASPIAN SEA

CENTRAL
ASIA
(5 PROVINCES)

Simferopol
KUBAN
PROVINCE
Stavropol

Novorossisk
Ekaterinodar
BLACK SEA
PROVINCE
TEREK
PROVINCE

BLACK SEA
Vladikavkaz
CAUCASUS
Temir-Khan-Shura
DAGHESTAN
PROV.

Kutais
Tiflis

Kars
Elisavetpol
Baku

Erivan

THE PROVINCIAL DIVISIONS
IN EUROPEAN RUSSIA, 1905

———— Boundaries of major administrative regions

Reprinted, by permission, from Pushkarev, *The Emergence of Modern Russia, 1801–1917*. Courtesy estate of Robert H. McNeal.

1
MEDICAL RUSSIA AT THE DAWN OF THE TWENTIETH CENTURY

At the beginning of the twentieth century, the Russian Empire was an extremely unhealthy place in which to live. This was especially true of European Russia, bordered by the Polish provinces to the west, the Ural Mountains to the east, and the Caucasus to the south—precisely the area in which most of the empire's inhabitants lived.[1] The lamentable state of public health was a favorite theme of both liberals and socialists, who maintained that significant improvements were impossible under such a backward and inefficient form of government as the Russian autocracy. Opponents of the tsarist regime, however, were not alone in criticizing the state of public health in Russia; some of the most trenchant criticism came from those who had themselves risen to high office. In June 1901, for example, Professor N. A. Veliaminov of the Imperial Military-Medical Academy in St. Petersburg, Chief Physician of the Imperial Household and Medical Inspector of the Ministry of the Imperial Court, sent to the then Minister of the Interior a memorandum on the need for a thorough reform of medical affairs throughout the empire.[2] Despite his many high offices, Veliaminov did not mince words; the opening sentences of his memorandum serve as a revealing summary of the problems the empire was facing:

What is the sanitary state of Russia?—In comparison with the states of Western Europe, and even with our own Finland, it has to be admitted that it is dismal in the extreme: the percentage mortality of the population is very high, the average life expectancy is short, and there is a great amount of contagious, epidemic and endemic disease.

It is axiomatic that the degree of sanitary welfare in a state depends on the level of culture of the population and its economic well-being, but it is impossible nevertheless to deny the enormous importance of a correct, systematic organization of medical-sanitary supervision. This last is, *de facto*, almost absent among us in Russia. Not long ago, wealthy Moscow and the big cities

1

along the Volga presented themselves as model antisanitary centers; in some wealthy southern *gubernii* with excellent climatic conditions, Poltava and Ekaterinoslav for example, the children are dying off from contagious diseases (diphtheria), while in the poor northern *gubernii* of Finland, with the most severe climate, they have succeeded in lowering mortality to 17–18%; that is to say, amid poverty, they have achieved what we [usually] meet only in the most cultured countries, such as Sweden, Norway, Denmark, and England. To this day, wealthy Odessa has nothing to celebrate with regard to hospital affairs, since it has, alongside excellent private hospitals, a notoriously bad civic hospital, housed partly in old casemates [fortified vaults]; it is only because of confusion and the lack of firm leadership that years have gone by without any improvement in the state of this hospital. If we approach the capital city, we see that in Tsarskoselskii *uezd*, in which are located two of the Imperial residences, the zemstvo has not one hospital for contagious diseases; in the Mariinskii water system, where hundreds of thousands of the poorest working people gather in the summer, there was until last year no medical-sanitary supervision; and just outside the capital city itself, in Shlissel'burgskii and Novoladozhskii *uezdy*, endemic typhus persists. Finally, in the capital city itself, we meet such institutions as the Saint Nicholas Hospital for Lunatics, where up to 800 of the sick occupy places meant for 400, and where the absence of the most rudimentary hospital appliances and the care [provided] remind [one] of the middle ages. All of these examples clearly demonstrate that a whole series of our difficulties in the sphere of medicine and sanitation frequently do not depend on the shortage of funds, but are a direct consequence of the absence of competent control and strict regulation, of a systematic structure of medical-sanitary administration; in this vast and crucial field of activity, the absence of a directing force . . . is felt with particular sharpness . . . [another example of existing shortcomings is the fact that] in those moments in the life of the state when a display of speed, proportion, and intensity of actions is called for, we usually resort to extraordinary measures or to private assistance, almost [always] without the participation of the medical personnel of the Ministry of the Interior.[3]

The Russian state's institutions of medical administration were, Veliaminov went on to point out, obsolete; the legislation on which they were based dated from the first half of the nineteenth century.[4] While these structures were aging into paralysis, the face of Russia had been changed by the Great Reforms of the 1860s, the coming of the railway, the growth of industry, and the development of commercial ties with the Orient; furthermore, he noted, the dimensions of state involvement in health issues had been changed by the growth of community medicine in Russia and by the sanitary reform movement that had enjoyed such successes in western Europe during the middle decades of the nineteenth century.[5]

One did not have to be a St. Petersburg professor to see the problems so clearly. Veliaminov's recitation of shortcomings was echoed every day in the minds of hospital interns, factory doctors, sanitary reformers, and rural midwives who frequently felt themselves overwhelmed by the sheer magnitude of the task of making Russia into a healthy country. Of course, the poverty and ignorance of the masses were the primary obstacles to be overcome, but many a factory or municipal physician could have corroborated Veliaminov's claim that the indifference of the wealthy and the lack of firm civic leadership had helped to make Russian cities and factories among the most unhealthy places in early twentieth-century Europe. Indeed, one had to go all the way to Dublin, on the western periphery of Europe, to find another major city in which epidemic disease took such a high annual toll as it did in St. Petersburg.[6]

To agree on a solution to the problem was, however, a great deal more difficult. Few of those involved in day-to-day medical and sanitary work among the Russian people shared Professor Veliaminov's optimistic belief that improvements could be made simply by introducing more systematic organization and regulation. Their skepticism derived not from ignorance of experience elsewhere—indeed, many Russian physicians knew about and admired what had been done in England and Germany in recent decades—but rather from a deepseated conviction that St. Petersburg bureaucrats, notorious for their untrustworthiness and incompetence, would simply botch any attempt to improve the existing state of affairs. In reality, the manifest failings of the bureaucracy were more often attributable to ignorance than to malevolence. Despite the conviction of many members of the intelligentsia, physicians included, that Russia was overgoverned, the opposite was in fact closer to the truth. A chronic lack of understanding of local conditions and aspirations was apparent in the stream of laws, rules, and instructions that constantly flowed from St. Petersburg only to provoke doubt, despair, ridicule, and occasionally rage on arrival at their destination.[7]

Admittedly, the government's record in the field of public health scarcely inspired confidence. The central government had sloughed off responsibility for public health and medical assistance at the local level onto the zemstvo institutions that had been created in 1864 to make up the void in local government caused by the emancipation of the serfs.[8] An indication of the extent of the government's concern is the fact that zemstvo expenditures for health and medicine were categorized as "optional," whereas expenditures for police and law enforcement were "obligatory." Zemstvo and municipal governments nonetheless became increasingly involved in health and sanitation and devoted a growing proportion of their budgets to hospitals, medical care, hygiene education, and the collection of health statistics. Little of this activity brought them plaudits from St. Petersburg; instead, they were berated for exceeding their proper jurisdiction, for hiring politically unreliable professional personnel, and for trying to create a role for themselves outside the state's bureaucratic structure. In 1890 and 1892, respectively, a new Zemstvo Statute and new Municipal Statute restricted the electorate, budgets, and pretensions of these local institutions. The government of Tsar Alexander III had shown itself to be no friend of local autonomy or of the aspirations of Russia's small but growing body of zemstvo professionals—among whom were physicians and various ancillary medical personnel. The terrible famine of 1891/92 and the ensuing cholera epidemic of 1892/93 provided chillingly conclusive evidence that the Russian government was considerably better at exacerbating than relieving the country's health problems.[9] Zemstvo physicians, who constituted an increasingly vocal one-fifth of all medical practitioners in the land, resolved in the wake of those terrible years to do everything they could to reduce the role and influence of the central government in local medical affairs. As a result, they firmly and successfully opposed a projected hospital statute that would have tied zemstvo hospitals and their staffs more closely to the state bureaucracy. By the end of the 1890s, the community physicians, as the zemstvo and municipal physicians called themselves, now the dominant group in the prestigious Pirogov Society of Russian Physicians, were moving—in the words of Nancy Frieden—"from social reform to political activism."[10]

THE CENTRAL MEDICAL ADMINISTRATION
Veliaminov, a proponent of administrative reform, naturally saw the situation from a quite different perspective. The burden of his criticism, apparent in the passage quoted above, was simply that *no one was in charge*—in matters concerning the health of the civilian population, no one official or institution was in effective control, either in St. Petersburg or throughout the country—and that many of the problems could have been reduced or averted by firm and purposeful leadership. To be sure, when it was a question of the health of soldiers or sailors, there was no administrative vacuum or confusion: both the army and the fleet had their own chief medical inspectors, responsible to the Ministers of War and the Navy, respectively, for the health of the troops, the state of the hospitals, and the careers of the medical personnel under their command. In the civil medical sphere, by contrast, all was confusion, overlap, disorder, and inefficiency. Virtually every important ministry maintained a medical establishment of some sort: health in schools came under the Ministry of Public Instruction; in prisons, under the Main Prison Administration, in factories and at

border crossings, under Finance; on railways and steamships, under Ways and Communications; on state lands, under Agriculture and State Domains; on the estates of the imperial family, under the Imperial Court, and so on. One of the largest civil medical establishments came under no ministerial authority: the Medical Department of the Institutions of the Empress Marie, which ran scores of hospitals and medical charities, was a part of the tsar's Imperial Chancellery.

To be sure, the law stated that there *was* a supreme head of civil medical affairs and described the Director of the Medical Department of the Ministry of the Interior (MVD) as "the General Staff Doctor of the Civil Branch,"[11] but the realities of tsarist government made such a grand title no more than a cruel joke. Not only could this official not direct the plethora of medical administrative offices outside of control of the MVD; he did not even run most of his own ministry's medical establishment. He was only an *ex officio* member of the Medical Council, which he could neither convene nor manage; he was only nominally the superior of the provincial and city medical inspectors, who were much more closely tied to their immediate superiors, the governors and *gradonachalniki;* he had no direct connection with physicians in government, zemstvo, or municipal service, exercised neither administrative supervision nor medical leadership over most of the empire's hospitals, and played no significant role in sanitary activities, which were increasinly under the control of zemstvos and municipalities. In reality, this "General Staff Doctor of the Civil Branch" dealt largely with forensic medical business, supervised prostitutes and apothecaries (both regulated by the state but obviously for different reasons), gathered statistics, ran the chancellery, and published a journal.[12] As Veliaminov pointed out, compared to the Medical Inspectors of the Army and the Fleet, the Director of the MVD's Medical Department was "neither a superior officer, nor a leader, nor an administrator, but a completely unknown quanity."[13]

There was an equally wide gulf between the actual role played by the Interior Ministry's Medical Council and its description in law as "the supreme scholarly medical body for reviewing questions regarding the protection of public health, the healing arts [*vrachevanie*], and forensic medical expertise."[14] Composed about equally of senior bureaucrats from many ministries and distinguished figures in academic medicine (in practice mostly professors from the Imperial Military-Medical Academy), the Medical Council was an advisory body whose advice was regularly ignored by everyone in government. Its president, although usually a distinguished medical figure, was an unpaid, part-time official without a staff; the council itself could neither initiate nor execute policy; consequently, ministers and senior Petersburg bureaucrats paid little attention to its deliberations. Its so-called indispensable members were busy officials from other ministries who rarely attended, whereas its advisory members—leading lights in the St. Petersburg medical establishment—either found its proceedings too boring to bother with or enjoyed the unique atmosphere of irresponsibility which marked its proceedings. For a brief moment in the 1880s, the Medical Council emerged from obscurity when a commission that it sponsored, headed by the eminent clinician S. P. Botkin, recommended that Russia set up a powerful central administrative agency to direct public health affairs.[15] This proposal aroused so much controversy, particularly among physicians, that during the next decade— despite the famine and cholera epidemic—the Medical Council lapsed back into its customary somnolence. Thus, by 1901, Veliaminov (one of its members) could state in all honesty that the council "has gradually lost its prestige and its significance, both in the eyes of state figures, and in the eyes of the medical world."[16]

The government itself tacitly admitted the failings of the existing medical administrative institutions in the late 1890s, when it set up a Special Commission for Measures against Plague. One might have thought this was the moment for giving serious consideration to Botkin's call for a centralized ministerial agency, but the imperatives that produced this special commission were quite different.

The experience of the cholera epidemic of 1892/93 pointed to the need for coordinated action involving all provinces and cities in the threatened region, but significant obstacles stood in the way. Joint action by the zemstvos in the affected provinces, although perhaps desirable from a strictly medical point of view, was politically out of the question, both because it would have involved permitting them to do something presently forbidden (holding regional or national congresses) and because it would have encouraged the aspirations of those who regarded the zemstvos as quasi-popular representative institutions separate from the state bureaucracy. A centralized government agency, such as had been proposed by the Botkin commission, was also out of the question because, to be effective, it would have had to trample upon the jealously guarded terrain of almost a dozen ministries, not least that of the powerful MVD itself. Moreover, the problem of finding a director for such an agency was almost insurmountable: to put a medical expert in charge was too great a concession to specialized knowledge, whereas not to do so virtually ensured rivalry and even conflict at the top administrative levels. What was required, then, was a response to the threat of epidemics that would satisfy critics of government inactivity, leave intact the powers and jurisdiction of all existing ministries and departments, and provide additional funds for antiepidemic measures while keeping both physicians and zemstvos in their places. The Special Commission for Measures against Plague filled all these requirements admirably.

Virtually the Committee of Ministers meeting under another name, the Antiplague Commission (as it soon came to be called) received petitions from local institutions in affected or threatened areas and allocated funds at its own discretion in response to those petitions. This process left initiative at the local level, encouraged each area to act on its own, and ensured that there would be vast discrepancies in the scope, nature, and effectiveness of antiepidemic measures from one locality to another. For Nicholas II, genuinely moved by the suffering that epidemics caused among his people, the illusion of activity by his government was sufficient: if he did not trust all his ministers completely, he nevertheless preferred their advice to the uniformly negative criticism of zemstvo physicians. Ministers and senior bureaucrats had nothing whatever to fear from the Antiplague Commission because they controlled its every move. Provincial and district zemstvos and their medical personnel were forced to go to the commission as supplicants, there to compete with each other for limited funds allocated by officials with no understanding of the problems involved in fighting epidemics. A triumph of tsarist statesmanship, the commission circumvented the political problems that the management of epidemics presented to the governance of Russia. That the commission was an ineffective response to the epidemics themselves was of little concern to anyone except physicians and potential victims of plague and cholera.[17]

If the tsar's ministers were less than lukewarm about establishing a ministry of public health, so also were the majority of Russia's community physicians, albeit for entirely different reasons. At the Second Pirogov Society Congress in 1887, participants agreed that the setting up of an agency such as that proposed by the Botkin commission was an enormously complex question that required thorough analysis and discussion,[18] but for almost a decade the idea was pursued no further. When it was raised again at the Sixth Congress in 1896, there was a sharp clash between the principal advocate of a ministry, A. L. Eberman, Director of the Imperial Philanthropic Society's hospital in St. Petersburg, and the most distinguished of the scheme's opponents, F. F. Erismann, Professor of Hygiene at the University of Moscow and one of the architects of the zemstvo medical services of Moscow province.[19] Erismann did not go as far as some of his followers, who charged Eberman with seeking ministerial office for himself, but he did state firmly what was to become Pirogov Society dogma on this issue: that it was entirely because of the zemstvos that Russian public health was improving and that to encourage the involvement of the government and its administrative officials would stop further growth and probably undo the progress that had been made thus far.[20]

Like S. Iu. Witte, the Minister of Finance who tried to persuade Nicholas II that zemstvo institutions were incompatible with autocratic government, Erismann believed that zemstvo medicine was incompatible with the formation of a ministry of public health. Nevertheless, the 1896 congress commissioned the Pirogov Society executive to canvas opinion on the issue among local medical societies and zemstvo medical-sanitary councils and offices and to report the results to the next congress in 1898.[21]

Dr. Eberman, a tireless campaigner for causes in which he believed,[22] decided to steal a march on the Pirogov Society by securing the widest possible support for the plan to create a ministry even before the idea was discussed at the next Pirogov Congress. He had several arguments for setting up a separate ministry: first, that the vastness of the Empire demanded central direction; second, that the MVD already had too many responsibilities to give health the attention it deserved; third, that both state and society would benefit from a healthier and more productive population; and fourth, that physicians' lives would be made easier because both their patients and the environment in which they lived would become healthier. Lest this mixture of geopolitics, pragmatism, neomercantilism, and professional self-interest not to be everyone's taste, Eberman was careful to specify that the new agency would regulate zemstvo and muncipal medical affairs only according to criteria agreed in advance by both representatives of local government and the physicians in their employ.[23] In January 1897, he put his arguments before the St. Petersburg Medical Society, which endorsed them unanimously, commended them to other medical societies, and created a committee (headed by Eberman) to work out a fuller and more detailed report on the subject. A copy of the full report was sent to the Pirogov Society executive, and an outline of its contents appeared in the society's *Journal* early in 1898.[24]

The Pirogov Society's executive refused to climb onto Eberman's bandwagon. The threat to zemstvo medicine was not the only reason for its hesitation: the question of a new ministry was arousing all kinds of controversy in both the general and the medical press.[25] Even its supporters argued about the reasons for having such a ministry, about its field of jurisdiction, about its structure, and about whether it should be headed by a physician. No aspect of Eberman's proposal was more controversial than his argument that a ministry was in the best corporate interests of the profession as a whole. Critics found this claim at best premature and at worst wrong-headed. Before the next Pirogov Congress, K. I. Shidlovskii, a member of the Society's executive, delivered a strong condemnation of the proposal in the Pirogov *Journal,* pointing out that Eberman's report was entirely one-sided in presenting only the case *for* a ministry and hence was a long way from the thorough analysis that had been called for in 1896.[26] Shidlovskii found it reprehensible that anyone should advocate such a step on the selfish grounds that it would enhance the interests of the medical estate and concluded with a ringing endorsement of the need for a decentralized structure to preserve and develop the institutions of community medicine. Perhaps not surprisingly in the wake of such a pointed condemnation, the 1899 congress refused to endorse not only Eberman's proposal but also the idea of the ministry of health in any form.[27] Ironically, the hostile attitude of the community physicians enabled bureaucrats who had their own reasons for opposing a health ministry to argue that the idea found little favor among the medical profession and hence should be dropped.

PLANS AND REORGANIZATION

The *pirogovtsy* were wrong about Eberman: anyone who cherished the ambition of becoming Russia's top medical official would have chosen a less public route by which to promote his interests. One such was Court Medical Inspector Veliaminov, who thought he saw his chance for personal advancement when the presidency of the Medical Council fell vacant in January 1901. Six months later, Veliaminov sent to Interior Minister Sipiagin the lengthy memorandum already referred to at the beginning of this chapter.[28] The greater part of the memorandum was devoted to outlining Veliaminov's plans for reform, which included both a revitalized and professionalized Medical Council and the transformation of the MVD's Medical Department into a powerful and efficiently organized main medical administration (an agency of quasi-ministerial status and powers).[29] Concluding with a twenty-two-point program of work to be undertaken as soon as possible, Veliaminov appealed to Sipiagin "to appoint one person Director of the [existing] Medical Department *and* President of the Medical Council, to confer on him at this point the rights of a Head [*nachal'nik*] of a Main Administration and Minister, and to allot him a certain period of time in which to put before [you] . . . the full proposal for organizing the main Medical Administration, so that it can be brought into existence by the customary legislative route."[30]

Veliaminov was not gauche enough to suggest himself for the job, but he narrowed the field by arguing that it would be inappropriate to choose someone whose specialty was anatomy, physiology, chemistry, or pathology because such work "has nothing in common with real-life medical and sanitary affairs."[31] Moreover, he stressed the need to make the head of the civil medical administration into as powerful a figure as the medical inspectors of the army and the fleet and noted that he himself had reformed the Court Medical Department along similarly hierarchical lines to maximize his own authority as inspector.[32] Sipiagin was not noted for his acumen, but he would have had to be dull indeed not to recognize Veliaminov's memorandum as a manifesto combined with a job application.[33]

Veliaminov's eagerness for higher office did not prevent him from putting his finger on the weaknesses in the existing arrangements (they do not deserve to be called a "system") for medical administration. Three aspects of his plans for reform are particularly noteworthy. First of all, he recognized that the Medical Department needed to be given more clout both within the MVD itself and in relation to other ministries and departments. Hence his plan to raise the department to a main administration and its head to the status of a deputy minister; hence his desire to limit the role of the Economic Department by making questions of medical economics (especially hospital budgets) subject to joint agreement before putting proposals before the minister; hence also his plan to require representatives of other ministries to attend general meetings of a reorganized Medical Council, presided over by the head of the Main Medical Administration, to discuss general issues of health and sanitation which affected areas of public administration beyond the immediate jurisdiction of the MVD. Second, Veliaminov understood the extent to which the existing administration was weak precisely because it had so little to do with what actually went on in the rest of Russia. Hence his determination that the power to hire and fire local medical inspectors should reside with the new head of the Main Medical Administration, rather than with the provincial governors or *gradonachal'niki*; hence his desire to make the head into a real boss who would visit the provinces, convene congresses of medical inspectors, hold conferences on particular issues, and inspect public hospitals; hence his wish to establish, through the local inspectors and the use of special emissaries (*chinovniki osobykh poruchenii*)[34] regular and direct contact with the medical councils, hospitals, and sanitary bureaus of provincial zemstvos. Third, Veliaminov appreciated, largely from his own experience, that the existing Medical Council wasted everyone's time and accomplished nothing of significance. Hence his desire to put it under the direct control of the head of the Main Medical Administration and to professionalize its operations by increasing its staff and employing advisory experts;[35] hence his ingenious plan to put all of its MVD business in the hands of a committee of six specialists[36] who would be paid and work full-time, while requiring its ex officio members to attend only occasional general meetings to deal with wider issues; hence his insistence that the medical establishments of every other ministry or department should be required to make an annual report to the Medical Council and that the council's president should make an annual report to the tsar.

Veliaminov's reform plan was much shrewder and more carefully thought out than Eberman's proposal; if the Pirogov Congress had known of its contents, it might have recognized that here, in these plans to centralize in St. Petersburg effective control over local medical administration, lay a potentially grave threat to zemstvo medicine and local autonomy. Nevertheless, Veliaminov's plan was bound to carry little weight with the minister, on whom such insight was lost; Sipiagin preferred nobles over professionals in the civil service and wanted to strengthen the administrative role of the governors in the provinces rather than the bureaucrats in St. Petersburg.[37] Deaf to Veliaminov's plea for a double appointment, Sipiagin simply left the presidency of the Medical Council vacant, and so it remained when he was felled by a terrorist's bullet on 1 April 1902. Two days later, V. K. Plehve was appointed Minister of the Interior. Plehve was to hold the position for an even shorter time than Sipiagin—he was assassinated on 15 July 1904—but during his brief tenure was to reorganize the ministry in such a way as to decrease even further the already low priority accorded to matters of public health, and physicians' views about them, within the government of Russia.

Plehve's plans for reorganizing his ministry centered on enhancing the stature within it of the Economic Department, so that it could take charge of relations with the governors, whose powers at the local level he, like Sipiagin, was determined to strengthen.[38] A foretaste of the new approach came only days after Plehve's appointment, when the Economic Department, acting entirely on its own and with no prior discussion with the Medical Department, sent a circular to all provincial governors asking them to comment on various proposals aimed at more effective administrative supervision over zemstvo and municipal medicine.[39] The current director of the Medical Department, L. F. Ragozin, who believed that physicians knew more about medicine than did bureaucrats, was unlikely to accept the growth of the rival Economic Department,[40] so Plehve speedily moved him to the vacant presidency of the Medical Council.[41] To replace him as Director of the Medical Department, Plehve chose one of the rising stars among St. Petersburg bureaucrats, V. K. von Anrep, a physician-administrator whose varied career included several positions in medical education as well as educational administration.[42] Von Anrep became ex officio a member of the Medical Council, so he and Ragozin had an institutional base of sorts from which to mount a counterthrust against the Economic Department.

Throughout 1903, a committee of the Medical Council chaired by

Ragozin worked on a new statement of the council's powers and duties.[43] The most important change proposed by the committee would have made it obligatory for all government departments, inside or outside the MVD, to submit any measure affecting medicine or sanitation to the Medical Council for its approval *before* the measure began to travel the usual legislative route. Other changes aimed at strengthening the council by increasing its budget, providing it with paid expert assistance, and establishing a research laboratory under its control. However, when the draft statute (*polozhenie*) was approved in March 1904, the scope of these changes was modified considerably:[44] only departments within the MVD were required to submit proposals for preliminary review by the council; other ministries and departments were to do so *only if they chose*, a concession that effectively destroyed any hope that the council's authority would extend to all government agencies. Although the new statute seemed to enhance the council's position *within* the MVD, this proved an illusory gain: other changes in the structure of the ministry left senior medical administrators virtually powerless.

The same session of the State Council which approved the new Medical Council Statute also approved two related and far more significant changes: the transformation of the old Economic Department into a main administration for local economic affairs and the transformation of the old Medical Department into a main administration of the chief medical inspector.[45] Although these changes nominally enhanced the status of both departments, the reality was that the Economic Department gained not only what the Medical Department lost but a great deal more besides. The new Main Administration for Local Economic Affairs was given jurisdiction over zemstvo and municipal economic affairs, roadbuilding, firefighting, insurance, public charity, and *local medical and sanitary affairs*. The chief medical inspector's office was left with the registration and inspection of medical personnel and, at least in theory, with "sanitary affairs of general state significance,"[46] although in practice this boiled down to antiepidemic measures, already the province of the Antiplague Commission (whose existence and role was ignored in all these changes within the MVD). The net effect of these changes was to ensure that the central medical administrative institutions would remain isolated from and irrelevant to the governance of Russia at both the national and the local level.

Ragozin and von Anrep were kept in the dark about the planned changes until, a few days before they were to be considered by the State Council, a copy of the proposal arrived—by accident—at the Medical Council. The council hastily conveyed both its outrage at having been bypassed and its unfavorable assessment of the proposed changes, which it found wrong-headed on two counts: on the one hand, local medical and sanitary affairs were to become the responsibility of an agency that had neither medical personnel directing it nor access to specialized knowledge; on the other hand, the trained medical personnel in the main administration of the chief medical inspector were made responsible primarily for matters of supervision and observation, "nine-tenths of which do not demand specialized knowledge."[47] Concluding that the proposal would in fact only multiply the shortcomings already apparent throughout the country, the council reiterated its conviction that all public health matters should be under the jurisdiction of an autonomous agency within the MVD run by specialists in medicine and sanitation.[48] In the medical press, the typical reaction to Plehve's changes was to claim that the bureaucrats were trying to exclude physicians from an effective say in public affairs at the national level, just as they were already trying to exclude them at the local level.[49]

Even before Plehve's assassination, his plans for reforming the provincial administration had run into difficulties: predictably, they aroused opposition both from other ministries, which disliked his plan to transform governors into powerful local agents of the MVD, and from the partisans of zemstvo autonomy, who correctly realized that a decentralized administration run by the MVD was an even greater threat than a bureaucracy that was, in the words of Edward M. Judge, "overcentralized, ill-informed, and unco-ordinated."[50] Nevertheless, Plehve's reorganization of the MVD itself proved to be enduring, bedeviling the efforts of would-be medical reformers for more than a decade. In an early Russian variant of *Catch-22*, plans to create a ministry of health now had to originate within agencies subordinate to the MVD, which in turn was strong enough to ensure that every obstacle would be placed in the way of realizing such plans.

LOCAL PUBLIC HEALTH ADMINISTRATION

The administration of public health at the local level was such a shambles that it almost defies description. As always, the tsar's local representative, the provincial governor or city *gradonachal'nik*, was theoretically omnipotent; he could give orders through the medical department (*vrachebnoe otdelenie*) on all aspects of medicine, sanitation, and public health. In practice, however, both his jurisdiction and his role were considerably more limited. For one thing, the same administrative diversity that prevailed in St. Petersburg also existed in the provinces, so that a governor had no real authority over matters of health in, for example, schools, railways, or prisons unless accorded it by the appropriate ministry. Moreover, the supervisory responsibilities of *guberniia* medical departments were so extensive that in practice many of them had to be ignored because of the shortage of personnel

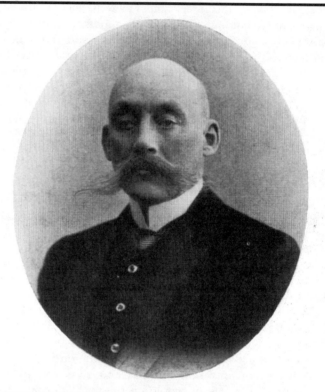

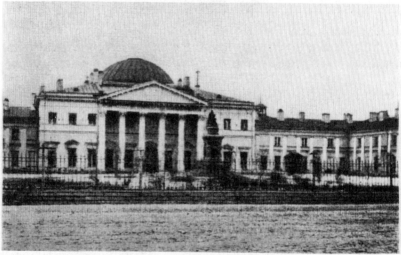

Fig. 1. Two pillars of the St. Petersburg medical establishment: Court Medical Inspector N. A. Veliaminov *(top)* and the Imperial Military-Medical Academy *(bottom)*.

and resources.[51] The medical inspectors were almost completely taken up with registering and monitoring local physicians, feldshers, and pharmacists, while the lower ranks of the government medical service—rural *uezd* and urban *gorodovoi* physicians—were preoccupied with the police and forensic medical work associated with crime, injury, death, and insanity. As a result, hospitals operated under little or no governmental supervision, foods and beverages were monitored only when there was a crisis, and little was done to raise the generally abysmal level of public understanding about personal hygiene and contagious disease. Indeed, it was largely because the administrative agencies did so little in the field of public health that many zemstvos went beyond providing elementary medical care to the rural population and began to pursue local sanitary improvements and to engage in popular hygiene education.[52] However, the resources, personnel, and enthusiasm that zemstvos were prepared to devote to public health work varied from province to province and even from district to district. In any case, many of the problems demanded concerted action at the regional or national level, something that the government was determined to prevent in order to contain the aspirations of zemstvo liberals, who hoped to create an alternative to, if not a replacement for, the existing government.

Jurisdictional confusion was only part of the problem, however: an equally significant obstacle to improvement was the fact that the government controlled the police, who were the only means of enforcing policy. Zemstvos and municipalities were legally empowered to regulate standards of cleanliness for public places, commercial and industrial institutions, and private homes; to ensure pure food and water supplies; and to prevent or eliminate epidemic or contagious diseases. Many zemstvos approved such regulations, but they depended on the police to enforce them. In any case, a new regulation required the approval of the governor or *gradonachal'nik*, who could refuse to endorse it for any number of reasons or insist on its being reviewed, either by the provincial administration or by officials in St. Petersburg.[53] In the end, whether these regulations were enforced depended not only upon the approval of the governor, but also upon the zeal of physicians in the government medical service, who might report violations or warn offenders, and ultimately upon the local police, who alone had the power to lay charges in cases where sanitary regulations had been contravened. The police did not, of course, see themselves as agents of the zemstvo and still less of zemstvo sanitary bureaus, so they were unlikely to take much interest in such matters unless encouraged to do so by local administrative officials. On the other hand, the police were empowered by their own regulations "to protect the salubrity of inhabited areas and to deal with anything harmful to public health,"[54] so they might well act without reference to zemstvo sanitary regulations. No matter what Russian liberals liked to think, the zemstvos' dependence on the tsarist police helped to make them almost indistinguishable in the popular mind from other organs of state administration.[55]

At the bottom of the apparatus of local medical administration stood the inspectors and the government's *uezd* and *gorodovoi* physicians. The capital city of St. Petersburg boasted no fewer than three inspectors: one, with a small staff, directed the provincial medical administration; another, with a staff of almost thirty, ran the much larger city medical administration; a third, operating out of the office of the *gradonachal'nik*, directed the special medical-police administration that was charged with supervising prostitution in the capital city. In Moscow, arrangements were somewhat different: the city and provincial administrations were united in one office run by a *nachal'nik* assisted by an inspector, whereas the medical-police administration was run by a staff of twenty-six police doctors who worked in the office of the chief of police. As might be expected, salaries in the big cities were high: the *nachal'nik* in Moscow earned 3,600 rubles annually, the St. Petersburg city inspector 3,100 rubles, and the other inspectors about 2,500 rubles.[56] The city of Warsaw had its own medical administration, and in 1902 Odessa was also accorded this special status, belated recognition of its population growth, industrial development, and location in the epidemiological danger zone of southern Russia.

In rural Russia, the administrative load was borne by the provincial inspectors and their assistants, a group whose responsibilities—at least on paper—were as big as their salaries were small. To become a medical inspector, one had to possess the advanced degree of *doktor meditsiny*, have served at least six years in the lower ranks of the government medical service, and have passed a series of examinations in forensic medicine, medical police, medical jurisprudence, veterinary police, epizootic diseases, and *materia medica*.[57] Although this was the only position in the imperial bureaucracy which required both an advanced degree and a special examination, neither salary nor working conditions made it attractive. Salaries had been fixed in 1876 at 1,800 and 1,000 rubles, respectively, for inspectors and their assistants. Although they improved somewhat during the 1890s in outlying areas, the salaries remained static in most of the central Russian provinces. By the turn of the century, populous, industrializing provinces such as Nizhnii Novgorod were forced (1903) to raise salaries for these positions to 2,500 and 1,500 rubles, respectively.[58]

As the chief medical officer of the provincial administration (*pravlenie*), the inspector's responsibilities theoretically included supervising all aspects of medical and public health work in the province. Yet, in performing these duties, he was, as Veliaminov pointed out, at the mercy of the governor and vice-governor (who were more likely to have noble backgrounds and social influence than a higher education) and was required to work with "half-literate chinovniki" who were usually paid more than he was and who frequently ignored his expert advice.[59] According to one report, an inspector was sacked in the wake of the 1905 Revolution when he refused to cooperate with the governor in an investigation of the political activities of local physicians.[60] Inevitably, vulnerability turned some inspectors into pliant timeservers: "neither knowledge nor energy is required of a medical inspector, but only the ability to please the authorities," commented one anonymous critic.[61] An inspector who ran afoul of the governor could expect no help from St. Petersburg; the MVD was virtually certain to uphold the authority of governors, no matter what the facts of the matter.

Inevitably, turnover was high in the medical inspectorate; on average, half a dozen inspectors had to be replaced every year. In 1893, a peak year after the epidemic of 1892, eighteen vacancies occurred, five through death and the balance because of resignations.[62] Understandably, some inspectors and many assistant inspectors looked elsewhere for more lucrative positions—in the army, perhaps, or as hospital pathologists or residents, or as factory inspectors. A few even became village physicians because in some provinces village physicians earned more than assistant inspectors. The highest turnover occurred, as one would expect, in the forbidding northern provinces; the epidemiologically sensitive southern provinces; the non-zemstvo provinces, where the administrative workload was increased, and the relatively few zemstvo provinces where migration and industrialization had led to increased health problems.[63]

The very lowest ranks of the government medical service consisted of *uezd* (or *okrug* in Siberia) physicians in rural areas and *gorodovoi* physicians in the cities. These had been established in the eighteenth and early nineteenth centuries, respectively, to provide basic medical care for the civilian population and to provide a first line of defense in the battle against epidemics. By the late nineteenth century, however, *uezd* physicians found their time almost wholly taken up with forensic medical work and the preparation of reports for various bureaucratic agencies; similarly, *gorodovoi* physicians, appointed in the 1830s to supplement the *uezd* physicians in the most populous areas, were by the 1890s almost entirely occupied with the surveillance of brothels and the inspection of prostitutes.[64] Instead of providing free care to the sick poor, therefore, government physicians were first and foremost engaged in chancery or police work; at worst, they simply did whatever they were told by the provincial administration.

With the exception of St. Petersburg and Moscow, which from 1902 onwards had three physicians for each *uezd*, the zemstvo provinces of European Russia had one government physician per *uezd*, no matter what their size or population. These physicians earned between 920 and 1,225 rubles annually; their counterparts in the Siberian *okrugi* did somewhat better: 1,000 to 1,500 in Western Siberia and 1,300 to 1,700 in remote Eastern Siberia.[65] In the non-zemstvo provinces, *uezd* physicians were quite unable to provide even minimum services to the populace; they were grossly overworked and always short of hospital beds, instruments, and medical supplies. In an effort to respond to criticism, the tone of which sharpened after the cholera epidemic of 1892/93, the government appointed a second *uezd* physician in all non-zemstvo provinces except Astrakhan and Archangel.[66] Needless to say, such a pathetically inadequate step did nothing to stem the tide of criticism from the zemstvo provinces. *Uezd* physicians were treated with disdain by provincial administrators; alone of all government employees, they were not given travel expenses in advance. In one notorious case, which took place in 1906, several *uezd* physicians became so indebted because of expenses incurred but not reimbursed that they had to remove their children from school and sell their cottages.[67]

The lot of the *gorodovoi* physicians was, if anything, worse. Objects of popular contempt and ridicule because of their role as supervisors of prostitutes and petty criminals, the *gorodovoi* physicians were also the perennial casualties of a jurisdictional battle between Russian cities and the central government. The central government took the view that the cities were rich enough to pay the salaries of the *gorodovoi*-physicians, while the cities claimed (especially after the Municipal Act of 1870) that they ought not to be required to pay for police and forensic-medical work. When the government, through a decree of the Senate, tried to force municipalities to pay for the *gorodovoi* physicians, the cities petitioned for their abolition. The government refused to back down, arguing that the responsibility for policing sanitary matters was too important to abandon.[68] A standoff ensued; on the eve of the outbreak of war in 1914, the government was finally considering a proposal to raise the salaries of the *gorodovoi* physicians.

THE ST. PETERSBURG MEDICAL ESTABLISHMENT

As an imperial capital, St. Petersburg had its medical establishment, an elite group of medically trained officials who regarded themselves as the link between the autocracy and the medical estate. St. Petersburg was not only the administrative center of the government, it was also the principal residence of the tsar, the court, and a goodly portion of "high society" and the seat of numerous institutions of medical teaching and research, as well as hospitals, asylums, and orphanages. The degree of influence which a member of the medical establishment could exert often had more to do with rank or ex officio position than with his reputation as a teacher, researcher, or healer. As one might expect in an empire founded by Peter the Great, military rank vastly outweighed mere civil office. Accordingly, the premier medical official in the empire was, in the eyes of the tsar (and hence in those of members of the medical establishment) the chief military medical inspector. The individual who held his office stood at the apex of the state medical service: he was head of the military medical administration; presided over the Military Medical Learned Committee (the most prestigious medical advisory body in the empire); was the commanding officer of more than 12,000 army doctors, phramacists, and feldshers and the inspector of all military hospitals;[69] he was also the immediate superior of the director of the Imperial Military-Medical Academy. Ex officio, he was a member of the Medical Council of the Ministry of the Interior, as was his somewhat less illustrious counterpart in the navy, the Chief Medical Inspector of the Fleet. For most of the period with which this study is concerned, the Chief Military Medical Inspector was A. Ia Evdokimov, a nonentity who reached his exalted position in 1905 after rising diligently through the upper ranks of the military medical service. His lack of imagination and foresight would become painfully apparent very soon after Russia entered World War I.

Next in seniority was the inspector of the Court Medical Branch, a position occupied from 1897 until the Revolution of 1917 by the Chief Physician of the Imperial Household, Professor N. A. Veliaminov. In addition to his not always honorific court duties, Veliaminov occupied two other influential positions: he was professor of surgery at the Imperial Military Medical Academy and director of the Maximilian Hospital in St. Petersburg. Ex officio, he served on both the Military Medical Learned Committee and the Medical Council of the MVD; he also acted as a consultant to both the Red Cross nursing school and the charitable institutions operated by the Department of the Empress Marie.[70] The latter body also had its own inspector of the medical section, but this position—held by N. N. Fenomenov—was neither as prestigious nor as rewarding as that of Court Medical Inspector.[71] These four inspectors—army, fleet, court, and Empress Marie—constituted, along with the Director of the Imperial Military-Medical Academy, the topmost layer of the medical establishment.

Below these senior officials, but still very much a part of the establishment, came the heads of the other three major centers of medical education and research: the Imperial Institute of Experimental Medicine (bacteriology and infectious diseases), the Women's Medical Institute (general medical education, emphasizing women's and children's diseases), and the Clinical Institute of Grand Duchess Elena Pavlova (advanced clinical training for medical students and qualified physicians pursuing a particular clinical specialty.) On a par with the heads of these institutes were the directors or chief physicians of the most important hospitals: the Imperial Foundling, the Clinical Military, Obukhov, Obuhkov Women's, Mariinskii, and Maximilian Hospitals. Those in this layer of officialdom, along with the senior members of the faculty at the Imperial Military-Medical Academy, constituted the pool from which were drawn both the members of the government's advisory committees and the executive officers of such quasi-official bodies as the Russian Red Cross Society, the Imperial Philanthropic Society, and the Russian Society of the Protection of Public Health. This last agency, for example, was headed for more than a decade by V. O. Gubert, chief physician of the Imperial Foundling Hospital. Among the senior faculty of the Military-Medical Academy, one encounters members of the establishment whose reputations rested on something more than administrative talents or bureaucratic timeserving: the great clinician V. N. Sirotinin, the eminent S. S. Botkin, the brilliant and controversial neuropsychiatrist V. M. Bekhterev, and the great Pavlov himself, who divided his time between the Academy and the Institute of Experimental Medicine. Eminence as a researcher, however, had little to do with salaries paid: in 1904, Pavlov earned 6,946 rubles, at first sight a healthy salary for a professor, but one that pales into insignificance beside the 15,196 rubles earned by Court Medical Inspector Veliaminov. And financial distinctions were not all: Veliaminov's position carried a higher rank in the Table of Ranks, was rewarded by a higher grade in the Order of St. Vladimir, and had brought him numerous foreign honors.[72] Pavlov's international reputation as a researcher brought him no closer to the imperial favor than his position at the Academy would allow, while Veliaminov, the polished physician-courtier, sat on all of the important government commissions.

After Evdokimov and Veliaminov, the most successful medical *chinovnik* in Russia at the dawn of the twentieth century was V. V. Pashutin, who had been director of the Imperial Military-Medical Academy since 1890. At the time of his premature death in January 1901, at the age of 56, he was also president of the Medical Council of the MVD, a member of the advisory council of the Ministry of Public Instruction, and president of the Russian Society for the Protection of Public Health. His career illustrates several noteworthy features of the St. Petersburg medical establishment: its admiration for the achievements of German academic medicine, its preference for theoretical as opposed to practical studies, and its predictable patterns of preferment and advancement.

One of Sechenov's most brilliant students, Pashutin received his Doctor of Medicine degree from the Imperial Medical Surgical Academy in 1870.[73] His dissertation was immediately published in Germany, and with Sechenov's encouragement he was able to spend most of the next three years doing further research in Western Europe. He spent time in Vienna, Graz, and Leipzig, where he worked under Carl Ludwig, the leading figure in German physiology in the second half of the nineteenth century. Ludwig encouraged his interest in the role of chemical factors in physiology, and he went on from Leipzig to Strasbourg where he worked with one of the founders of physiological chemistry, Felix Hoppe-Seyler. Pashutin also paid a short visit to Paris, but he returned to Russia a disciple of the German approach to physiology, with its emphasis on physical and chemical analysis. In 1874, he obtained a post teaching general pathology at the University of Kazan, where he created a sensation by teaching pathology as an experimental subject, sending his students to the (woefully inadequate) laboratories and publishing his own textbook to offset the pathetic resources of the library.

Pashutin's *Lectures in General Pathology* appeared in 1878,[74] just in time to be useful to those in St. Petersburg who believed that it was high time to introduce experimental pathology there; when a post fell vacant in the following year, the adherents of clinical pathology were defeated and Pashutin was offered the job. Once again he had to campaign for funds to build better laboratory facilities, but at least he had a better library at his disposal. Fresh experiments and publications followed in short order. By this time, Pashutin was clearly becoming a force to be reckoned with in Russian medicine.

In 1885, he began to climb, with almost breathtaking rapidity, the ladder of official success that soon led him to occupy top positions in medical education. First he was made learned secretary of the Military-Medical Academy; then he was approached by the Ministry of Public Instruction to evaluate candidates for professional appointments in university medical schools. In 1876, he undertook a review of the whole field of medical education as a member of the ministry's advisory council. Two years later, he was made a member of the Medical Council of the Ministry of the Interior and—with almost unseemly haste—became its president seven months later. Less than a year after this elevation, he was appointed head of the Military-Medical Academy, an administrative position that meant abandoning his professorship, but he was the recipient of compensating honors: elected academician in 1890 and honored professor in 1894, he was made privy councillor in 1896. The many honors perhaps helped to offset his relatively low salary: as he pointed out in an autobiographical fragment, despite his work for three ministries (War, Interior, and Public Instruction), he earned only about 4,500 rubles from his administrative position at the Military-Medical Academy.[75]

As befitted one of the leading figures in St. Petersburg—and Russian—medicine, Pashutin was also active in medical societies. He played a major role in the first three conferences of the Pirogov Society during the late 1880s; he was president of the (disciplinary) court of honor of the St. Petersburg Physicians' Medical Society of Mutual Assistance, and after many years on the executive of the Russian Society for the Protection of Public Health he became its president in 1898, only to be honored by it and dozens of other medical societies when he died in 1901. His former student S. M. Lukianov, who delivered a moving tribute, praised his ability "to stimulate lively interest in pathology as such, beyond its direct and indirect connections with clinical medicine."[76] In a country such as Russia, with its great poverty and ill health, he went on, there was always a danger that theoretical subjects would be overshadowed by practical needs; Pashutin, on the other hand, had spent his life convincing Russian physicians of the need to study the theoretical and scientific foundations of medicine.[77]

In fact, of course, as Pashutin's career shows, the tsarist regime and the St. Petersburg medical establishment were always ready to provide promotion, rewards, and honors for medical scientists whose work was more theoretical than practical. German physiology, with its emphasis on the human organism entirely abstracted from real social conditions, always found a congenial home in St. Petersburg; physicians and scientists interested in the social and environmental aspects of disease and in the prevention of disease through social change could make little headway in the capital city. Of course, Pashutin reached the eminence he did not because he was simply an adherent of German physiology, but because he was a brilliant exponent of German medical science. He was so hailed by his professional contemporaries. But then, so was Pashutin's contemporary and von Pettenkofer's brilliant student, the hygienist Friedrich Erismann, yet he was never offered rank or position in the St. Petersburg medical establishment. Erismann made his career with the zemstvo of Moscow province, where his views on sanitary education and disease prevention were appreciated by overworked clinicians and enthusiastic social reformers.[78]

The regime was careful to identify and promote those who could be trusted not to upset the political applecart. In turn, those academics who expected to benefit from the regime's patronage were careful to keep their charmed circle free of anyone who might be too loud, zealous, or persistent in supporting unpopular causes.

An example of how this informal accommodation with the regime worked in practice can be seen in the way senior appointments were made at the Military-Medical Academy. As we have already seen, Pashutin's advancement within the Academy came after he had proved himself to the satisfaction of the regime on a number of governmental commissions. Those who put him forward for more responsible offices were the sort of people who had proved themselves both in the world of science and in the world of government service. Like not only hired, but also promoted like and sought to ensure that the attitudes, assumptions, and tone of the group were maintained. Sometimes, appointments revealed the extent to which this unofficial search process actually influenced proceedings, as happened in 1890 when it was necessary to find a new holder of the chair of hygiene upon the death of A. P. Dobroslavin.[79] Like Pashutin, Dobroslavin had made his reputation as a laboratory scientist and was thus in the forefront of the transformation of hygiene into an experimental science during the second half of the nineteenth century. Initially, five candidates entered the lists for the vacant position, including the celebrated Erismann from Moscow and the equally well-known M. Ia. Kapustin, Professor of Hygiene at the University of Kazan. Aware that Kapustin would probably benefit from the Academy's propensity to appoint its own graduates, Erismann withdrew; no doubt he would have been happy to see Kapustin, the author of a fine critical study of zemstvo medicine,[80] occupy the chair. But two other candidates withdrew as well, leaving Kapustin in competition with S. V. Shidlovskii, his junior in age, academic seniority, and scientific achievements. Where Kapustin was already something of a tribune on the subject of public health, Shidlovskii, a younger version of his mentor Dobroslavin, had already proved himself both a dedicated laboratory scientist and a cautious and reliable consultant on various government commissions. Not surprisingly, therefore, the academy committee charged with reviewing their credentials found Shidlovskii to be as suitable a candiate as Kapustin. In the ballot conducted among members of the academic conference, Shidlovskii was the overwhelming choice (eighteen for, two against).[81] The subsequent careers of the two men revealed the differences in temperament which were perhaps a subconscious factor in the 1890 decision: Kapustin became openly critical of the government during the famine and cholera epidemic of 1892/93 and emerged in 1905 as a public figure playing a significant role at Pirogov congresses and becoming one of the founders of the moderate Union of 17 October; Shidlovskii, meanwhile, avoiding all but the most guarded comments on public health and municipal sanitation, worked doggedly towards his lifetime goal—the creation of a first-class institute of hygiene—which was not to be achieved until the early Soviet period. The St. Petersburg establishment found certain kinds of scientific enquiry, certain assumptions and preoccupations, to be more congenial than others, and the regime rewarded those whose possessed these qualifications and qualities with the means of patronage at its disposal. It was almost foreordained, therefore, that a sort of antiestablishment, stressing the social and environment aspects of disease causation, would grow up in Moscow in opposition to the biological, experimental orientation that predominated in St. Petersburg.

DEGREES OF SUBSERVIENCE

The professional status of all Russian physicians, whatever the nature of their employment, was defined by laws that they, as a group, had taken no part in framing. In contrast to their colleagues in many western countries, Russian physicians entered the twentieth century lacking any form of corporate organization with legally recognized powers over the licensing of practitioners. Under the Medical Edict,[82] the title (*zvanie*) of physician (*vrach*) could be awarded only to persons who possessed both recognized degrees and the legal right to practice. Thus, intending practitioners were required first to obtain a degree (*lekar* for men, *zemshchina-vrach* for women) from the medical faculty of a Russian university, from the Imperial Military-Medical Academy, or from the Women's Medical Institute. After an additional and extremely arduous year of study and the writing of a dissertation, those possessed of a first degree could be awarded the degree of M.D. (*doktor meditsiny*) or M.S.D. (*doktor meditsiny i khirurgii*). Degrees did not by themselves confer the right to practice; this could be obtained only by applying to the medical inspector in the area where one intended to practice. Effectively, therefore, the final licensing body for most of the empire—the borderlands had their own rules—was the main administration of the chief medical inspector, to which all guberniia medical departments were theoretically subordinated. These rules applied to all physicians in government service, in the employ of public or semipublic agencies (such as the Red Cross), in the employ of zemstvos and municipalities, and in private practice. Physicians in military service were licensed by the medical inspector of the army or the fleet. Physicians who possessed degrees from foreign universities could practice only after their qualifications had been approved by the Medical Council of the MVD. The important point in all this is that the decision to license a practitioner was made not by an autonomous, chartered body such as a college or chamber of physicians, but by an agency of the civil or military administration.

Physicians had no more control over matters of professional responsibilty and discipline than they did over licensing. The main administration of the chief medical inspector was charged with the investigation and prosecution of persons who engaged in unlawful medical practice.[83] Physicians were legally required to attend the sick whenever called upon to do so, and the Medical Edict set out fines and further punishments—including exile or imprisonment—for those found derelict in their duty. Medical memoirs of the period—especially Veresaev's well-known *Notes of a Physician* [*Zapiski vracha*][84]—abound in stories of physicians whose days and nights were disrupted by patients, both rich and poor, who treated doctors as if they were lackies. No aspect of professional life came under so much criticism in the medical press and at medical conferences as the cavalier attitude of all levels of Russian society towards physicians. Things were different elsewhere, they knew; as Veresaev observed, "In England, France and Germany, the laws obliging medical men to appear at the patient's first call and to attend the poor gratis have long been repealed."[85] That they were still in force in Russia, and indeed still enforced, testified to the extent to which the state, and not physicians, controlled the terms of medical practice.

Russian physicians were all servants of the state, but the form of their employment largely determined the degree of subservience in which they worked. Worst off were physicians employed in the army and the navy. The ship's surgeon in Eisenstein's *Battleship Potemkin* who refused to concede the presence of maggots in obviously rotten meat exemplifies the tyranny that military life imposed upon medical judgment. Nancy Frieden has graphically described the plight of physicians in the army, professionally impotent before an officer corps whose code of honorable behavior included beating up the regimental doctor for an evening's amusement.[86] Physicians in the army or the navy were required to serve for at least two years; after this they could, at the state's discretion, be transferred to the reserves for a further sixteen years. In the event of war, reserve medical personnel were the first to be called up; exemptions were granted only to senior hospital physicians or to those teaching courses "designated as important" in a medical school.[87] Army physicians were subject to the absolute authority of the Military-Medical Administration; its rules included absurdities such as a prohibition against attending concerts and a rule that spurs must be worn at all times. Nevertheless, a career in military medicine had some financial rewards;[88] these presumably had to serve as compensation for the complete absence of professional autonomy and self-respect.

The responsibilities of physicians in the civil sector were set out in law according to whether they were in government service, in zemstvo or municipal service, employed by public bodies such as the Red Cross or by private hospitals, or working as "voluntary" (i.e., private) practitioners.[89] Both zemstvo physicians and private practitioners had to secure official permission to practice; in addition, zemstvo and municipal appointments were subject to the confirmation of the governor or *gradonachal'nik*. Jewish physicians could practice only in the provinces of the Pale of Settlement, unless they held doctoral degrees, in which case this restriction was lifted.[90] Private practice, though tolerated, was scarcely encouraged by the government; because it brought few financial rewards, medical graduates went into it as a last resort if they failed to secure a salaried position in government or public service or in a hospital.[91] In the eyes of the government, every physician was actually or potentially in state service; hence the state retained extensive rights of co-optation. Zemstvo physicians and private practitioners could be ordered to perform prison, police, or forensic medical work if no *uezd* physicians were available or even to take on military medical responsibilities, particularly examining recruits, if no army physician could be found or spared. In the event of an epidemic, zemstvo physicians and private practitioners could be conscripted (at fixed rates of payment) for state service wherever they were needed. Failure to notify the authorities in cases of epidemic disease could result in fines or even suspension of the right to practice. All medical practitioners were legally obliged to submit monthly to the local medical inspector a list of all persons treated, no matter where such treatment occurred. One did not escape the overwhelming presence of the Russian state by going into private practice; neither could one completely escape it in the zemstvos, but with congenial colleagues and an understanding local zemstvo board—not, of course, found everywhere—zemstvo service offered the greatest degree of professional autonomy that a physician was likely to find in tsarist Russia. For this reason, it was inevitable that supporters of community medicine would sooner or later clash with both the medical establishment in St. Petersburg and the tsarist regime itself.

This overview of government medical administration in imperial Russia reveals several noteworthy features of the country's political and social structure. In the first place, it is obvious that civil administration took a back seat o the interests of the army and the fleet. Even where civil administ ators did function, their work was almost entirely devoted to routine paperwork of a regulatory nature. Second, despite the growth of a sense of professional identity among zemstvo physicians, there were clear and seemingly unassailable obstacles in the way of its further development. Control over finances and the police made it relatively easy for the government to keep the zemstvos and municipalities on a very tight leash. As long as the state regarded all physicians as servitors who could be called upon whenever necessary, a huge gulf would separate the assumptions of St. Petersburg bureaucrats from those typical of community physicians. In any case, the regime's overwhleming but frequently ineffectual presence in medical affairs was maintained both by the physicians who were recruited into the medical establishment in the capital and, inadvertently, by the community physicians, whose opposition to the establishment of a health ministry helped to perpetuate the overlapping powers and jurisdictions of the St. Petersburg bureaucracy.

2
PHYSICIANS, POLITICS, AND THE 1905 REVOLUTION

During the 1905 Revolution, community physicians challenged both the political legitimacy of the tsarist regime and the professional dominance of the St. Petersburg medical establishment. No longer were they willing to play the subordinate role to which they had been condemned by the laws, social customs, and political structure of tsarist Russia. Rallying around the slogan, "making Russia healthy" (*ozdorovlenie Rossii*), the community physicians and their sympathizers began to criticize virtually every institution and office in the tsarist medical structure on the grounds that their powers were both morally indefensible and an affront to the dictates of medical science. The authority of office was challenged by those who asserted the authority of knowledge. In hospitals, all-powerful chief physicians were challenged by collegial boards; wherever epidemics struck, the government's Sanitary-Executive Commissions—creatures of the Antiplague Commission—were challenged by zemstvo medical institutions.

One constant theme ran throughout these conflicts: that the essential condition for improving the health of the Russian people was a substantial political reform that would reduce the authority of the state bureaucracy and encourage the growth of local autonomy and spontaneous public activity (*obshchestvennost'*) among the citizenry. Understandably, a new urgency affected the continuing debate over medical professional organization. The genteel and cautious quest for corporate status encouraged by the St. Petersburg medical establishment held little or no appeal for the increasingly militant community physicians who, during the 1890s, had become the dominant force in the Pirogov Society.[1]

Both of these challenges—the political and the professional—became stridently public at the extraordinary Pirogov Congress held in Moscow in March 1905. Having approved a series of strongly political resolutions, participants went on to form a radical union that would proselytize physicians and other medical workers on behalf of their vision of a remade Russia. Caught up in the revolutionary turmoil that enveloped the country in the spring and summer of 1905, the community physicians, along with the liberal and revolutionary intelligentsia, were confident that a stronger, healthier, democratic Russia was just around the corner. They were wrong. The regime proved to be more durable than its opponents had expected and survived 1905 with minimal concessions. In the aftermath of failure, erstwhile advocates of political and professional radicalism were hounded from their jobs by the agents and allies of a vengeful government; they were also subjected to the recriminations of their disappointed and disillusioned colleagues.

THE AUTHORITY OF KNOWLEDGE VERSUS
THE AUTHORITY OF OFFICE

In its institutions of medical education and research, the tsarist regime welcomed the development of scientific medicine within certain unstated but nevertheless real limits. Medicine was encouraged because it was seen as a source of knowledge about the inner workings of the human organism, not as a source of knowledge about human society which could yield scientifically correct principles of social organization. Still less was medicine seen as a source of proposals for social reform advocated on the basis of the alleged dictates of science. Anyone rash enough to advance the claims of knowledge as a source of authority was bound to run up against a social and political structure founded upon the assumption that authority derived from office. Consider the authority of the tsar himself: Nicholas II became tsar not because of his acknowledged skill in governing but because circumstances had dictated that he should succeed his father; his authority was sacred, mysterious, almost defiantly irrational. The tsar's agents— ministers, governors, *gradonachal'niki*, bureaucrats—exercised their authority because he so willed it: imperial favor was the sole source of their authority. Because Nicholas II's predecessors had willed it, the whole edifice of tsarist government had grown over the centuries into a ramshackle cluster of offices and jurisdictions whose powers reflected a host of historical, accidental, and personal factors. It was a regime that almost defied description, let alone understanding. Its institutions—the Antiplague Commission, for example—could be explained in their own terms but often appeared senseless to those whose expectations were based upon quite different assumptions.

Medical knowledge grew so rapidly in the late nineteenth and early twentieth centuries that its scope and pretensions were inevitably carried beyond the limits tolerated by the tsarist regime. As physicians' understanding of health and disease increased, they were less and less content to see problems ignored or defined and dealt with inappropriately, when the scientifically correct solution or course of action was already apparent. Physicians began to medicalize particular problems by establishing expert committees or conferences to study them and produce proposals that would solve or at least contribute to solving, them. For example, the age-old drunkenness of Russians, hitherto a problem of morality in the eyes of churchmen and of public order in the eyes of the police, became in the eyes of physicians the "alcohol problem"; in 1898, the Russian Society for the Protection of Public Health set up a special commission to study it.[2] Similarly, prostitution, long a matter of greater concern to the police than to the church, became, as knowledge about the forms and transmission of veneral diseases increased, an appropriate object of medical attention and a problem about which physicians could have opinions based on scientific knowledge.[3] From this stage it was but a short step to the next, in which physicians believed their expertise extended to pronouncing upon how to reduce or eliminate alcoholism or venereal disease. At this point, those possessed of the knowledge had to approach those whose possession of office gave them the authority to effect change and urge change upon them through advice, requests, recommendations, and petitions.

And if those in authority would not listen, what then? Out of the ensuing frustration came the complaint common to most educated experts and professionals in late imperial Russia: "all the wrong people are in charge." This was of course the cry of the self-confident and the impatient; it would not take long before some of them began to seek political changes that would rid them of "the wrong people" and the institutions through which they clung to authority. Founded upon the authority of office, the tsarist regime was bound to resist the claims of those who based their authority upon knowledge; with equal resolution, impatient and idealistic physicians joined in the Revolution of 1905 as declared opponents of the regime. Before analyzing the overtly political activity of physicians during the 1905 events, I will explore the frustration that put so many physicians in the revolutionary camp. Two examples will serve to illustrate the process at work: first, among a group of hospital physicians who sought to introduce rational principles of hospital management, and second, among bacteriologists who sought to base antiepidemic measures on sound scientific advice.

THE STRUGGLE FOR HOSPITAL REFORM IN ST. PETERSBURG

Russian hospitals, both civil and military, were run along strictly authoritarian lines. Each was run by its chief physician (*nachal'nik*), who was both medical director and administrative head. This pattern slowly began to change in the late nineteenth century. In many provincial zemstvo hospitals and a few civic hospitals in Moscow, chief physicians began to share their powers with a collegial body representing hospital physicians and occasionally the lesser medical and non-medical staff. Indeed, collegial decision-making became one of the hallmarks of zemstvo medicine; collegiality (*kollegial'nost'*) became one of the professional goals towards which the Pirogov Society directed its labors.[4] The old ways naturally continued in the non-zemstvo provinces and above all in St. Petersburg, where the chief physicians of the many hospitals were very much a part of the medical establishment. Even in hospitals funded by St. Petersburg's notoriously parsimonious municipal Duma, authoritarian government was the rule.[5] The chief physicians, through an informal council, also controlled relations with the municipal Duma's hospital commission; hence they took the brunt of criticism from residents and interns who suffered the consequences of persistent underfunding throughout the 1890s.

After several lean years, a group of dissatisfied hospital physicians decided in 1900 to organize themselves. Thus was born the Society of Hospital Physicians of St. Petersburg, which grew to a membership of almost 200 in its first year of existence.[6] The society's immediate goal was to provide a forum in which physicians could discuss the economic and administrative aspects of hospital management, in the hope that their views would carry more weight with the municipal Duma and with the government itself; members seemed to cherish the belief that they would soon be able to raise the status of all hospital physicians, to obtain increased funding for hospitals, and to replace the autocratic system of administration with a collegial one.[7] As one member pointed out, with the blithe confidence characteristic of the naive, "the correctly understood interests of hospital physicians coincide with the interest of hospital affairs, just as in general the correctly understood interests of the medical estate [*soslovie*] coincide with the interests of public health."[8] In the first flush of enthusiasm, the members proposed to study no less than forty-two separate topics, touching every aspect of hospital location, construction, organization, and management—everything from the influence of climate on urban morbidity to recreational programs for ancillary staff.[9] The ultimate goal was of course to enhance the authority and prestige of hospital physicians not only within the institutions themselves, but in the larger society of St. Petersburg.

The most striking aspect of this program was its complete faith in science as both the source of positive knowledge about society and the instrument through which social institutions could be reformed.[10] Members of the society regarded hospital administration as a simple matter of harmonizing the structure and operation of hospitals with the dictates of reason and science. Institutions for the sick, they believed, ought to be differentiated into categories based on the typology of disease; the order prevailing in them ought to be derived from the principles of hygiene; planning for the future ought to be based on statistical information and scientific analysis.[11] The whole thrust of their program was to place hospital administration on a foundation of science, independent of all historical, accidental, and personal factors to whose unchecked operation they ascribed the present unsatisfactory situation. There is nothing disingenuous about their belief that their own status and authority must be increased. This was the only way, they believed, to liberate these institutions from the baleful effect of an outmoded form of government.

They wanted science to be in charge, and they therefore sought to put themselves in charge because they were the appropriate and competent interpreters of the dictates of science. Hence they expected to become the informants and advisers of the civil authorities who provided operating funds; they also proceeded to draw up the regimen that ought to prevail for patients and staff alike within the walls of the institutions. And because—or so they believed—an impersonal science would speak with equal clarity to all of its trained practitioners, there was no need for hierarchy; decisions would be made collectively, with all physicians having an equal voice, thus avoiding the mystique of a system of authority based—inappropriately, in their view—on age, rank, or office.

Not surprisingly, the society's self-righteous attitude, as well as its open espousal of collegiality, earned it the enmity of hospital administrators. Chief physicians and their senior colleagues (who were also their most likely successors) saw no reason to cooperate with a society that wished to eliminate their positions and that advocated sweeping and expensive changes likely to be unpopular with the city's taxpayers and its government. They refused to provide information or statistics and in some cases prevented members of the society from carrying out investigations on its behalf.[12] What is remarkable is not the understandable hostility of the chief physicians but the startling presumption of the society's members, who believed that all doors would be opened to them because they claimed to be acting on principle and not out of personal animus towards any individual.[13] In Moscow, it was claimed, the situation was different; there hospital physicians were already enjoying some unofficial influence with members of the municipal Duma and its Hospital Commission.[14] The chief physicians of St. Petersburg, however, were a bastion of the old order; with so many administrative positions available in the ministries and departments of the government, they saw no reason to jeopardize their careers by conciliating the would-be reformers.

Three years of fruitless effort taught the society a lesson about the strength of the existing system. As its president, A. N. Rubel', told a general meeting held on 30 January 1903, "very soon the conviction grew that without a wholesale reform of the entire administrative and financial structure of hospitals, any improvement . . . would be impossible; without a complete overhaul of the existing system *in toto,* all attempts at improvement would remain fruitless palliatives, inconsequential half-measures."[15] From here it was but a short step to recognizing that the fate of hospital reform was intimately connected to the fortunes of zemstvo and municipal institutions because only in community medical circles was collegial decision-making beginning to be-

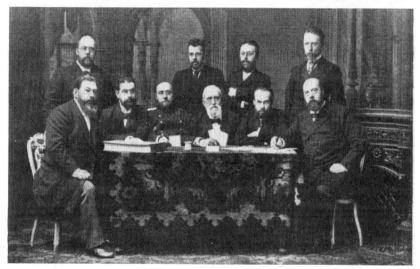

Fig. 2. Dr. A. L. Eberman *(center)* with the executive of the St. Petersburg Physicians' Mutual Assistance Society in 1895.

come established practice. Rubel' went on to condemn as "narrowly professional" the "mistaken point of view that the interests of physicians can be separated from the interests of public [*obshchestvennye*] institutions"; the hospital, he concluded, is but "one of the links in the long chain of public institutions in general."[16] Thus, by 1903, this group were beginning to recognize that the future progress of science and society, as well as their own future as workers in that cause, was bound up with the struggle of zemstvo activists to obtain both greater autonomy and a larger role for those institutions in the governance of Russia.

The next two years brought fresh disappointments. Plehve's term as Minister of Interior did nothing to advance the cause of zemstvo au-

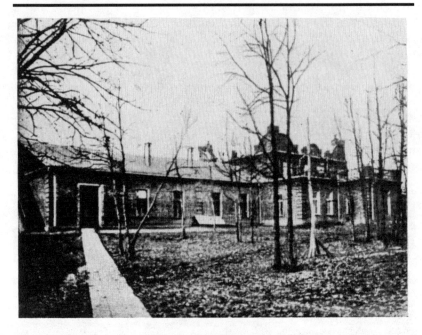

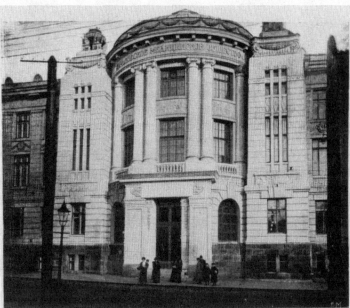

Fig. 3. Russian medicine came of age rapidly in the late nineteenth century. In Khar'kov, for example, the local medical society moved from its previous cottage-like premises *(top)* to an imposing new building *(bottom)* in 1911.

tonomy, while his reorganization put hospital financing in the hands of the Main Administration for Local Economic Affairs, beyond the reach of medical advice. Recognizing that larger issues were now the first priority, the frustrated hospital physicians of St. Petersburg virtually suspended their own agenda; instead, aroused and inspired by the resolutions of the Ninth Pirogov Congress (which met in St. Petersburg in January 1904), they joined in the banquet campaign organized by the liberal opposition to the tsarist regime.[17] More than a dozen members of the Hospital Physician's Society would attend the Pirogov "Cholera" Congress in March 1905.[18] Among them were former executive members A. N. Rubel' and G. I. Dembo, both by then ardent advocates of political reform as the *sine qua non* for medical reform.

BACTERIOLOGISTS AND POLITICS

Frustration with existing institutions and policies also drove Russian bacteriologists into the ranks of the political opposition. The leading lights of Russian bacteriology—G. N. Gabrichevskii, V. K. Vyskovich, L. A. Tarasevich, P. N. Diatroptov, D. K. Zabolotnyi, and N. M. Berestnev— helped to organize and direct the 1905 "Cholera" Congress, which endorsed a series of political resolutions demanding a constituent assembly and the granting of basic civil freedoms. Indeed, bacteriologists and epidemiologists were to play a crucial role in the struggle for medical reform throughout the entire period with which this study is concerned and continued to play important roles well into the 1920s.[19] Leading Russian bacteriologists of the early twentieth century strongly supported social and political reform; they stood in sharp contrast to Robert Koch and his associates in imperial Germany, where the government itself sponsored the development of the subject and where Koch himself held high positions in both the imperial civil and colonial services.[20]

Bacteriologists are not born radicals; in Russia they were made so by events.[21] When the bacteriological revolution broke upon Russia in the 1880s, its enthusiasts—especially I. I. Mechnikov and his students— encountered the hostility and suspicion of community physicians who feared that the fad for bacteriology would diminish or even undermine social and environmental explanations of health and disease.[22] The unofficial theoretican of zemstvo medicine, F. F. Erismann, had studied with von Pettenkofer in Munich and was a thoroughgoing environmentalist in his views on public health; his magisterial pronouncement at the 1887 Pirogov Congress that bacteriology could be "no more than a useful weapon in certain circumstances" was meant to puncture the balloon that Mechnikov and the other "bacteriology-fanatics" had inflated so enthusiastically.[23] While Erismann was warning young zemstvo physicians in Moscow to beware of bacteriology, in St. Petersburg the new discipline was establishing itself at both the Military-Medical Academy and the Institute of Experimental Medicine. For a time in the early 1890s, it seemed that, in Russia as in Germany, bacteriological research would enjoy the sponsorship of the government and the medical establishment.

A decade later, this prospect had altered dramatically. Once the clinical applications of the new subject were perceived and once it was clear that bacteriology did not threaten to supplant preventive medicine or sanitary reform, Moscow quickly outstripped St. Petersburg as the most congenial environment for the further development of bacteriology. Most of the credit for this startling transformation must go to G. N. Gabrichevskii, Professor of Pathology at the University of Moscow, whose emphasis on the therapeutic applications of clinical bacteriology led to the founding of the Bacteriology Institute, of which he became director. His therapeutic successes—notably with diphtheria serum during the epidemic of 1893/94—aroused interest among community physicians who began to take courses at the institute. At the same time Gabrichevskii threw himself energetically into the activities of the Pirogov Society, serving as chairman of its Malaria Commission; its 1903 report, as Nancy Frieden has pointed out, emphasized the importance of strong institutions of local self-government to the success of antiepidemic measures.[24] Gabrichevskii's achievement was to make bacteriology palatable to the increasingly firm political opinions of the community physicians.[25] No longer a fad to be dismissed nor a weapon to be feared, bacteriology was now championed by community physicians who saw it as a tool to be used for the benefit of the people.

By the turn of the century, further advances in understanding the causative mechanisms of plague and cholera had taken place; malaria and other contagious diseases were being studied intensely by other researchers. From a scientific point of view, it began to make sense that bacteriologists should be assigned a leading role in planning and carrying out antiepidemic measures. Yet it was at this very moment that the government, for the reasons explained in the previous chapter, chose to create the Antiplague Commission, the composition and mandate of which made no scientific sense whatever.[26] By adding measures against cholera to the commission's jurisdiction, the government compounded its previous error by giving incompetence and amateurism an even larger terrain over which to blunder.[27] The commission's new rules for combating cholera, published on 11 August 1903, were the predictable result; in calling for the creation of new Sanitary-Executive Commissions (SECs) composed of minor local officials (and virtually excluding qualified medical opinion), the Antiplague Commission simply replicated at the local level its own uniformed and anachronistic approach to epidemic prevention.[28] By contrast, during that same summer of 1903, the Pirogov Society's Malaria Commission praised the effectiveness of antiepidemic measures mounted by zemstvo medical organizations and condemned the backwardness of public health organization in the non-zemstvo provinces and the borderlands.[29] The Malaria Commission included some of the best minds in Russian medicine and biology; community physicians therefore assumed that its conclusions, based upon the results of sponsored research expeditions, rested incontestably upon the authority of knowledge.

Nevertheless, the Antiplague Commission and its SECs possessed the authority of office. The SECs were given extensive emergency and police powers; they could order that their decisions be carried out immediately, a necessary requirement in areas where no zemstvo medical or santiary organization existed but a prescription for conflict where they did. The local officials who made up the SECs behaved with the arrogance typical of *petis fonctionnaires*, compounded by the Russian bureaucrat's double disdain for zemstvo professionals. Not only physicians were affected; zemstvo board members were outraged that SECs could order whatever they liked and insist that the costs be borne by the local zemstvo. From the moment the 1903 rules were passed, the medical press was filled with examples of incompetent or ill-advised decisions and actions taken by SECs.[30]

Many zemstvos, often on the advice of their medical councils, concluded that the rules were "poorly thought out, unsuitable, awkward, and often completely unworkable."[31] The Ministry of the Interior was deluged with petitions asking that the rules be scrapped and that zemstvos and municipalities be officially recognized as the appropriate agencies to manage antiepidemic measures. All of these protests were fruitless, however; the government had both practical and theoretical reasons for sticking to its guns. The greatest epidemiological threats to European Russia came from the Caucasus, the Don region, and Central Asia—all regions where zemstvo institutions were lacking; emergency measures in these areas were necessarily in government hands. The Don Army *Oblast'* was in fact a military district where local government was the responsibility of the Ministry of War, which was notoriously unwilling to join forces with the zemstvos of neighboring provinces to combat epidemic disease. In any case, the government could not, on such an important issue, concede that local professional experts knew best; such an admission would then have required it to increase both the powers of local government institutions and the status of physicians and other professional experts. Hence the MVD rejected all requests that the 1903 rules be abolished and persisted in its support of the SECs despite the growing fear in early 1905 of a summer cholera epidemic.

Here again, as in the case of the struggle for hospital reform, the regime's intransigent defence of the authority of office drove those who asserted the authority of knowledge into the ranks of the political opposition. As will be shown, bacteriologists played a leading role in the Pirogov Society's extraordinary "Cholera" Congress in March 1905, the resolutions of which firmly aligned the community physicians with the liberal and radical opposition to the tsarist regime. Bacteriologists were also associated with the founding of a physicians' union, a militant and openly political organization that challenged not only the legitimacy of the tsarist regime but also the genteel and subtle dominance exerted by the St. Petersburg medical establishment upon the forms of professional organization.

THE STRUGGLE FOR PROFESIONAL UNITY

During the last decades of the nineteenth century, Russian medicine grew in stature both at home and abroad; the number of licensed physicians was growing steadily and so was their sense of identity as a distinctive group in Russian society.[32] New medical societies were founded, and the medical press grew apace. Not surprisingly, Russian physicians began to chafe under the restrictions imposed on them by the Medical Statute, and to look enviously at the achievements of their professional colleagues in western Europe. The first congress of the Moscow–St. Petersburg Medical Society (later the Pirogov Society) in 1885 discussed a report on the medical organizations already in existence in England, France, Belgium, and Germany; its author argued that Russian physicians ought to organize themselves to achieve the social status and material position of their colleagues elsewhere.[33] One physician who felt most strongly the need for a protective and benevolent society was A. L. Eberman; largely as a result of the tireless campaign mounted by him, the Third Pirogov Congress in 1889 established a committee to draw up an appropriate constitution and bylaws; these received official approval in May 1890.[34] Eberman was elected the first president of the St. Petersburg Physicians Mutual Assistance Society (SPMAS), which set out to assist needy physicians and their families, to defend the legal interests and improve the legal status of physicians, to act as guardian of the ethical standards of the profession, and to provide unemployed physicians with information about vacant positions.

Physicians had enjoyed so few opportunities to improve their material welfare and working conditions that the new SPMAS aroused great interest. Within a decade, membership had reached more than 1,000;

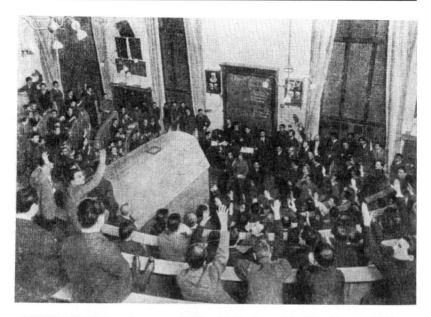

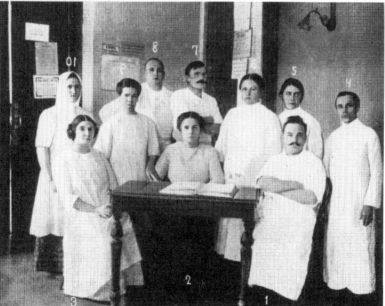

Fig. 4. "Beautiful words and noble impulses": medical students at the University of Moscow *(top)* voted to join striking workers during the 1905 Revolution. Radical leaders of the medical union aimed their message at overworked but idealistic young people such as the members of this hospital medical team in Khar'kov *(bottom)*.

branches were formed in Moscow and in thirty-five other cities and towns as far away as Tiflis and Irkutsk. A fund was estalished to enable the society to make small interest-free loans to members and outright awards—albeit modest ones—to needy physicians and their families.[35] The society put before the government petitions that sought improvements in the legal status of physicians. An unofficial court of honor was set up to settle disputes among members and to establish by its decisions the basis for a code of ethics. In 1900, the executive of SPMAS sponsored a series of informal "friendly discussions" to explore further ethical issues and to define, to their own satisfaction, the professional responsibilities of physicians.[36] Soon there were suggestions that SPMAS, with its many branches, might become the nucleus of a corporate professional organization. If all physicians were required by law to join such a body, then its executive—and not the MVD—would become the administrative and disciplinary organ for the entire profession. In an article written for the first issue of the society's journal in 1902, the president of SPMAS—the psychiatrist M. N. Nizhegorodtsev—reviewed the whole question of professional organization. Conceding that eventually legislation would be required to create a medical corporate body, he argued that the time was not yet ripe for such a step to be taken. Instead of compelling all physicians to join one body, he preferred to wait until "estate (*soslovie*) consciousness, conscientious moral discipline, and fraternal agreement" had impelled physicians to join voluntarily; at that point, legislation would simply confirm reality.[37] For the present, Nizhegorodtsev wrote, the society should concentrate on increasing its membership by making itself more attractive to those who had not yet joined.[38]

There is little doubt that Nizhegorodtsev and his colleagues in SPMAS had taken as their model the form of corporate professional organization which had prevailed in Germany since 1887, when Chambers of Physicians were established by law in every province of the Empire. Composed of representatives elected by and from the physicians of a province, the chambers were legally entitled to regulate medical activity, to protect the corporate interests of physicians, to further the interests of public health, and to make representations to the government on all these subjects.[39] Each chamber was subject to the authority of the *Oberpresident* of the province, while in Berlin a Council of Chambers of Physicians served as a link among the individual chambers and between all of them and the government.[40] Nizhegorodtsev specifically referred to Bavaria and Saxony as examples of the situation which ought eventually to prevail in Russia, wherein physicians would enjoy "rights, acknowledged by the government, of participation through the elected representatives of the [recognized medical] Society and its branches, in the consideration of both sanitary and medical-estate questions in the supreme medical governmental institution."[41] In fact, as Nizhegorodtsev well knew, not only SPMAS but also (and more importantly) the MVD were far from ready to implement such a scheme in Russia.

At bottom, these ideas about corporate organization raised the question of transforming Russian physicians into a self-governing professional estate, a status that had been granted to barristers during the reforms of the 1860s. The Court Reform of 1864 had forced the government to concede that certain aspects of public affairs fell outside the corporate institutions of the traditional estates of Russian society (clergy, gentry, merchants, townspeople, and peasants) and that new arrangements would have to be devised to accommodate barristers, whose participation in the business of running the country was admitted to be both "necessary and useful."[42] Confronted by the need to share power but determined to retain control of those with whom power was shared, the reformers set up district (*okrug*) councils of barristers as the corporate institutional structure of the new estate. The barristers' councils were empowered to control admission to the estate (*soslovie*), to carry out its legitimate business, and to establish disciplinary procedures for its members. This autonomy was, naturally, not unconditional: the government retained for itself the right to scrutinize the work of the councils to ensure that appropriate standards of truth, honesty, and responsibility were observed by barristers in their dealings with both the government and their clients.[43] Such controlled autonomy may have set limits upon the extent and rate of professionalization among Russian lawyers, but from the government's point of view the new arrangements served its purposes reasonably well.[44]

There is no evidence that reformers within the government regarded the barristers' councils as model organizations that could be adapted to suit other professions, but that did not stop some physicians from believing that they too could attain the status of a professional *soslovie*. In their view, it was a worthwhile goal that promised Russian physicians a measure of autonomy, perhaps less than was enjoyed by physicians in Germany, but certainly far more than Russian physicians enjoyed at present. To be sure, *soslovie* status implied that their obligations to the state and to society at large would be spelled out in detail and scrutinized with rigor. Physicians, no less than barristers, would be expected to behave responsibly, and the government would be watching to see that they did. Hence Nizhegorodtsev felt it imperative to warn that there would be no place in a medical corporate organization for young hotheads: he wanted as members only those who would weigh their words and actions carefully, not "adolescents, with only beautiful words and noble impulses."[45] Physicians would achieve their goals, he concluded, not by phrase-mongering but by hard work: he was prepared to work for change, but only within the limits of the law and the dictates of professional responsibility.

To be sure, *soslovie* status also implied a certain accommodation between the medical profession and the tsarist regime, a certain willingness to accept the political rules of the game. It therefore appealed to those physicians who believed that orderly change within the existing system was the most desirable goal. Nizhegorodtsev stressed that the quest for *soslovie* status could succeed only if physicians worked within strictly legal avenues and were careful never to exceed their own sphere of competence.[46] In his view, tenacious and effective advocacy, coupled with responsible behavior, would inevitably yield positive results; hence he urged SPMAS to submit well-researched petitions to the government and to take an active role in defending physicians who found themselves involved in legal proceedings or public disputes. *Soslovie* status involved demonstrating that physicians were prepared to work with the regime as a precondition for reaching an accommodation with it.[47]

SPMAS had been founded as an offshoot of the Pirogov Society, but Nizhegorodtsev's faith in gradualism and responsible behavior found little support among the community physicians whose concerns now dominated the parent society. The "lessons of experience and [good] sense" which had counseled moderation to Nizhegorodtsev and his colleagues in SPMAS evoked quite different responses from physicians who were becoming impatient and frustrated in their efforts to set Russia on the road to medical and social progress. A growing number were coming to believe that their principal enemy was a regime that kept the people in poverty and ignorance, and some had already concluded that the duty of conscientious physicians was to work for fundamental political reforms, if not the destruction of the tsarist regime itself. A few were beginning to raise questions about the relationship between public health and political economy.[48] Pirogov Society meetings and congresses, as Nancy Frieden has shown, moved from an attitude of resistance to the regime in 1902 through the aggressiveness and determination of 1903 to the militant opposition of 1904.[49] The *pirogovtsy* of these years rejected the whole idea of seeking *soslovie* status for physicians: at the time when fundamental reforms appeared increasingly necessary and, by 1904, even probable, these physicians had no wish to become part of the legal, social, and political structure of the unreformed autocracy. They were repelled by everything that Nizhegorodtsev and SPMAS stood for: stodgy respectability, a cautious and excessively dignified approach to political lobbying, an obsession with ethical and legal problems, and an evident distaste for any form of political or professional militance. This does not mean that the goal of professional unity was abandoned along with the quest for *soslovie* status; on the contrary, the radicals had their own ideas about the form that professional unity should take and endeavored to put them into practice during the Revolution of 1905.

THE HEYDAY OF RADICALISM

The events of 1905 clearly revealed the differing complexions of medical radicalism in St. Petersburg and Moscow. Given the entrenched strength of the medical establishment in St. Petersburg, it was almost inevitable that opposition to the status quo would be led by junior hospital physicians and interns and would be directed against chief hospital physicians. During the spring and summer, the Hospital Physicians' Society organized in all of the large city hospitals campaigns for improved wages and working conditions, as well as better treatment for junior hospital physicians. Staff at the Obukhov hospital petitioned the city administration to eliminate the position of chief physician and substitute instead an elected council representing the staff and the city.[50] In October, frustration finally erupted into turbulence at Nikolai Chudotvorets Hospital; rebellious junior staff put the chief physician in a wheelbarrow and dumped him ignominiously just outside the grounds of the hospital.[51] In Moscow, on the other hand, where opposition was led by community physicians—some of them with ties to left-wing political groups—radical activity went well beyond the wheelbarrow stage. Already in late 1904, P. I. Kurkin, head of the sanitary statistical bureau of Moscow *guberniia* zemstvo, had organized a discussion group composed of zemstvo physicians who were broadly sympathetic to the aims of the revolutionary movement. Few were party members, and their sympathies ran from left Kadet (Constitutional Democrat) to Bolshevik, but they helped to spread revolutionary propaganda and to circulate illegal literature. According to Mitskevich, already a member of the Moscow Bolshevik underground, Kurkin told him in January 1905 to "make use of us in the interests of the revolutionary movement."[52]

For a brief moment in early 1905, Mitskevich and a handful of other Bolshevik physicians took advantange of the sense of outrage which virtually all educated Russians felt in the wake of the Bloody Sunday massacre. When the government announced the establishment of a commission to investigate discontent among urban workers, Mitskevich successfully persuaded the Moscow Society of Factory Physicians to boycott its proceedings.[53] He also organized municipal physicians into a political discussion group that included his fellow Bolsheviks V. Ia. Kanel', I. V. Rusakov, and S. M. Shvaitsar; as its members became better versed in the nuances of party politics, some gravitated naturally towards the Bolshevik cause, but others located themselves in the Menshevik and still others in the Socialist Revolutionary camp.[54] The importance of this handful of Bolsheviks should not, of course, be overestimated: frustration with an apparently obsolete regime and outrage over its ham-fisted attempts at repression did far more to raise the political temperature among community physicians than did Mitskevich and his associates in the revolutionary underground. Nevertheless, the earnestness and omnipresent shrillness of this handful of radicals seemed to suggest that the medical opposition to the regime had moved even further to the left than the liberal-constitutionalist demands espoused by the 1904 Pirogov Congress—as indeed it had, although not so far left as Mitskevich would have liked.

In the end it was the frustrated bacteriologists, rather than the dedicated Bolsheviks, who were responsible for organizing that great forum of medical radicalism in 1905, the Pirogov Society's "Cholera" Congress. Had it not been for the shock waves generated by Bloody Sunday, it is questionable whether official permission would have been granted for holding such a meeting. Although the fear of a summer cholera epidemic was real enough, officials must have realized that the bacteriologists and community physicians would use the occasion not to plan how to coordinate the work of zemstvo and government agencies, but rather to demand that their own plans and organizations take over leadership in the struggle against cholera from the official agencies. Nevertheless, official permission was granted, on the basis of a program that seemed to be entirely concerned with scientific and medical rather than social and political issues.[55]

The Congress was scheduled to meet in Moscow from 21 to 23 March, at the very time when the liberal constitutionalists and revolutionary sympathizers in the opposition front organization known as the Union of Liberation were endeavoring to organize white-collar employees into unions having both professional and political goals.[56] Although there is no evidence that Gabrichevskii or his fellow members of the Pirogov Society executive deliberately planned to use the congress as a forum in which to stage political demonstrations or to organize such a union among physicians, there can be little doubt that many—perhaps most—of the more than 1,600 physicians who converged on Moscow for the congress expected some kind of political fireworks. Inevitably, rumors of what might happen reached St. Petersburg; officials at the MVD had a last-minute change of heart and tried to prevent the congress from taking place. They were too late, however; as the organizers pointed out, many would-be participants were already en route to Moscow. In the end, the MVD had to give in, but the Moscow city governor (gradonachal'nik) was ordered to police the proceedings to ensure that there were no public sessions, no unauthorized participants, and no inflammatory speeches "touching political or public issues."[57] Not surprisingly, this task proved impossible.

There is no need here to recapitulate the debates that occurred at the "Cholera" Congress; they have already been described in detail by Nancy Frieden.[58] What might usefully be underlined, however, is the extent to which speaker after speaker recognized the tsarist regime as the principal obstacle to the improvement of public health. Naturally the Antiplague Commission and the SECs were denounced at every opportunity; as one speaker put it succinctly, "we need cooperative action, not chancery red-tape."[59] The bureaucrats were, of course, by no means the only enemies of ozdorovlenie; both the police and the clergy were also condemned repeatedly for "spreading fantastic and wicked rumors about the intellectual segment of the population among the ignorant masses."[60] Instead of stirring up the people against physicians and the educated classes, argued P. P. Rozanov, the government ought to be doing its utmost to help workers and peasants whose poverty and ignorance made them most vulnerable to disease in general and cholera in particular.[61] Inevitably, these sweeping condemnations of the government and its agents helped to raise the political temperature among congress participants and to ensure overwhelming support for an explicitly political resolution that defied official restrictions and sounded the call for action.

The culmination of these opposition sentiments was the resolution hatched apparently by a group of like-minded physicians and introduced at the final plenary session by D. Ia. Dorf.[62] Its lengthy prologue accused the government of administrative abuse, financial mismanagement, and military adventurism; it spoke feelingly of "torrents of blood" flooding the fields of Manchuria and of "citizens murdered en masse" in St. Petersburg and several other cities. Faced with a cholera epidemic, the government sought the help of physicians while undercutting their efforts by its administrative incompetence and by its attempt to arouse the people against physicians and medical knowledge.

While such abuse continues [the resolution continued], we cannot dream of normal conditions in which to carry out our medical work, of normal conditions of life in general.

Therefore the Pirogov Congress declares that it is necessary for physicians to organize themselves for an energetic struggle hand in hand with the toiling masses against the bureaucratic structure, for its complete elimination and for the convocation of a constituent assembly.

This assembly should be summoned on the basis of universal, equal, direct and secret suffrage, without distinctions of sex, religious faith, and nationality; [its convocation] should be accompanied by a speedy end to the war, the transfer of the police into the hands of public institutions, and the introduction of the principles of inviolability of persons and property, freedom of conscience, speech, press, assembly, unions, and strikes, and the liberation of all those who have suffered for their political and religious convictions.

After calling for ministerial responsibility to a unicameral legislature and a long list of legal, social, and economic reforms,[63] the resolution concluded with a grand flourish:

Only if these preliminary conditions are realized will it be possible to organize a fruitful and planned struggle against the poverty of the people and against epidemics; only then will our country no longer face the fearful plague, cholera, or any other kind of epidemic.

In particular, concerning the struggle with the impending cholera, the Congress finds it impossible for physicians to participate in the Sanitary-Executive Commissions, or to fulfil their directives . . . The Congress considers it reprehensible that physicians continue in the service of those institutions—both public and government—which will demand the fulfillment of [SEC] instructions . . .

Having refused to work in the SECs, physicians at the same time shall not, of course, refuse to join the struggle against cholera in the capacity of private physicians.

For voting purposes, the resolution was divided into two parts. The general statement of political demands passed unanimously, and the call to boycott the SECs was overwhelmingly approved, with only three dissenting votes recorded.[64]

With the corridors and hallways full of students, journalists, and spectators—not to mention the police, who had not been able to contain the proceedings—there was an atmosphere of revolutionary defiance about the closing session of the congress. In this heady atmosphere, a paper was already circulating through the hall advocating the formation of a physicians' union that would join the growing popular opposition to the tsarist regime. The final act of the congress was to give unanimous approval to a hastily drafted resolution establishing an All-Russian Union of Medical Personnel that would work towards realizing the political demands and social reforms already approved.[65] After a short break, congress participants reassembled as members of the union for a short meeting that ended, according to Mitskevich, with cries of "down with the autocracy" and the singing of several revolutionary songs.[66] This moment was to be the high point of medical radicalism in 1905; though there were further manifestations later in the year, none of them equaled the high emotions of the night of 23 March. Ironically, it was also a night's work that would soon come back to haunt those who participated in it.

For the moment, however, all was optimism. The radicals who organized the union believed that this body would attract not only physicians, but all medical personnel—pharmacists, midwives, dentists,
and feldshers—who understood that political reform was the key to
the improvement of public health. The contrasts between this union
and the *soslovie* organization sought by Nizhegorodtsev and his SPMAS
colleagues are instructive: the radicals wanted not an exclusive guild
of physicians, but a more egalitarian organization of medical workers;
not an accommodation with the sociolegal structure of the tsarist regime, but the formation of a new society based on individual equality
and civil rights. Where conservatives such as Nizhegorodtsev had defined medical ethics solely in terms of the relationship between physicians and individual patients, the radicals who promoted the union
believed that all medical professionals, both individually and collectively, had ethical obligations to society as a whole as well as to their
individual patients. Hence they proposed not secret courts of honor to
deal with particular violations of professional standards, but frank and
open criticism of physicians whose social and political behavior violated what the union asserted to be their obligations to society. In
these aspirations lay a radically different conception of the relationship between medicine, society, and the political order, one that reflected the fact that the union's supporters sought to express both a
political and a professional commitment to social change. Because
they expected physicians to play a great role in shaping the new Russia, it was important that the medical union should itself embody the
principles that would guide that new and better society.

The union's program was sketched out in the resolution that brought
it into being.[67] First and foremost, it was to work for the establishment
of a representative form of government in Russia and for the realization of the many reforms called for by the "Cholera" Congress. This
would involve forming as many branches as possible, organizing concerted action by those branches, and cooperating with organizations
that shared similar goals. Within two months, membership in the
union had reached 2,000; by August, it was close to 25,000, including
some twenty local branches in European Russia.[68] To establish a working relationship with other professional-political unions, the medical
union sent delegates to the May Congress of the Union of Unions,
where Mitskevich's radicalism apparently frightened the moderate
constitutionalists from the zemstvo liberal movement.[69] The union's
second major task was to support its members and supporters against
victimization and persecution, and a defense fund was speedily established to aid those suspended or dismissed from employment because of their political activities. At the union's first (and only) congress in August 1905, delegates voted to establish an employment

bureau to assist dismissed colleagues to find other work and called upon physicians to boycott vacancies created by politically motivated dimissals.[70] The original program also committed the union to engage "in the moral evaluation of the public-political misdemeanors of physicians" and suggested that "appropriate measures" would be taken to deal with them, but there is no record of any formal attempts to realize these objectives outside the intense political debate that raged throughout Russian society during 1905.

The revolutionary optimism so evident in March lasted until the union's August congress, after which the radicals began to find themselves overtaken by events. It was easy to persuade congress participants to condemn the government's sole concession of the revolutionary movement, the consultative legislative body proposed by Minister of the Interior Bulygin, as an attempt to dupe the people and strengthen the bureaucracy.[71] But what was to be done to force more substantial concessions from the government? The August congress, still under the spell of earlier rhetoric about struggling alongside the toiling masses, decided that a strike would be the appropriate weapon and approved in principle a proposal that its members should, if necessary, join a strike to achieve their political goals. As it happened, the government made sufficient concessions in the tsar's Manifesto of 17 October 1905, promising a proper legislative assembly and the introduction of civil liberties, that the strike resolution never had to be implemented. Doubtless this was just as well, because a strike by community physicians could have shut down the hospitals and dispensaries operated by zemstvos and municipalities, a result that probably only the union's most dedicated supporters would have been able to justify by asserting the primacy of social over individual obligation. In the wake of the tsar's concessions, political parties were established to contest the forthcoming elections; once they were on the scene, the highly politicized professional unions created during the revolutionary days seemed quickly to become irrelevant. In contrast to its pompous proclamations about evaluating physicians' "sociopolitical misdemeanors," the medical union soon proved unable to cope with the fact that physicians were not unanimous in supporting any one political party or ideology. Though all might agree that the autocracy was an obstacle to the improvement of public health, the fact was that *ozdorovlenie* was a broad enough goal to encompass a range of political opinion that ran all the way from the center of the spectrum to its extreme left. As parties grew and party political debate began, the medical union—like others of that ilk—began to disintegrate.[72] Militant radicalism among Russian physicians had blossomed, flowered, and wilted in a matter of months.

The October manifesto altered the political terrain by supplying the moderates with enough concessions to form a respectable compromise and by diverting the energies of the liberals from illegal to legal opposition. Under the respective banners of the Union of 17 October and the Constitutional Democratic Party, moderates and liberals organized to fight the elections that were to be held for the newly formed legislative body, the State Duma. When the government in April 1906 published new Fundamental Laws that took back much that the October manifesto had granted and yet survived unscathed, it was clear that the revolutionary tide had ebbed considerably. In these changed circumstances, the radicals of 1905 quickly became not the leaders of a crusade but the targets for recrimination. The "Cholera" Congress was soon transformed from an asset into a liability for community medicine because of the overtly political resolution it had adopted and because of the radical union organization to which it had given birth. Taking fresh courage from the survival of the tsarist regime, conservative physicians and zemstvo assemblies soon began to isolate and repudiate the radicals of 1905. To be sure, physicians such as Nizhegorodtsev and his colleagues in the St. Petersburg medical establishment had taken no part in the "Cholera" Congress or the union; now they took the position that the radicals, who had isolated themselves by their own rash behavior, ought to be abandoned to their fate.[73] Exactly what that fate would be gradually became apparent during 1906, as a wave of reaction against liberalism and especially against radical professionals swept through the zemstvos. The next few years were to be a period of ordeal and torment for Russian community medicine.

3
COMMUNITY MEDICINE
IN DISARRAY,
1907–1913

The failure of the 1905 Revolution provoked the Russian intelligentsia to engage in a lengthy, intense, and agonizing self-appraisal. Community physicians had shared the intelligentsia's populist enthusiasms, democratic aspirations, and reformist assumptions; they were consequently devastated by the events of 1906/07. The idea of *ozdorovlenie* and the program of reform which community physicians associated with it took a battering from the gentry reaction in the zemstvos. An immediate casualty was the working alliance between *zemtsy* and community physicians which had lasted for a decade. Meanwhile, the government of Premier P. A. Stolypin resorted to punitive expeditions to restore order in the countryside; instead of zemstvos at the *volost'* level, the government established field courts-martial. Far from extending public participation in politics, Stolypin scrapped plans for local government reform, thereby allowing the gentry to consolidate their grip on the countryside and, in what amounted to a coup d'état, changed the electoral law to give them an artificial prominence in the State Duma. The very events that many had expected to cripple the tsarist regime had, in fact, served as a restorative tonic. Recognizing that the government was a more formidable foe in 1907 than it had been in 1904 or 1905, members of the intelligentsia found themselves drinking deeply from the cup of bitterness and despair.

For community physicians, the reappraisal naturally began with the social and political assumptions underlying zemstvo medicine. Within six months of Stolypin's coup, the Pirogov Society's *Journal* carried an essay by S. N. Igumnov which asked whether the new political realities of post-1905 Russia had made *obshchestvennost'* into an anachronism.[1] Soon a barrage of criticism was directed at the populist (*narodnik*) ideology of the Pirogov Society and of zemstvo medicine, criticism that was the more searching and devastating because it came from community physicians themselves. Some argued that it no longer made sense for physicians to try to shape the education and political reorganization of the Russian people and that the times now demanded a narrower and more rigorous professionalism. Others argued that present political conditions made the social mission of community medicine more important than ever; they despaired over the apparent loss of public spirit among younger zemstvo physicians who dared to refuse work if they found salaries or working conditions undesirable or to supplement their salaries by making housecalls to the rich on a fee-for-service basis. What had become, more than one writer was to ask, of the selfless dedication that the older generation had learned from Pirogov himself?

The so-called crisis of zemstvo medicine, which loomed so large in the medical press from 1908 onwards, was, however, but one aspect of the disarray in which community medicine found itself. To be sure, both the political reaction and the generation gap were real enough, but of greater significance for the future were developments within medicine itself which threatened the aspirations and assumptions that Russian community physicians had held in the years before 1905. Those who were affected by these new developments began to question not only the strategy and tactics of zemstvo medicine, but its ideology, which they increasingly believed was lacking in scientific rationale and integrity.

Russia was by no means unaffected by those forces that were changing the face of European medicine at the turn of the century. The knowledge gained in the course of the bacteriological revolution set off a struggle between physicians and bacteriologists in every country that shared in these discoveries.[2] As scientific knowledge proliferated, specialization began to strain the traditional organization of medical knowledge, education, and practice.[3] In Germany, where Bismarck's social insurance legislation had given rise to workers' hospital funds and to the new field of occupational medicine, there was a lively debate about the nature and content of social medicine—*sozialmedizin*—which spilled over into Russia.[4] Russian medicine, like medicine everywhere in the West during these years, was in a state of ferment; what turned this ferment from creativity into disarray was the pervasive and uniquely Russian ideological dimension that cast its shadow over every new development and intruded upon every debate. Pirogov traditionalists, fearful of anything that would undermine zemstvo sanitary services or make sweeping social reforms unnecessary and clinging with grim determination to Erismann's environmentalism, revived their earlier criticisms of bacteriology. The same group greeted the growth of medical specialties not with optimism but with distaste, fearing that specialization would both undermine the Pirogov Society and alter drastically the delivery of zemstvo medical services. When such innovations as hospital funds and factory medicine (industrial hygiene) made their appearance in Russia, Pirogov traditionalists barely tolerated their presence outside the zemstvo medical structure.

THE PIROGOV SOCIETY IN THE STOLYPIN ERA

The political resolutions passed at the 1905 "Cholera" Congress made the government so angry that it refused to grant permission for the regular Pirogov Congress that should have been held in 1906. Thus the society did not meet until the early spring of 1907. In the more than two years that had passed since the "Cholera" Congress, the Union of All-Russian Medical Personnel had become virtually defunct; its erstwhile leaders met again before the 1907 Pirogov Congress to see if anything could be salvaged from the wreckage. While they would have liked to keep alive some of the ideals of 1905, they had to face the fact that the Ministry of the Interior would refuse to legalize any organization suspected of radicalism. Moreover, the union's doctrinaire stance on ethical issues in 1905 and its apparent support for strike action had alienated moderate physicians, who were now chary of direct political action. In the circumstances, the most sensible course of action was to tie the idea of a revived medical union to the reform of local government which, it was thought, Stolypin was about to introduce. Despite growing evidence of a gentry reaction in the zemstvos against the liberal goals of 1905, members of the intelligentsia still expected the new premier to broaden public participation in government, initially by introducing zemstvo institutions at the *volost'* level.[5] In these proposals for change, the advocates of a medical union were able to see opportunities for the continuing involvement of physicians with social issues and popular education.

The result of these deliberations was the proposal, put before the Tenth Pirogov Congress in April, to form an All-Russian Medical Union that would pursue both professional and public (*obshchestvennye*) goals. Its main tasks would be "to prepare the ground for the imminent crowning reform in local self-government [the *volost'* zemstvo]; to prepare the people to take an active part in this reform, and in their own future autonomy; and to respond to their most pressing questions and needs."[6] To allay the fears of moderates, supporters of the proposal argued that this would not be a political body like the 1905 union; instead, it would engage in nonpolitical "public work" while the political battles were fought out in the State Duma. The structure proposed for the union was a bizarre, if faithful, reflection of its sponsors' faith in both the Pirogov Society and local autonomy; there were to be autonomous branches at the *raion, uezd, guberniia,* and *oblast'* levels, while the union's "All-Russian Bureau" was to be composed of a dozen members chosen by Pirogov congresses, as well as of the entire Pirogov

Society executive. Inasmuch as *raion* branches were given sweeping responsibilities, it is less than clear what role was envisioned for the bureau, let alone for the three intermediate levels of organization.[7] As it happened, however, structure was a secondary issue: participants at the congress wanted first to discuss the character of the proposed union.

Opinion was sharply divided.[8] Some argued for a very narrow, professional body on the grounds that the less the union had to do with larger issues, the more likely its success; such a gradual, professional approach, they claimed, would "correspond to the situation in which zemstvo physicians find themselves, since . . . in the majority of cases they have no close connection with the population."[9] Defenders of the proposal, on the other hand, argued that a narrowly professional organization would not be trusted by the people and hence would increase the isolation of physicians; they also warned that zemstvo physicians must not be reduced to "artisans, drained of their community ideals and spirit."[10] A straw vote on the preferences of those present produced 215 votes for the proposal and 205 for the alternative of a "purely professional" organization.[11] Some of the 205 may well have sympathized with the idea of a broadly based union but believed its formation to be unwise in present political circumstances. None of those who spoke against the union proposal seem to have thought of returning to the quest for *soslovie* status which had been led by the St. Petersburg Physicians' Mutual Assistance Society before 1905. Participants in the 1907 Pirogov Congress were obviously a chastened group, but they were not yet in despair. They sought not an end to their conflict with the autocracy but a truce. In the end, the congress assigned the task of producing a revised constitution for the union to a specially chosen committee of twelve; it also asked the Pirogov Society's executive to make recommendations concerning the union's ultimate relationship with the society and to circulate these to all interested societies and institutions so that everything could be settled at an extraordinary congress to be convened especially for that purpose.[12]

Momentous events occurred in the weeks after the congress. Under pressure from the provincial gentry, Stolypin abandoned his plans to introduce *volost'* zemstvo institutions and referred the whole question of local government reform back to the MVD. If community physicians had looked forward to the reform because they expected it to give them a big role in the shaping of Russian society, conservative gentry feared it for precisely the same reason; they did not wish the countryside to be taken over by a rural intelligentsia they suspected of being the tool of "Jewish interests."[13] On 3 June, the premier carried out his coup against the State Duma, altering its electoral law so as to give an artificial predominance to voters who owned significant prop-

erty, provided they were also of great Russian stock and of the Orthodox faith. Taken together, Stolypin's actions constituted a repudiation
of the influence of professionals in Russian life; they were to be permitted almost no role whatever in public affairs, whether in the villages
or in the State Duma.

For the physicians who had tried to keep alive the spirit of the 1905
medical union, Stolypin's change of course was a disaster. Everything
that they had envisioned for the reorganized union was based on the
expectation that the government would begin to broaden the composition, expand the powers, and increase the revenues of the zemstvos.
The enthusiasm for "public work" had come from those who envisioned the reorganized union working with local, popular zemstvo institutions to rebuild Russian society. Stolypin's accommodation with
the gentry reaction meant that, although there might be further tinker-
ing with local government, nothing would be done that would allow
zemstvo professionals to rebuild their relationships with the people.

Stolypin's actions not only took all the momentum out of the attempt to revive the medical union, it also threw into question the place
of professionals, particularly public-spirited professionals such as
physicians, in Russian society. For six months after the coup, while
stunned observers tried to work out the implications of what had been
done, the medical press was virtually silent on public issues. Then, all
at once, began the laments, the recriminations, the soul-searching that
would dominate its pages for the next six years. By pulling the rug out
from under the expectations of the *pirogovtsy*, Stolypin unwittingly
precipitated a reconsideration of the entire enterprise known as zemstvo medicine.

THE CRISIS OF ZEMSTVO MEDICINE

The first person to attempt an assessment of what had happened tried
to strike a positive note. In a long article in the Pirogov Society *Journal*
in January 1908, G. A. Berdichevskii considered the future of community medicine in the wake of the collapse of the revolutionary movement and the triumph of reaction in the zemstvos.[14] Without using the
words themselves, he argued that it was time for small deeds rather
than senseless dreams: in his view, the situation was far from hopeless, and zemstvo physicians should by no means throw up their
hands in despair. Now was the time, he proposed, to stand back and
take a long look at the delivery of rural medical care, to make it more
efficient, and to improve both its quality and its acessibility to the
population. As examples of what might be done, he proposed restrict-
ing the number of clinics for which an *uchastok* physician was responsible, setting limits to the working day, and screening the patients
seen, with feldshers routinely dealing with less serious cases.[15] It was

high time, he implied, that the outdated idealism of traditional zemstvo medicine was replaced by a more flexible, pragmatic, and realistic
approach. For Berdichevskii, the fact that the 1905 Revolution had
failed seemed almost a blessing in disguise.

Predictably, this line of argument aroused the fury of dedicated
narodnik physicians, one of whom—S. N. Igumnov—took up his pen
to reply.[16] What particularly galled Igumnov was that Berdichevskii was
proposing to throw overboard, in the name of realism, the best traditions of zemstvo medicine. His views on the role of the clinic were a
case in point: from Igumnov's point of view, they were an attack on the
heart and soul of the encounter between physician and patient.

> The old zemstvo physicians attached enormous importance to the clinics. For
> them, the clinic was not only a place for selecting the sick for bed-rest and
> for operations, but an independent area for systematic care . . . For them
> the clinic was not only an office . . . but an auditorium of a kind, in which
> the physician preached hygienic and medical knowledge in concrete cir-
> cumstances, demonstrated the need for systematic care, and trained [his pa-
> tients] in it.[17]

Igumnov could see clearly what was coming if Berdichevskii had his
way. The roles of preacher, demonstrator, and teacher would be for-
saken, and physicians would put in no more than a perfunctory appearance at the clinic, where they would hastily select patients for
hospital care. From such a prospect he recoiled with horror.

> He [the zemstvo physician] is a community physician, who satisfies the needs
> of broad strata of the population and who studies its sanitary condition, and
> not a clinician who shuts himself in his chamber or operating room; he is a
> physician-sociologist who has the broad masses of the population for the ob-
> ject of his study and activity, and not a physician-individualist, who is inter-
> ested only in a particular sick organism.[18]

Thus, he argued, Berdichevskii's proposals aimed not simply at shedding the idealism of earlier generations, but at a fundamental transformation of zemstvo medicine.

Nevertheless, Igumnov did not claim that everything about zemstvo
medicine was sacrosanct; he was prepared to grant that "in the hopes
and aspirations of former zemstvo physicians there was no small
amount of sentimentality and naive faith" and that the shedding of
those illusions was probably beneficial. He was prepared to see a thoroughgoing exchange of opinions on the principles, structure, and
character of zemstvo medicine because he felt that the present atmosphere was indeed one of internal crisis.

All is not well in zemstvo medicine: its development has been complicated by big new tasks, and their solution has been made more difficult by influences which go against its former tendencies, the alteration of which, it is acknowledged, is untimely. All this, in addition to other—political and social—conditions, is creating a situation in which it is difficult to foresee its speedy resolution or to point to the way out. Perhaps it will be a fatal blow to the old answers offered by zemstvo medicine, perhaps new people will bring forth a new answer . . .[19]

popular
nostalgia

Igumnov's stance typified that of the older generation of zemstvo physicians in the wake of 1905. They knew that the end of an era had arrived and that zemstvo medical life would never again be the same; they were nostalgic for the past, uneasy with the present, and fearful for the future.

The exchange between Berdichevski and Igumnov opened the floodgates; soon every number of the medical press carried at least one article on the theme of a crisis of zemstvo medicine. Virtually every aspect of zemstvo medical work was analyzed and criticized: salaries and working conditions; relations between physicians and zemstvo boards; the alleged loss of public spirit among younger physicians, reflected particularly in the growth of private practice among zemstvo physicians; the lack of direction and the obvious disunity apparent at the 1907 Pirogov Congress. The debate had scarcely begun when bacteriology and laboratory research were once again held up as symbols of all that had gone wrong with community medicine, a turn of events which demonstrated that the accommodation between bacteriology and the Pirogov Society was more fragile than had appeared to be the case in 1905. A predominantly Marxist minority endeavored to expand the focus of the debate beyond medicine itself to include the social tensions and political conflicts of post-1905 Russia, but on the whole physicians preferred to concentrate on the uniquely medical and professional aspects of their situation. Hence the obsession, shared by so many contributors to the debate, with physicians' inability to create a strong, unified professional organization. Supporters of unity seized on the idea of forming an All-Russian Pirogov Society and converted it into a kind of Holy Grail, which could be attained only by those of the purest heart and noblest character. Soon this debate over the future of zemstvo medicine became a debate about appropriate ideals and moral standards, a physicians' counterpart to the debate then raging among the intelligentsia as a whole in the wake of the publication of *Vekhi* (*Landmarks*) by a group of repentant Marxists and idealist philosophers.[20]

"Everything youthful, courageous, and noble is fleeing from the zemstvo," lamented N. A. Vigdorchik in a review of the events of 1908, because "the glorious temple of zemstvo medicine" no longer holds the attraction that it once did.[21] Because of firings, repression, or bureaucratic formalism, he went on, the zemstvos were losing their best workers; those who were dismissed and those who feared to remain began to escape from the countryside to the largest cities. There was, however, little work to be found because municipal dumas were also cutting back on medical and sanitary services; many of these "refugees" remained unemployed or at best found some temporary employment fighting cholera with a Red Cross medical team. Shortage of work strained collegiality to its breaking point. Vigdorchik noted that one now found an attitude of *sauve qui peut* where there was once only support and mutual assistance.[22] A few physicians, it was

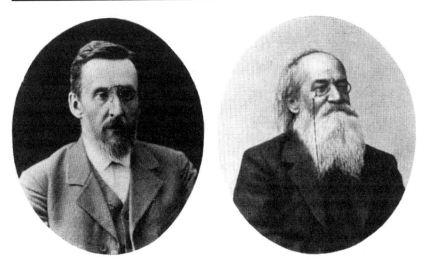

Fig. 5. The defenders of traditional community medicine: S. N. Igumnov *(left)* and D. N. Zhbankov *(right)*.

rumored, had even sought the protection of such right-wing organizations as the Union of the Russian People and the Union of Michael the Archangel.

Evidence from the provinces confirms many of the impressions which Vigdorchik had formed in Moscow and St. Petersburg. A. V. Amsterdamskii, who reviewed the scene in 1911, noted that many zemstvos had been forced to raise the salaries of *guberniia* and *uezd* physicians between 1908 and 1911, but that these actions had merely slowed, rather than stopped "the flight of physicians from zemstvo service."[23] Typically, salaries were increased from the 1,200–1,500-ruble range to the 1,500–2,000-ruble range, with possible increases to as much as 3,000 rubles after ten or fifteen years of service. Perm *guberniia*, for example, found it necessary to raise the salaries of its physicians to make them closer to what it paid its engineers and to introduce changes that would make long service financially attractive.[24] In Saratov, the problem was not so much one of attracting young physicians but one of retaining their services after an initial year or two.[25] Various expedients were tried, such as regular periodic salary increases, reducing the qualification period for a service pension, and credit for previous work with another zemstvo, but these were no more than stopgap measures. Zemstvos in more remote—especially northern—areas had even greater difficulty in attracting and retaining physicians.[26]

Even physicians who remained in the countryside shared in this growing indifference towards zemstvo medical work. One persistent example was the frequently noted absence of *uezd* physicians from the meetings of provincial sanitary councils. In Kaluga in 1910 and Ufa in 1912, *uezd* physicians boycotted such meetings; in Tauride *guberniia*, the council was forced to pay travel costs and per diem allowances to secure representation from Yalta.[27] Other zemstvos also found it necessary to pay physicians' travel costs, but even these incentives failed to stop the growth of absenteeism, especially in those provinces where the zemstvo board was notorious for ignoring the recommendations of its sanitary council. Absenteeism became chronic in the provinces of Moscow, Voronezh, and Riazan. Amsterdamskii commented that, "Evidently among zemstvo physicians there is . . . suppressed dissatisfaction with their status, the insufficiency of their work, a diminishing of past excitement and a loss of faith in the broad public significance of their work."[28]

The alleged indifference and materialism of physicians provoked complaints from zemstvo board members and cries of despair from those who remembered the "selfless dedication" of an earlier generation of zemstvo physicians. The most flagrant example of this new materialism was the rise of private practice among zemstvo physicians. Private practice in any form had been regarded as a mortal sin by the *narodnik* ideologists and propagandists of community medicine, who saw it as their duty to save Russia from the commercial entrepreneurship that, they alleged, dominated European and Anglo-American medical practice. For any Russian physician to operate on a fee-for-service basis was, in their eyes, lamentable, but for a zemstvo physician—the bearer of the Russian service ethic—to do so was despicable. That many zemstvo physicians did nevertheless engage in varying amounts of private practice was a fact well known to the Pirogov Society; its prevalence was usually ascribed to inadequate salaries and occasionally to individual greed. Traditional attitudes were reasserted in late 1910 at a congress of Moscow *guberniia* zemstvo physicians, when a resolution was passed which condemned private practice in no uncertain terms, stating flatly that real medical work in the hospitals and *uchastki* was suffering because of it.[29]

Two months after the congress, *Obshchestvennyi Vrach* carried a long and thoughtful article on the subject by K. G. Slavskii, himself a Moscow *uchastok* physician with a wide experience of zemstvo medicine in several provinces.[30] Slavskii began by admitting that virtually all zemstvo physicians took a fee for making a house call but that some never earned more than a few rubles a year in this fashion while others earned as much as a thousand. He rejected both low salaries and personal greed as explanations for the phenomenon and argued instead that its prevalence was primarily due to the imperfections of zemstvo medicine itself. With refreshing candor, Slavskii pointed out that there were people who preferred to avoid zemstvo hospitals and dispensaries, not because they were aristocratic snobs, but because they knew very well that "the typical 2 or 3-minute examination that occurs there is no way to make decisions about the state of the human organism."[31] If zemstvo physicians or members of their families became ill, he admitted, they did not join the queue at the dispensary, but instead sought a talented colleague, as Slavskii himself had done when his daughter was stricken with typhoid fever. More was at stake, however, than the quality of medical care; there was also the fact that physicians did not want patients who were suffering from contagious or epidemic diseases to come to zemstvo hospitals anyway. Ideally, such people should have been sent to the isolation barracks, although in reality it was impossible for zemstvo physicians to see all these patients in their homes for preliminary diagnosis. Hence physicians were likely to go either where they knew a fee would be waiting or where they risked a legal complaint if they failed to respond.[32] Thus he concluded that private practice by zemstvo physicians would die out only when substantial improvements had been made in the quality of hospital, dispensary, and home care.

Instead of the moralizing that was typical of many spokesmen for community medicine, Slavskii had taken a pragmatic view, arguing that zemstvo physicians should be judged by the quality of the work they did while on duty and not by some "relentless" standard that would condemn them for how they spent their off-duty hours, "whether it is in reading learned journals, playing cards, or engaging in private practice."[33] In a final salvo, he predicted that he would be condemned as a heretic by the upholders of "zemstvo orthodoxy" (*zemskoe pravoverie*), who would not share his view that "the time is already pressing for a review of many of the principles of zemstvo medicine."[34] Nevertheless, he urged his readers to rethink attitudes that were so inflexible that they lacked human feeling and ignored real questions about the quality of medical care—the very attitudes, by the way, which physicians were quick to condemn in St. Petersburg bureaucrats.

Slavskii's article quickly drew hostile responses, the most important of which was written by D. N. Zhbankov, the administrator of the Pirogov Society.[35] Zhbankov methodically worked his way through all of the arguments that he had ever heard advanced on behalf of private practice and questioned or dismissed every one of them. In his view, the problem had developed neither because of low salaries nor because of shortcomings in the structure of zemstvo medicine but as a consequence of the conservative tide that had swept through the zemstvos after the Revolution of 1905. Lamenting the passing of those fine days when dedicated physicians taught the *zemtsy* what was really meant by public service, Zhbankov deplored the lack of concern displayed by the new generation of *zemtsy*. The growth of private practice was, he claimed, a symptom of the decline in idealism among zemstvo physicians. To explain it was not to condone it, however; he insisted that clear limits would have to be set, lest its growth "demoralize the whole family of zemstvo physicians and destroy their influence in the zemstvos and among the population."[36]

Warming to his theme, the old *narodnik* stressed the need for physicians to behave in an exemplary fashion, so as to retain the loyalty of the wealthy minority who paid the lion's share of the physician's salary through zemstvo taxes.[37] Inevitably, he followed this with a eulogy of the "true" zemstvo physician, one whose ideals, temperament, and psychology were modeled as closely as possible upon the character and career of Pirogov himself, as if invoking the master's name would somehow ward off any temptation to depart from his high standards. The populist, even Slavophile quality of Zhbankov's world view is especially apparent in his frequent references to zemstvo physicians as a family and in the remarkable analogy that he drew between this "family" and the peasant commune. Replying to one critic who had said that many of the zemstvo physicians who engaged in private practice were themselves adornments to zemstvo medicine, Zhbankov scoffed, "this is like calling an *otrubnik* [one who had separated from the village commune under the Stolypin land reform] the protector of, and an adornment to, the Russian commune."[38] From a *narodnik* such as Zhbankov, there could be no greater pejorative; those who separated from the commune violated that mystical sense of Slavic *sobornost'* which, populists believed, gave the commune its vitality; violated it,

moreover, in the immoral and ultimately sterile pursuit of western in-
dividualism and financial gain.

This first phase of this debate over zemstvo medicine served to reveal the extent to which its development had rested on the ideology of
populism. Igumnov's attack on narrow clinicians proceeded from the
same *narodnik* assumptions about the social role of physicians as did
Zhbankov's condemnation of the evils of private practice. It was all
very well for Igumnov to suggest that the present crisis might only be
resolved by new people with new answers, but the fact is that he and
Zhbankov were establishing themselves as the custodians of the moral
purity of zemstvo medicine. New people such as Slavskii knew very
well that their new answers would evoke hostility from the defenders
of zemstvo orthodoxy (*zemskoe pravoverie*). Igumnov and Zhbankov
became the most articulate spokesmen for Pirogov traditionalists, stak-
ing out the moral high ground for what was to become a protracted
defense of populist values against the forces of medical innovation.

THE PROBLEM OF SPECIALIZATION

Central to the development of community medicine was the idea of
the zemstvo physician as a generalist. Diagnostician, therapist, surgeon, ophthalmologist, and sometimes midwife as well, the zemstvo
uchastok physician was idealized in the publications of the Pirogov Society as a heroic jack-of-all-trades. The founders of community medicine—Osipov, Molleson, and Erismann, along with the great Pirogov
himself—were celebrated as much for the range of their interests as
for their devotion to the people's welfare. When sanitary bureaus and
sanitary physicians were introduced during the 1890s, it was not with
the idea that they would specialize in public health matters while the
uchastok physicians spent more of their time in hospital work; on the
contrary, sanitary physicians were meant to complement the generalism already inherent in zemstvo medical work. Where *uchastok* physicians used clinics not only for therapeutic but also educational purposes, sanitary physicians used them to obtain the raw material from
which to analyze morbidity and mortality in the locality. Thus the sanitary physician was functioning not only as a hygienist but also as a
statistician, topographer, anthropologist, and even ethnographer. The
essential purpose of these studies was to provide *uchastok* physicians
with information that would enable them to function more effectively
in their various roles; hence the first *guberniia* sanitary physicians
were not newly minted medical school graduates who knew nothing
of rural practice but rather zemstvo physicians with several years' experience.[39] It soon became an article of faith that every sanitary physician ought to have served a period of duty as an *uchastok* physician.

Among Pirogov traditionalists, such generalism was applauded at every turn.

Just as the ideology of community medicine discouraged specialization, so the Pirogov Society itself discouraged the formation of separate groups of specialists at the national level. It was all right for zemstvo or municipal physicians to meet at the *uezd*, *guberniia*, or municipal level or even for the hospital physicians of St. Petersburg or the obstetricians and gynecologists of Kiev to meet together, but at the "All-Russian" level the Pirogov Society strove to encompass all of the various professional interests of Russian physicians. Hence the eclectic programs of its congresses, with sessions on everything from surgery and ophthamology to the prevention of epidemics and "medical life" (a euphemism for discussion of salaries, working conditions, and legal and social status). What the society did not want to see was the formation of other national bodies of physicians united either by specialty (e.g., forensic medicine) or by type of employment (e.g., factory physicians), bodies that would claim to speak for their own members and that might try to cast the Pirogov Society as only the mouthpiece for zemstvo and municipal physicians. Hence the Society's leaders always behaved as if all salaried physicians in the empire—whether employed by the state or by public or private charities—had interests identical to those of the community physicians and wished to pursue them under the banner of the Pirogov Society. Elements of this universalist approach can be seen in the 1907 proposal for an All-Russian Medical Union; in a modified form, it survived in the dream of forming an All-Russian Pirogov Society. Hostility towards the formation of specialist groups contributed to the disarray in which community medicine found itself between 1907 and 1914.

The problem surfaced first within the Pirogov Society itself over the seemingly intractable problem of professional unity. Partisans of both a "professional" and a "public" union kept the argument alive in the medical press, hoping no doubt to influence the special commission that had been established at the 1907 Pirogov Congress. The commission finally published its proposal for an All-Russian Pirogov Society in March 1908.[40] Although the goals proposed in this draft statute were broad enough to please almost everyone, the proposal itself was stillborn.[41] Thanks to the tide of reaction, there was no longer any significant support for the idea of a professional association. The fact was that, as one commentator put it, 1908 had been a "dry and fruitless year" for both community medicine and the Pirogov Society.[42] Interest in the old questions of community medicine declined, attendance at medical society meetings fell off, and membership in the Pirogov Society itself plummeted to a point where both the salaries of its staff and the budget for its publication program were threatened. The government added to the society's problems by arresting temporarily its administrator, D. N. Zhbankov, confiscating three numbers of its *Journal*, and interfering with the operation of its standing committees.[43] Morale among community physicians was, it seemed, at an all-time low.

The events of 1905–1908 led some supporters of a united medical profession to reconsider the whole idea. M. M. Gran', who had earlier been one of the strongest supporters of a public-professional union, published an article in 1909 to which he gave the provocative title, "Are Physicians Capable of Uniting?"[44] His conclusion was, almost predictably, pessimistic: given their differences in social background, educational level, medical specialty, political allegiance, and circumstances of employment, Russian physicians could never organize themselves into one national professional association. As if to dramatize his argument, the Eleventh Pirogov Congress, which met in St. Petersburg in April 1910, was a spiritless and indecisive affair that made few decisions and avoided politically dangerous topics. Almost embarrassingly, the All-Russian Pirogov Society proposal had to be dealt with; in the general mood of apathy, fear, and government intimidation, the congress hastily buried this relic of 1907 with a vote not to change the constitution at this time "because of universal apathy about the stagnation of the state."[45] In the wake of this glaring admission of failure, Zhbankov and other diehard supporters of the idea of an All-Russian Pirogov Society were reduced to campaigning for the establishment of a Pirogov memorial building in Moscow, but even this drastically modified objective ran into difficulties.[46]

Unable to unify Russian physicians into a national professional association, the Pirogov Society was forced to reconsider another of its aspirations, that of providing a roof under which specialized interests would be content to shelter. For almost two decades, this policy of containment had worked well; the psychiatrists were the only group who had gone their own way in the face of suspicion and hostility from somatic physicians, including those who dominated the Pirogov Society.[47] However, in the difficult years after 1907, the society was no longer strong enough to stand in the way of the growth of legitimate professional specialties. Both factory medicine and bacteriology were by this time more than ready to blossom on their own, and so, concurring in the inevitable, the Pirogov Society lent its support to the holding of separate congresses by these groups of specialists, beginning in 1909. (Russian psychiatrists held a national congress in 1911, but they proceeded without the support or encouragement of the Pirogov Society; some specialties were clearly more acceptable than others.) As these specialists began to voice their own concerns and aspirations, it became clear that more of the cherished assumptions of community medicine would have to be revised or abandoned.

The professional situation of factory physicians had been discussed at the 1907 Pirogov Congress just before the optimism of the revolutionary years had been totally dissipated. At that time, participants were almost patronizing in their assumption that factory physicians had everything to gain from a closer association with zemstvo medicine and the Pirogov Society. Discussion centered on their financial plight; most had to take on additional work to make ends meet; professional leaves of absence and pensions were both virtually unknown.[48] Stirrings of protest against this situation were already apparent; it was reported that an organized group of factory physicians in Moscow was already planning a national society and the establishment of a mutual aid fund and that it was ready to battle against those employers who regarded physicians as lackeys or even as policemen who should assist in the administration of the factory.[49]

Factory physicians soon had a chance to flex their own muscles at their first All-Russian Congress, which met in Moscow in April 1909.[50] Its packed agenda revealed the breadth of their interests; sessions were held on such themes as workers' housing and sanitation, illness and accidents, social diseases (alcoholism, tuberculosis, and syphilis), the position of factory medical personnel, and factory inspection. Several papers were devoted to analyzing the government's recently formulated proposals on sickness and accident insurance. Three papers and a lengthy discussion were devoted to the question of what relationship, if any, ought to exist between factory medical care and zemstvo medicine. During the course of these sessions it became clear that, contrary to the assumptions of the *pirogovsty*, many factory physicians were not in favor of transferring factory medicine to the jurisdiction of the zemstvos.[51] They were as aware as their colleagues in zemstvo medicine that there was continual tension between zemstvo boards and their employees, that budgets for medical and sanitary work were already insufficient, and that zemstvo *uchastok* physicians were notoriously overworked. Even if the government gave zemstvos additional funds to defray the cost of factory medical work, factory physicians were skeptical that these funds would actually be spent as intended, given the many other expenses that zemstvos already faced for medical care. Their clear preference was for the establishment of employee-managed hospital funds, paid for largely by employers but free of control by either employers or the government. Recognizing that this was probably an impossible goal in the existing circumstances, some factory physicians were prepared to accept—but only as the lesser of two evils—zemstvo or municipal supervision over the administration of hospital funds.

These views and preferences were forcefully reiterated a year later during a session on factory medicine at the 1910 Pirogov Congress.[52]

Many longtime *pirogovtsy* were astonished to discover that factory physicians had their own ideas about the future and that these did not include factory medicine becoming a poor relation of zemstvo medicine. At the same time, other participants suggested a persuasive financial reason for reconsidering the desirability of a zemstvo "takeover" of factory medicine: if the government turned factory medicine over to the zemstvo without forcing employers to pay for this care or without providing additional funds, then the costs would be staggering and might well further imperil zemstvo medical and sanitary work.[53] In the wake of this discussion, many *pirogovtsy* began to question their earlier belief that all forms of medical assistance would inevitably attach themselves to the zemstvo medical structure. When the government proceeded to introduce workers' sickness and accident insurance legislation in 1912, the gap between factory physicians and community physicians only widened.

If factory physicians raised legitimate questions about the scope and jurisdiction of zemstvo medicine, bacteriologists questioned the effectiveness of its public health work. The 1911 Conference on Bacteriology and Epidemiology opened up what was to become a central issue in Russian medicine during the prewar years: the scope and direction of zemstvo sanitary services.[54] Even before the conference met, there were indications that zemstvo sanitary activities were in considerable difficulties. A year earlier, Shingarev had tried to blame their sorry state on the shortage of funds made available by zemstvos and by the state treasury and on administrative interference and arbitrary behavior, arguing that zemstvo medical budgets must be reformed and grants from the state increased.[55] Part of the difficulty, however, stemmed from the fact that the radicals who deplored Stolypin's change of course had tried to keep alive the conception of a small zemstvo unit in the form of the "sanitary guardianship," a campaign that had more to do with education and social improvement than with sanitary reform per se.[56] At least one critic saw this endeavor as wasteful, dismissing sanitary guardianships as "a pitiful, insignificant palliative which has no solid foundation in the contemporary life of the masses."[57] In the end, the congress took no clear position; it was easier to blame others for existing shortcomings than it was to try to find appropriate solutions.

During the interval between the 1910 Congress and the 1911 Bacteriology Conference, two very important articles appeared that paved the way for the searching discussions that followed. One, by Dr. T. M. Brok, a zemstvo physician in Kherson *guberniia*, was a blistering attack on zemstvo medicine for being out of date, in a rut, and unscientific.[58] Pointing to all of the discoveries in bacteriology, chemistry, physics, and radiography, Brok attacked zemstvo physicians for still relying primarily on the stethescope, the thermometer, and the bottle of pills. Without microscopes and laboratory facilities, he pointed out, they could not possibly keep abreast of recent research on blood, urine, and stomach juices; hence their diagnoses were based on guesswork and imprecision when mathematical accuracy was both desirable and possible. Zemstvo medicine, he concluded, needed to broaden its public health work and drastically revise its methods of individual care, "arming medical wisdom with the weapons of research and the laboratory."[59]

A parallel argument about the deficiencies in zemstvo antiepidemic measures was put forward by the new director of the Nizhnii Novgorod *guberniia* sanitary bureau, A. N. Sysin.[60] He placed the blame for zemstvo medicine's poor performance in fighting the 1910 cholera epidemic (see chapter 4) not on the shortage of funds or on administrative interference but on organizational shortcomings and the failure to take appropriate measures. In particular, he pointed to the absence of an effective antiepidemic program at the *uezd* level. Even where *uezd* sanitary physicians existed—a rarity in most provinces in 1910—an *uezd* zemstvo office was, he argued, simply unfitted to cope with a cholera epidemic because it did not have the time, the personnel or the requisite expertise. Without local agents who could feed it accurate information at top speed via telegraph, the *guberniia* sanitary bureau was also in no position to coordinate the battle; Sysin compared its situation to that of a surgeon operating with his eyes closed.[61] Trained personnel with appropriate plans and rapid means of communication were absolutely essential if the struggle against epidemics was to become effective at the *uezd* level. Ironically, Brok and Sysin had between them produced an indictment of zemstvo medicine and sanitary services on precisely the two grounds upon which its supporters had always prided themselves: the care of patients and the struggle against epidemics. After years of ridiculing the government for the low level of medical care in the non-zemstvo provinces and scoffing at the efforts of Sanitary-Executive Commissions, traditionalists were dismayed to find the supposed strengths of zemstvo medicine now exposed as weaknesses by knowledgeable insiders.

Pressure for an increased emphasis on laboratory research came from two quarters: (1) hard-pressed *uchastok* physicians who agreed with Brok's argument that their diagnostic and therapeutic skills would be enormously assisted by the availability of laboratory tests and verifications and (2) younger sanitary physicians who were dissatisfied with the constraints imposed by the traditional emphasis on sociological and statistical research. Although these groups could agree with each other about the need to build and fund laboratories, their different emphases contained the seeds of future disagreement over the content of the research program: ought the laboratory to be primarily at the dispoasl of *uchastok* physicians or the staff of the *guberniia* sanitary bureau? Or was it conceivable that laboratory work could serve both groups at the same time? Before these latent difficulties could reach the surface, the supporters of laboratory research had to withstand a counterattack from Pirogov traditionalists, whose self-appointed spokesman on this issue was S. N. Igumnov.

Head of the Khar'kov *guberniia* sanitary bureau and a fervent admirer of Erismann, Igumnov was convinced that the community direction (*obshchestvennost'*) of zemstvo medicine was threatened by the growing emphasis on laboratory work in bacteriology. At the 1910 Pirogov Congress, he lamented the fact that the old sociological emphasis of zemstvo sanitary work was giving way to the "fad" of specialization, especially in bacteriology.[62] He noted that a two- or three-month exposure to bacteriology might now be decisive when zemstvos came to choose one candidate over another for a vacancy among sanitary physicians. This kind of "narrowing," he argued, ought to be opposed in the name of the "public tasks" of zemstvo sanitation.[63] He was prepared to admit that changing conditions associated with industrialization required some reconsideration of the qualifications necessary for work at the *uezd* level but was nonetheless determined that any changes should only strengthen the dedication of zemstvo physicians to the principle of *obshchestvennost'*. The weakness of his position was obvious: although he admitted that change was necessary, he had no proposals of his own and condemned those of everyone else. In what the Soviet historian Strashun has called the battle between the "pen" and the "test tube," Igumnov was the pen's most consistent and articulate defender.[64] Nevertheless, his traditionalist emphasis was already out of date; perhaps to his surprise, his speech failed to evoke strong support. Many participants at the 1910 Pirogov Congress took the less extreme view that bacteriology was not a threatening new direction and that greater specialization in it was both inevitable and desirable.[65]

When the issue was discussed again at the 1911 Bacteriology Conference, Igumnov took a somewhat more conciliatory tone. On this occasion the principal contribution had been a report by E. I. Iakovenko of the Kherson *guberniia* sanitary bureau, describing the organization and goals of the hygienic-bacteriological laboratory run by his bureau.[66] Iakovenko had sought to establish common ground by arguing that hygiene and sanitation should employ *both* bacteriology *and* statistics and that in this process neither the demands of science nor the aspirations of hygiene would suffer. Igumnov found much to praise in this report, in particular Iakovenko's belief that research must not be confined to purely clinical matters but should range over broad ques-

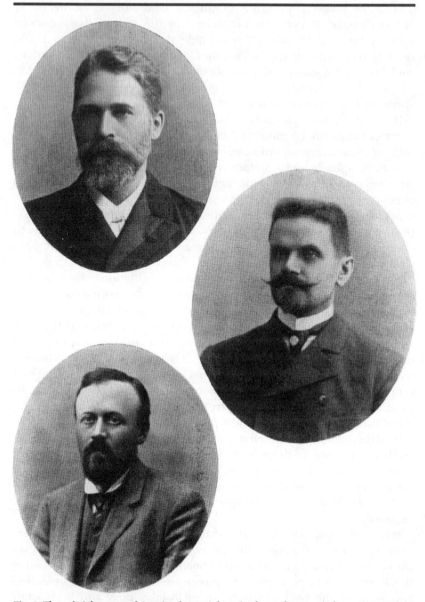

Fig. 6. Three bright stars of Russian bacteriology in the early twentieth century. *Top to bottom;* P. N. Diatroptov, L. A. Tarasevich, and D. K. Zabolotnyi.

tions such as housing, living and working conditions, commercial and industrial activity, water supply, and food products.[67] Unable to turn back the clock, Igumnov had apparently decided to moderate his position so as to preserve his role as a critic of the direction of bacteriological research.

Within a year, yet another innovation seemed to the traditionalists to challenge everything they valued about zemstvo medicine: this was a new approach to sanitary reform called sanitary engineering. (Russians called it the "sanitary-technical direction" [*sanitarno-tekhnicheskoe napravlenie*], but "sanitary engineering" is a more felicitous English term.) The leading exponent of sanitary engineering was A. N. Sysin, who had already attracted attention because of his criticisms of zemstvo antiepidemic measures. He had taken no part in the squabbles between the defenders of the sociological approach and the champions of bacteriology, but in 1912 he launched a new offensive aimed at putting zemstvo and municipal sanitary improvements on an entirely different footing.

At a joint meeting of the Conference of Sanitary Physicians and the Second Conference of Bacteriologists and Epidemiologists held in 1912, Sysin delivered an important report in which he outlined the role of sanitary engineering in zemstvo work.[68] In his opinion, the most challenging task of the sanitary physician was to work towards providing communities with a dependable supply of pure water. To do this, he argued, sanitary physicians should work with other professional and technical employees of the zemstvo, especially engineers, agronomists, fire fighters, and insurance officers. Their work ought to be coordinated and directed by a special hydrotechnical bureau, which would function as a department of the zemstvo *uprava*, working closely with the sanitary bureau itself.[69] The hydrotechnical bureau, headed by an engineer, would employ geologists, hydrographers, and engineers to carry out surveys of districts and provinces and develop plans, budgets, and construction schedules for new schemes of piped water, sewage disposal, and sewerage.

Sysin's sanitary engineering approach created an even bigger stir in community medical circles than did the controversy over bacteriological research. Impressed by his dynamism and originality, the Moscow *guberniia* zemstvo lured him away from Nizhnii Novgorod in 1913 to become head of its sanitary bureau.[70] He carried his message to a wider audience at the 1913 Pirogov Congress and began to attract some outspoken supporters—notably N. A. Kost' and A. A. Tsvetaev—who acted as publicists for sanitary engineering.[71] Only 38 years old at the time of his appointment in Moscow, Sysin soon became a symbol of youthful vitality for the generation of physicians who came of age in the wake of 1905 and who had evidently had enough of what they saw as hand-wringing and sermons about the need to revive the idealism and self-sacrifice of earlier generations.

Although Sysin tried to link his approach with the traditional responsibility of the sanitary physician to improve public health in his district, there is no doubt that his brand of sanitary engineering implied a fundamental transformation in zemstvo sanitary work. Sysin's ideal sanitary physician was neither the sociologist-statistician-topographer of Pirogov tradition nor the experimental hygienist at home in the laboratory; instead, he was a technical specialist who, along with others like himself, pooled his expertise to fulfil grand schemes of public works. This new breed of sanitary physician was more likely to rub shoulders

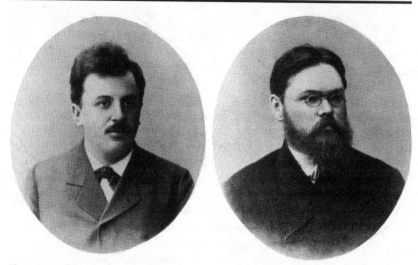

Fig. 7. Two of those who rose above the "pen versus test tube" controversy: V. Ia. Kanel', an early Russian exponent of German social medicine *(left)*, and N. I. Teziakov, a pioneer in the study of child hygiene *(right)*.

with engineers, architects, and town planners than with clinicians, *uchastok* physicians, or laboratory researchers. Although the common people were to be the beneficiaries of his improvements, he himself had little or no contact with them.

It was precisely this professional, exclusive aspect of sanitary engineering that traditionalists feared most. Their ideal sanitary physician was in constant contact with the people, meeting them as healer, teacher, adviser, and confidant. The propaganda and educational material produced by the Pirogov Society's Commission for the Diffusion of Popular Hygiene Education had been used by sanitary physicians to simplify the principles of hygiene, to break down barriers between physicians and ordinary people, and to demystify both medicine and the medical practitioner.[72] Sysin's sanitary engineering threatened to undermine all of these endeavors by turning sanitary improvement into a highly technical subject, comprehensible only to a minority of highly trained experts. Even more menacing was the fact that these improvements in water supply and sewerage were carried out, as it were, behind the scenes; there was no need to enlist the people as active participants in improving their own health. Improvements could be made by anyone who understood the technology; there was no assurance, as there was in the case of popular hygiene education, that the physician/teacher believed in the individual dignity, freedom, and autonomy of his citizen-pupils. Improvements in water supply and sewerage were politically neutral; indeed, as will be shown in chapter 4, they could be promoted by the most ardent servant of the autocracy.

It was one thing to recognize the threat that sanitary engineering could pose to community medicine; it was another thing to fight against it. For one thing, although technology might be politically neutral, its advocates were not; on matters of social and political reform, Sysin, Kost', and Tsvetaev were all radicals. One could scarcely argue that they were any less committed to democracy and revolution than the populist traditionalists. Moreover, supporters of sanitary engineering could point to results already achieved outside Russia by the introduction of systems of water filtration and sewage treatment and to consequent reductions in morbidity and mortality from water-borne diseases, particularly cholera and typhoid fever.[73] These results were impressive enough to disarm traditionalists. Finally, there was the undeniable fact that sanitary engineering was attractive; it offered tangible, measurable improvements within a relatively short period, whereas popular hygiene education was a never-ending and always problematic enterprise. Sysin and his supporters had all the best arguments on their side.

Pirogov traditionalists of *narodnik* sympathies were not the only ones to lament the new emphasis on sanitary engineering. A Bolshevik physician such as E. G. Munblit could share their concern that opportunities for educational work and popular discussion were being cast aside by the new-style engineers. In a particularly strong attack on the consequences of specialization in Moscow *guberniia*, Munblit pointed out that sanitary physicians no longer had close contact with the population, the connection between *guberniia* and *uezd* organization had been lost, and there was no coordination between the work of *uchastok* physicians and that of the sanitary bureau.[74] What he called "broad *uchastok* activity" (*shirokaia uchastkovaia deiatel'nost'*) was in decline throughout the province; zemstvo physicians were paying fewer home visits to the sick, while sanitary physicians pursued the new technology at the expense of their traditional role in combating epidemics, supervising schools, and organizing sanitary guardianship committees.[75] Igumnov took a somewhat different tack, conceding defeat in Moscow but endeavoring to stop the rot from spreading to other provinces. In a review of the whole subject after a 1912 conference of sanitary physicians, he put forward the argument that Moscow *guberniia* was unique because of the degree of its industrialization and the consequent heavy emphasis on industrial hygiene and sanitation; this left him free to argue that the rest of Russia needed not specialists in sanitary engineering and occupational hygiene but traditional "general tasks" sanitary physicians.[76]

Igumnov's reaffirmation of the traditional goals of zemstvo sanitary work overlooked the fact—well attested to in the literature—that, before the advent of sanitary engineering, many zemstvo sanitary physicians had spent more time writing reports for the board (*uprava*) than they had directing sanitary improvements.[77] If a province were foolish enough to appoint as sanitary physician someone with no understanding of sanitation or training in sanitary engineering, the typical result was that this individual tried to cover up his ignorance by placing additional demands on already overworked *uchastok* physicians.[78] In a forceful criticism of existing procedures, N. A. Kost' argued that all sanitary physicians ought to be trained specialists, not seconded *uchastok* physicians, and that they ought to spend their time directing sanitary improvements, not writing reports for the zemstvo *uprava*.[79]

Given the remarkable achievements of zemstvo medicine in the Russian countryside, it is scarcely surprising that there was a good deal of nostalgia for what Zhbankov and Igumnov saw as the "golden age" of the 1890s. In the end, however, the traditionalists could halt neither the evolution of medical science nor the transformation of the Russian countryside and the new needs that were imposed by industrialization, urbanization, and population growth. Indeed, as the debates at the 1910 and 1913 congresses demonstrated, the traditionalists were unable to rally a majority of the participants to oppose the alleged threats posed by bacteriological research and sanitary engineering. The 1910 congress, in fact, elevated two of Russia's most distinguished bacteriologists—L. A. Tarasevich and P. N. Diatroptov—to membership in the Pirogov Society executive. Grumbling about the undesirable consequences of sanitary engineering did nothing to arrest the meteoric career of A. N. Sysin, who was also elected to the executive and who, like the other two, joined the editorial board of *Obshchestvennyi Vrach*. Zhbankov and Igumnov seemed to be fighting a losing battle to maintain the traditions of zemstvo medicine. Nevertheless, one should not jump to the conclusion that their *narodnik* ideology had been abandoned by most zemstvo physicians for, on the most important

issue of all—the role of the state in the improvement of public health—
the *pirogovtsy* showed no signs whatever of abandoning the anti-
statism that was inherent in Russian populism.

COMMUNITY MEDICINE AND THE STATE

Russia's community physicians did not seriously begin to confront the
question of the proper relationship between medicine and the state
until after the failure of the Revolution of 1905. Both populism and the
liberationist movement of the early 1900s had encouraged the assumption that the autocracy and its state apparatus would vanish from the
scene, either by collapse from within or, more likely, by revolution
from without. In the wake of 1905, these hopes were obviously illusory:
a slightly reformed autocracy, aptly dubbed by one historian "a demi-
semi-constitutional monarchy,"[80] had not only survived but seemed to
be rejuvenated by Stolypin's firm hand at the helm. Instead of remak-
ing the world to their liking, the *pirogovtsy* now had to find ways to
accommodate their aspirations to the continued existence of the autocracy. This was to prove a difficult, if not impossible task.

A major reason for this difficulty was the fact that the ideologists of
community medicine—like the intelligentsia of which they were a
part—had never come to terms with the existence of the state or the
exercise of state power. The ideology of community medicine, reduced
to its essentials, consisted of a few homilies that were repeated over
and over again without ever being subjected to serious investigation:
central government is bad, local government is good, private practice
is wicked, public practice is noble; zemstvo medicine is the envy of the
civilized world and must be kept from the profaning hands of St.
Petersburg bureaucrats. To be sure, the government had frequently
acted in a ham-fisted fashion. Nevertheless, the community physicians
continually ignored the fact that the Russian state had created both
the zemstvo institutions and the conditions that gave rise to zemstvo
medicine. The "we-they" mentality of the *pirogovtsy*, forged in the
battles against the Hospital Statute of 1894, the Sanitary-Executive
Commissions, and the Antiplague Commission, made it impossible for
them to separate the idea of the state from the activities of the bureaucrats whom they saw as their enemies. Consequently, they found
it impossible to discuss the role of state and local governments in
the protection of public health without lapsing into a posture of
confrontation.

Community physicians carried this "zemstvo versus autocracy"
mentality over into their understanding of developments elsewhere in
the world, with the result that their perceptions were selective, contra-
dictory, and distorted. England they hailed as the ideal to be imitated
because of its sanitary reforms, the success of which they ascribed en-

tirely to the fact that parliament had left these matters to the jurisdiction of local government; France they denigrated for its backwardness, which they attrbuted (naturally) to the excessive centralization of its government.[81] The simple-minded picture of the world overlooked the fact that England was a stronghold of the very private practice and corporate elitism that they themselves so regularly denounced. Moreover, the powers enjoyed by local governments in England were the result of compromises between headstrong centralizers such as Edwin Chadwick and entrenched local interests such as vestries and poor law guardians (of which there were few counterparts in Russia). The legislators who established the General Board of Health and (later) the Local Government Board did so because they believed that in England sanitary improvement must necessarily accommodate itself to established local interests. Yet, without these forceful initiatives at the national level, the English sanitary reform movement would never have enjoyed the successes that it did.[82] When the *pirotgovtsy* looked at England, however, they saw only what they wanted to see: a sanitary revolution carried out by local governments. They were equally wide of the mark in their assumption that centralization had bedeviled the cause of sanitary reform in France; according to one recent study, this was the reverse of the truth.[83] Moreover, the French situation was complicated by the difficulty of finding a place in the conservative Second Empire and Third Republic for the radicalism that had permeated the French hygiene movement since the early nineteenth century.[84] Russia's community physicians ignored these subtleties, the better to confirm their prejudices against state involvement.

In 1910, rumors began to emanate from St. Petersburg that the government, or at least the Ministry of the Interior, was considering yet another substantial reform in the administration of public health, leading perhaps to the establishment of a separate ministry. The Pirogov Congress held in April, noteworthy for its apathetic attitude to medical-political issues, ignored these rumors; all it did was to endorse a proposal by the leading Kadet physician, A. I. Shingarev, that the government ought to spend far more money on health care by granting larger subsidies for this purpose to zemstvos and municipalities.[85] Among leading *pirogovtsy* it was taken for granted that, outside the ranks of the career medical bureaucrats, there would be no support for opening up once again the question of medical reform. It was therefore both a surprise and an embarrassment when one of Russia's leading bacteriologists, N. F. Gamaleia, announced his support for the idea of establishing a ministry of public health. His views were published first as an editorial in his journal *Gigiena i Sanitariia;* this was subsequently reprinted in pamphlet form to reach a wider audience.[86]

Gamaleia's argument proceeded from a thorough review of the role of central state institutions of public health in the major European states, England, the United States of America, and Japan. He was particularly impressed by the role played in Germany by the *Reichsgesundheitsamt* and in England by the Local Government Board in taking the lead in establishing the best methods of sanitary improvement and then overseeing their implementation by local authorities.[87] Where Pirogov Society publicists had been uniformly negative, Gamaleia stressed the creative, positive role played by central agencies and the debt that was owed to them by local government bodies. Reviewing the sad state of affairs in Russia against the backdrop of what had been achieved elsewhere, he found that Russia's highest priority was "the establishment of a supreme sanitary organ to work out the sanitary laws which are lacking, and also to provide instruction, leadership and control in matters of public health."[88] He was emphatic that this organ ought to be an autonomous government agency, subordinate neither to the office of the Chief Medical Inspector nor to the Medical Council of the Ministry of the Interior and endowed with ample funds and the necessary legal power to do its job. Attached to it as its research arm would be a State Institute for Social Hygiene. Its principal tasks, Gamaleia proposed, were the following:

1. The teaching of sanitation and sanitary technology, with appropriate state examinations.
2. The elaboration of sanitary legislation for consideration by the State Duma.
3. [To serve as a repository of] expertise in sanitary questions on the basis of familiarity with local conditions and laboratory verification.
4. The control of local sanitation through statistical information, personal observation, and leadership in setting up a network of sanitary districts (*okrugy*) with bureaus and sanitary physicians.
5. Participation in the introduction of reforms necessary to the state by making reports to the State Duma concerning required appropriations and expenses.[89]

To facilitate communication and reduce duplication of effort, Gamaleia proposed that there be a common board of management for both the supreme sanitary organ and the institute, with the director of the institute serving as a member of the board of the supreme organ. Gamaleia considered it one of the merits of his proposal that the institute could be placed alongside the existing structure of medical administration without requiring substantial changes: even zemstvo and municipal sanitary activity could continue, he claimed, because it was based on "the correct principle of autonomy," although he hoped that his scheme would serve as "a corrective to their sometimes all too evident neglect of the interests of the poorest class" by establishing central control over local activity.[90] Autonomy was evidently an advantage so long as local governments chose to do what the central government wanted, but it was not a license to neglect what needed doing.

Gamaleia's stature in Russian medicine made it virtually impossible for the Pirogov Society to ignore his pleas for the establishment of a central administrative agency. Moreover, *Gigiena i Sanitariia* was an influential journal that counted among the thirty-one members of its editorial board several of the leading lights in Russian medicine, a number of whom were also members of the Pirogov Society.[91] Throughout 1910 and 1911, Gamaleia's journal returned again and again to the need for a thoroughgoing reform of Russian medicine, for the publication of a comprehensive new law on public health, and for the establishment of a strong central supervisory agency. Not all of these contributions echoed that of Gamaleia, either in tone or content. Dr. I. V. Poliak, for example, argued for a substantial role for zemstvos and towns in such areas as water supply and vaccination campaigns and conceived of a central agency whose role was more one of observation and cooperation than of direction and control.[92]

Not until the end of 1911, however, did a leading *pirogovets* attempt to grapple with the issues raised by Gamaleia. Ia. Iu. Kats first reviewed the history of state medical administration in Russia since the days of Catherine II and then turned his attention to contemporary advocates of a larger state role, in particular Gamaleia.[93] The weakness in Gamaleia's position, Kats argued, was his "curious" belief that a new ministry or central agency could work wonders when the poverty, ignorance, and backwardness of Russia demanded that economic and social reforms precede sanitary reform. Advocates of better housing, he pointed out, seemed not to realize that it was more than a question of disinfectants: land use policy, state credit, and the enforcement of housing standards were also involved. Advocates of pure water were missing the point in a Russia where peasants consumed alcohol in such large amounts. Dirt, he contended, could not be eliminated by police measures; what was required was to raise the general level of popular welfare.[94] According to Kats, all attempts to deal with sanitary reform through central government action would be self-defeating because they would result only in additional interference by bureaucrats in the work of physicians, hospitals, and community medical services.

Kats' argument was a predictable recitation of Pirogov grievances against the tsarist government. He even invoked the now familiar Pirogov shibboleths—the Hospital Statute and the Sanitary-Executive Commissions—to back up his claim that government supervision and interference would become even more "trivial and audacious" if the state were to play a greater role in public health administration.[95]

Kats' argument underlines the extent to which the ideoligists of zemstvo medicine shared the Russian intelligentsia's distrust of the state. It was manifestly absurd to assume that all aspects of health reform—housing, water supply, hygiene, epidemic prevention, and the rest—could be handled by zemstvos and the municipalities if only they had more power and more money.[96] Without a central directing agency, there was little likelihood of a concerted assault on any of these problems. To suggest that the state had no role to play except to dole out the money and then ignore how it was spent—the essence of Kats' position—was both politically unrealistic and out of keeping with contemporary practice in western Europe. Nevertheless, blind opposition to the state remained the standard response of the *pirogovtsy*, as A. I. Shigarev discovered when he tried to provoke a rational discussion of public health administration at the 1913 Pirogov Congress.[97] He found himself confronting a hostile audience that agreed with Kats that the state had no substantial role to play in these matters. On this subject, opinion had apparently not changed since 1898.

Russian intellectuals were fond of attacking the tsarist regime for inhibiting free enquiry in the interests of maintaining an outmoded political ideology. In fact, however, they sometimes did the same thing themselves: the response of Pirogov traditionalists to developments in medicine during the prewar years is a striking example of this self-imposed censorship. Every innovation in theory or practice was tested to see whether it was compatible with the ideals of traditional zemstvo medicine; if not, it was unlikely to receive support. physicians who began to strike out in new directions ran the risk of being berated for suggesting that anything could be superior to Russian community medicine. Traditionalists were particularly suspicious of any new approach that assumed that national as well as local governments had a role to play in public health. In an era when medical opinion abroad increasingly supported the idea of rational state planning for the improvement of health, the Pirogov Society set itself firmly against anything that would advance this doctrine in Russia. Every important question was approached from the premise that St. Petersburg was the enemy, a prejudice that corroded the discussion of medical and scientific *desiderata* and that led a few formerly active *pirogovtsy* to dissociate themselves from the society. Thus, it can be said that the disarray of these years resulted not only or even principally from the cynicism engendered by the political reaction in the zemstvos but from the tensions created by ideological dogmatism for those who wished to explore, to experiment, and to innovate.

4

THE GOVERNMENT
AND
MEDICAL REFORM

The community physicians liked to think that only they cared about the state of public health in Russia, but in fact a host of official commissions and conferences addressed the problem of medical reform throughout the reign of Nicholas II. The persistence of epidemics was a major reason for the government's concern; morbidity and mortality rates were far too high for a country with pretensions to the status of a great power and constituted a source of weakness at home and embarrassment abroad. The empire could ill afford the wastage of human and financial resources consequent upon repeated epidemics; neither could it contemplate with equanimity the repeated displays of popular discontent that epidemics brought with them.[1] Cholera riots threatened not only the lives of physicians but also, and far more importantly from the regime's point of view, authority itself. When the people refused to do as they were told, their rulers had no recourse (in the absence of an effective police force) but to call in the army. Such disturbances exposed the fragility of legitimate authority and left its bearers wishing that these exasperating and frightening events would not be repeated.

Even if persistent epidemics had not threatened the civil order, ministers and bureaucrats in St. Petersburg would still have pursued the goal of medical reform as part of their continuing efforts to define, in the wake of the Great Reforms of the 1860s, the relative powers and spheres of influence of central and local government. St. Petersburg had not foreseen the enormous growth of zemstvo medical and sanitary services in the 1890s. The government's forced and abrupt retreat in the face of zemstvo opposition to the proposed Hospital Statute of 1894 indicated that the tail was becoming strong enough to wag the dog.[2] An overall reform became even more necessary after the establishment of new legislative institutions in 1905. On the morrow of the

October Manifesto, probably no one in St. Petersburg could have said for certain which of the profusion of agencies that shared responsibility for the administration of medical affairs would take charge of drafting legislative proposals for the consideration of the Duma.

The proliferation of jurisdictions in the imperial government, described at the beginning of the present work, was a major obstacle to reform. No one ministry, not even the Ministry of the Interior, was in a position to design and direct a reform of civil, let alone military, medical affairs. Thoroughgoing reform would require the establishment of an interdepartmental commission, an instrument so cumbersome and potentially fractious as to deter all but the most dogged reformers. Because any reform had to confront both the existence and the future of community medicine, discussions of medical reform inevitably turned into rehearsals of all the arguments about whether local self-governing institutions were compatible with the preservation of autocracy.[3] Partisans of the three main positions mounted their predictable offensives: diehard supporters of autocracy argued that the powers and pretentions of zemstvos and towns must be curbed; a much larger group of pragmatic conservatives argued that the zemstvos must be given more to do at the local level to wean them away from meddling in issues of state significance; a tiny handful of reformers argued that the zemstvos must be given more to do not only at the local but also at the state level to prepare the way for eventual self-government under a real constitutional monarchy.

Would-be reformers always ran up against the MVD, which already had the lion's share of control over civil medical affairs and which was determined not to yield this power to any other ministry, certainly not to a new ministry of public health. Yet while the MVD could hinder reform efforts elsewhere, it could not direct them itself because its senior bureaucrats could not agree on whether medical or economic considerations should dictate the nature of the reforms. This was Plehve's legacy, for he had cut in two the old Medical Department of the MVD; his innovations, though intended to reassert the power of the MVD, hampered reform efforts for a decade and virtually ensured that success would come only to someone who was prepared to bypass the MVD. As discoveries in bacteriology and immunology began to make possible a systematic assault on infectious diseases, there were those who argued that the government should mount such an assault to reap the political benefits; no such campaign could be mounted effectively, however, so long as the MVD insisted on retaining separate administrative agencies to deal with the medical and economic aspects of its work and on treating epidemics as events to be responded to with piecemeal emergency measures. Institutions that had been designed primarily to control and restrict zemstvo activities in the sphere of public health could not easily be converted into agencies capable of mounting a rational, planned, and sustained program of antiepidemic work. Reformers within the government were therefore every bit as hostile to the Antiplague Commission and the Sanitary-Executive Commissions as the community physicians themselves, although they had quite different ideas about what institutions should replace them. The MVD was thus criticized both by community physicians who sought to expand the health services of local self-governments and by those who wished St. Petersburg to design a systematic, modernized, and streamlined policy for the improvement of public health. Yet the MVD's institutional structure survived unscathed, not because it worked well, but because of the fundamental political differences that made it impossible for conservative monarchist reformers in St. Petersburg to work with democrats, populists, and socialists in the community medical institutions. Moreover, during the crucial years from 1906 to 1911, its structural integrity was protected by a minister who was also chairman of the Council of Ministers.

The other major problem that confronted reformers within the government was what to do about the medical profession. The awkward reality was that the advance of scientific medicine, which made possible increasingly effective action against disease, also converted public health from a branch of general police administration into a field of scientific knowledge fully understood only by specially trained physicians. Inevitably, therefore, reform meant giving more power to physicians to design, direct, and even evaluate state action to improve health. Yet how could such power be delegated and its exercise controlled in a manner compatible with the survival of the tsarist regime? How was the empire to profit from the increasing effectiveness of medicine without legitimizing a new standard of judgment—science—on the basis of which the autocracy, the estate (*soslovie*) structure of society, and the sacred values espoused by the Orthodox Church might be declared obsolete or even harmful? Could the empire be made healthy and still survive as the empire? In 1905, outspoken physicians had identified themselves with the cause of revolution against traditional authority. How could those who had supported the resolutions of the Pirogov Society's "Cholera" Congress and joined the Union of All-Russian Medical Personnel be made to abandon their subversive notions and to behave like loyal servitors of the state? How could the state fight epidemic disease effectively when medical professionals claimed that the dictates of science demanded sweeping political change? Efforts at reform from above continually foundered on the

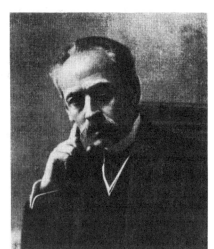

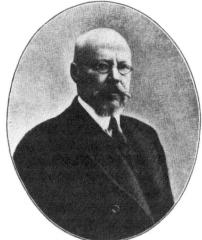

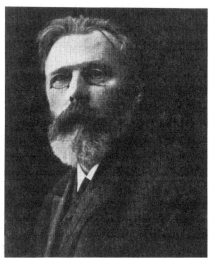

Fig. 8. Three advocates of a strong government role in Russian medicine. *Top to bottom:* Chief Medical Inspector L. N. Malinovskii; V. K. von Anrep, who held a succession of high medical offices in the MVD; and M. S. Uvarov, editor of *Vestnik obshchestvennoi gigieny, sudebnoi i prakticheskoi meditsiny.*

rock of medical professionalism; only when this problem was confronted directly was there a real chance that reform would succeed.
The man who did this—Professor G. E. Rein—was himself a physician,
and he understood better than laymen how to cut the ties between
medical professionalism and political radicalism; this insight made
him the most imaginative and, from the point of view of community
physicians, the most dangerous of the tsar's advisers.

THE MEDICAL COUNCIL AND THE MVD

Russia was by no means exempt from the trend, evident throughout
Europe at the end of the nineteenth century, towards the creation of
special state institutions to administer public health.[4] Everywhere,
those who employed scientific and medical arguments to elevate the
status of public health administration were forced to convince or out-
flank traditionalists who viewed public health as simply one branch of
the general administrative or police responsibility of the state.[5] In Russia, the creation of a separate ministry or agency for public health was
rendered particularly difficult by the fact that the Medical Council,
where most of the supporters of such an agency were found, was
housed within the MVD, and the Ministry itself viewed such an innovation with considerable suspicion. Indeed, because the Medical
Council could propose legislative changes only through the Minister
of the Interior, it was possible for the latter to block reform proposals
almost indefinitely. This is not to suggest that the MVD was a bastion of
reaction; indeed, as Daniel Orlovsky has shown, the MVD was, during
much of its existence, a far more innovative agency than has generally
been appreciated.[6] It was, however, in the business of extending, not
curtailing, its authority, so it remained hostile to any attempt by the
Medical Council to assert its control over public health administration.[7]

In 1886, after an embarrassing discussion of the state of the Russian
Empire at the International Sanitary Conference a year previously, the
Medical Council appointed the distinguished clinician S. P. Botkin to
compile a report on ways to reduce mortality and improve sanitary
conditions.[8] The Botkin Commission recommended the establishment
of a main administration (*Glavnoe upravlenie*)—an autonomous administrative body with powers comparable to those of a ministry—to
organize and direct public health administration. Although the proposal gave rise to a flurry of comment in the medical press, Botkin's
death in 1889 deprived the Medical Council of its foremost advocate of
change. The disastrous famine and cholera epidemic of 1892/93 dramatically underlined the economic and social consequences of the
government's failure to take coordinated preventive measures. In its
wake, no effort was made by the Medical Council to revive Botkin's
proposal; undoubtedly one reason for its inactivity was the unfavor-

able reaction of the Pirogov Society. Both the epidemic of 1892/93 and the conflict over control of zemstvo hospitals in 1894 had strengthened the community physicians' conviction that local autonomy was vastly preferable to centralized direction.[9]

During the 1890s, the theoretically broad legal powers of the Medical Council were ignored in practice. A startling example of its weakness was the creation, in July 1901, of the Special Commission for Measures against Plague as a ministerial agency independent of both the Medical Council and the Medical Department. On the eve of major advances in vaccine and serum therapy, the Medical Council had been effectively deprived of the possibility of supervising and funding emergency measures. These responsibilities were now assigned to an agency dominated by bureaucrats who had no medical understanding whatever and who conformed to the ministry's traditional reliance on generalists rather than "narrow" specialists.[10] The disbanding of the Antiplague Commission became a necessary prelude to the centralization of public health administration sought by reformers such as von Anrep and Rein; its demise was also, though for quite different reasons, an objective of the community physicians.

Plehve's reorganization of the MVD further weakened the influence of physicians within the bureaucracy. Many of the responsibilities for public health were transferred from the Medical Department to the new Main Administration for Local Economic Affairs; those that remained were reorganized under the Main Administration of the Chief Medical Inspector.[11] The individual most affected by these changes was the Director of the Medical Department, V. K. von Anrep, who in 1904 suddenly found himself named Chief Medical Inspector, his staff reduced, and his salary pointedly fixed below that of the director of the rival Main Administration for Local Economic Affairs.[12] Von Anrep had not joined the MVD to see his career wither on the vine; he had already headed three important medical institutions (the Clinical Institute of Grand Duchess Elena Pavlovna, the Women's Medical Institute, and the Imperial Institute of Experimental Medicine) and served as warden of the Khar'kov and St. Petersburg Educational Districts. A career medical *chinovnik* and a firm believer in the virtues of centralized administration, he was unlikely to abandon the field without a fight, especially as the reorganization had been carried out without his prior knowledge. He was not without allies because members of the Medical Council had also been kept in the dark about the proposed changes and learned of them only in time to make a strenuous, if unavailing, protest.

Von Anrep's opportunity for a counterattack came later in the year, when an epidemic of cholera broke out in the provinces of the lower Volga and the Caspian littoral. After traveling through the affected area, he returned to St. Petersburg convinced of the need for sweeping reforms that would enable the empire to fight such epidemics more effectively. The place to start, he argued in a subsequent report to the Medical Council, was with the outdated and almost useless Law on Medical Police (ustav meditsinskoi politsii), a relic of the late eighteenth century wholly unsuited to twentieth-century problems. Although von Anrep was impressed by zemstvo medical efforts and supported greater rights of initiative for these institutions in protecting public health at the local level, he also believed that money and effort would be wasted without an overall plan and system run from St. Petersburg. Accordingly, he argued, as had Botkin before him, for the creation of a central organization specially charged with planning and overseeing sanitary reform throughout the empire.[13] The Medical Council responded favorably to his proposal and asked him to chair a special subcommission that eventually recommended that one autonomous and independent department be established to manage all governmental activity concerning medicine and sanitation. By the time the subcommission reported, the tsar's Manifesto of 17 October 1905 had been issued, a development that von Anrep seized on as yet another reason for the adoption of his proposal, so that one government agency would be charged with formulating proposals for the consideration of the new legislative institutions.

Once the Medical Council began to press for reform, however, it ran up against the obstacle of its subordinate status within the MVD. The proposed new department could not become independent of the MVD without the support of the minister, and such support was not forthcoming. Stolypin, who became Minister of the Interior in April 1906, recognized the necessity for overhauling Russia's outdated medical and sanitary legislation but saw no reason why this enterprise required the creation of an agency independent of the MVD. A former provincial governor before he became minister, Stolypin undoubtedly recognized that von Anrep's proposal would create enormous practical difficulties at the guberniia level by moving matters of public health into a separate jurisdiction and imposing yet another chain of command—rivaling that of the MVD—on the governors and their provincial administrations.[14] At the very time when Stolypin was considering broad reforms in local government, von Anrep's proposal would have forced the recently created Main Administration for Local Economic Affairs to give up many of the powers it had so recently assumed and would have placed local health affairs beyond the control of the MVD.[15] Moreover, the political activities of many community physicians in 1905 suggested that, for reasons of state security, zemstvo and municipal employees ought to remain firmly under the control of the MVD. Whatever arguments von Anrep advanced to justify the creation of an independent agency, Stolypin could find more convincing reasons for opposing it.

In 1907, von Anrep suddenly resigned from government service to stand for election to the Third Duma, to which he was subsequently elected as an Octobrist deputy. Perhaps he had concluded that the Medical Council could not by itself overcome Stolypin's opposition and was gambling that pressure from a Duma dominated by moderate reformers like himself would force the premier to give way. If so, he overestimated both the urgency with which his new party colleagues would treat the issue of medical reform and the extent of their influence on Stolypin.[16] His position as Chief Medical Inspector was filled by his former assistant, L. N. Malinovskii; under the latter's direction, the subcommission that was supposedly drafting proposals for reform quickly became bogged down in conflicting proposals for reviewing and updating the empire's antiquated medical legislation.[17] Stolypin refused to intervene, and it appeared that von Anrep's proposal for a separate ministry had been trapped in the web of the St. Petersburg bureaucracy.

A NEW BROOM: THE APPOINTMENT OF G. E. REIN

In the summer of 1908, Stolypin received from the tsar a formal request that his government take decisive measures, not merely to combat epidemic diseases, but to eliminate them.[18] Still firmly of the opinion that everything necessary could be done within the structure of the MVD, Stolypin seized the occasion of making a new appointment to the Presidency of the Medical Council as an opportunity to demonstrate to the tsar that he was indeed taking the request seriously.[19] This did not, of course, mean that he would seek out Russia's leading epidemiologists to offer them the position; such behavior would have contradicted the MVD's traditional disdain for narrow specialists. In any case, the search might well have produced the names of Diatroptov, Tarasevich, or Zabolotnyi, all of them politically unacceptable in the wake of the 1905 Revolution. Nevertheless, the position—a senior one in the bureaucracy, carrying the third rank, equivalent to a deputy minister—had by law to be filled by a physician. Shrewd politician that he was, Stolypin knew that he needed to find someone whose loyalty to the throne was unquestionable, whose scientific credentials were impeccable, who would bring new but not dangerous ideas, and who if at all possible could be presented as a public figure (*obshchestvennyi deiatel'*) with both scientific and zemstvo connections. His choice—a brilliant one, in the circumstances—was Professor G. E. Rein of the Imperial Military-Medical Academy, who was appointed President of the Medical Council on 21 November 1908.[20]

Neither the Pirogov Society nor Russian university professors had distinguished themselves by their loyalty to the regime in 1905, but Rein was an exception; in academic as well as medical circles, he belonged to the minority vocal in its support for the tsarist regime. This is not to say that Rein was either a blind reactionary or a sycophant; his career before his appointment, as well as his tireless pursuit of the cause of reform in the years that followed, make it clear that he was both a dynamic figure in the evolution of Russian medicine and something of a thorn in the side of the government. To be sure, he made no secret of his politics, having sat as an Octobrist deputy in the stormy Second Duma, where he joined the conservatives in denouncing political terrorism. Nevertheless, he was a prominent figure in St. Petersburg medical circles well before his excursion into party politics. Stolypin may have selected Rein primarily because of his energy and his loyalty, but he came to the premier's notice only because his peers in university and medical circles had already recognized his stature as a scientist, teacher, and organizer.

That Rein had a promising career ahead of him seemed likely when he took the gold medal at the Imperial Medical-Surgical (later Military-Medical) Academy in 1874.[21] After obtaining his M.D. degree and serving at the front in the war against Turkey, he returned to the Academy as a *privat-dotsent*. He soon left St. Petersburg again for an extended research trip to western Europe. Most of his time was spent in Strasbourg studying microscopic anatomy and embryology and in Paris studying histology, but he also visited scientific institutes and clinics elsewhere in France, Germany, and Italy. While in England to attend an international medical congress of physicians, he familiarized himself with Lister's recently successful antiseptic techniques. Returning to Russia, his further research in the physiology of sex, embryology, and surgical obstetrics gained him the chair of obstetrics and gynecology at Kiev University in 1883. He made an immediate impact because of his insistence on antiseptic surgery; mortality from obstetric operations and childbed fever was dramatically reduced. For seventeen years he remained in Kiev where, in addition to his academic duties, he founded the Kiev Obstetrics and Gynecology Society, edited its *Transactions* (*Trudy*), raised money for the construction of a new clinic, and attended local, Pirogov, and international medical congresses. When he left in 1900, it was to return to the capital to occupy the Chair of Obstetrics and Women's Diseases at the Imperial Military-Medical Academy.

Rein's career in academic medicine kept him well away from most of the concerns of Russia's community physicians. Where they were disposed to regard the growth of zemstvo medicine as the great beneficial innovation of the nineteenth century, Rein held precisely this view of antiseptic surgery. Although he attended Pirogov congresses, it was not the sections on community medicine which interested him, but those on physiology, surgery, and obstetrics. He was a medical society man but an organizer of scientific specialists, not of physicians as an occupational group. For the legal and material difficulties experienced by his colleagues elsewhere in the profession he showed little sympathy; the practical problems that faced zemstvo physicians in small rural hospitals were beyond his comprehension. In Kiev, thanks to private donations, new facilities, and hard work, he had been able significantly to reduce maternal mortality; how could he not be skeptical of those physicians who claimed that only sweeping changes in the country's political, economic, and social structure could reduce Russia's high mortality rate? In Rein's view, most of the propagandists of community medicine were little better than merchants of doom.

During the years from 1900 to 1905, the very time when liberal and radical sentiments were growing apace among the community physicians, Rein was settling comfortably into the academic and medical establishment in St. Petersburg. Within a year, he had been elected Academician, and in 1905 was chosen an Honored Professor of the Academy. Continuing the work begun in Kiev, he became president of the St. Petersburg Obstetrics and Gynecology Society, edited its journal, and planned the curriculum for the Academy's new Obstetric Clinic. By the time that revolution broke out in 1905, he had become a member of several bodies advisory to the government, including the Medical Council of the Ministry of the Interior, the Learned Committee of the Military-Medical Academy, and the Commission to Reform Higher Educational Institutions. While the Pirogov Society was joining ranks with the opposition, Rein was forging ever closer ties with the tsarist regime.

In addition to his professional life as a scientist and academic, Rein was also a landowner; he had acquired a substantial estate (3,600 *desiatina*) in the Ostrozhskii district of Volhynia province. Here again, Rein was atypical; very few physicians had country estates. About one-fifth of the empire's physicians were employed by zemstvos (and numerous others had had zemstvo experience at some point in their careers), but Rein's contacts with the zemstvo were of a different order; he had served as an elected deputy (*glasnyi*). His political outlook had more in common with that of his fellow landowners than with that of zemstvo physicians and other third-element employees. These facts help to explain why, when Rein ventured into the Second Duma in 1907 as a deputy from Volhynia, he gravitated not to the Constitutional Democrats, where so many academics and professionals found a congenial home, but to the more conservative Octobrists. A middle-aged conservative in an assembly of young radicals, Rein could scarcely have enjoyed his experience as a deputy and took little part in the Duma's proceedings. He made the ritual denunciation of terror, pleaded that the disparity of the empire be recognized by those engaged in devising solutions to the agrarian problem, and provoked the wrath of the left by suggesting that Jews were especially adept at evading military service. He did not stand in the elections to the Third Duma and, when Stolypin invited him to become President of the Medical Council, he seized the opportunity with relish.

There can be little doubt that Rein emerged from his excursion into party politics thoroughly frightened by meeting revolutionaries in the flesh and sadly disillusioned with popular representative institutions. Stolypin's invitation to assume the Presidency of the Medical Council helped him to work out his own future role in Russian society. Combining his loyalty to the tsar, his penchant for public service, his scientific expertise, and his organizational ability, he would put himself at the disposal of Nicholas II to bolster the sagging prestige of the autocracy. By employing the best measures that contemporary science could suggest to reduce mortality and improve living conditions, he would help to defeat the liberals and revolutionaries by proving them wrong. Like the community physicians, Rein was beginning to understand the relationship between politics and public health. As he was to argue in a report submitted to the tsar in 1910, cholera and other epidemics resulted not only in the deaths of hundreds of thousands of people, but also in the wasting of financial resources, the destruction of the economy, the loss of international stature, and—perhaps most importantly—the undermining of the people's trust in their rulers.[22] To be sure, cultural, economic, and educational improvements would in time help to promote public health, but Rein understood that the political situation was too precarious for sensible persons to reply on such long-term measures.

What, then, could a loyal, concerned scientist do? A great deal, according to Rein, who, as a pioneer of antisepsis, easily appreciated the scope that the bacteriological revolution offered for decisive intervention by the state. He began to emphasize the importance of improving drinking water, eliminating impurities from all water supplies, supervising the quality of food products, and improving housing conditions. He was able to make his point forcefully in 1909, when the Medical Council was called upon to deal with a serious outbreak of cholera in St. Petersburg. Rein immediately rushed off abroad to learn about ozone water purifiers and, on his return, persuaded the city administration to install one quickly; as a result, he claimed later, "pathogenic microbes were virtually eliminated from the water that went through it."[23] This event provided him with precisely the sort of example he needed to demonstrate that intervention by the state, employing the latest technology, could result in dramatic success. Contrasting his own performance with the inactivity of the City Duma, which had allowed the problem of impure water to reach catastrophic proportions, and with the indifference of the Third State Duma, Rein was confirmed in his belief that little could be expected from elected bodies. He had also satisfied himself that the so-called experts in community medicine simply did not know what they were talking about.

CHOLERA AND MEDICAL REFORM

Rein's growing appreciation of the possibilities for state action was sharpened by his experience during the cholera epidemic in southern Russia in 1910. The epidemic began in June in the Donets basin, one of Russia's most important coal-producing areas.[24] Within a month, production had been seriously affected, and the Congress of Mining Industrialists of South Russia, the mineowners' organization, began to panic at the prospect of financial loss. Their petition to the government, calling for the invocation of extraordinary measures, was presented to the Minister of Trade and Industry, S. I. Timashev, by one of Russia's leading industrialists, N. S. Avdakov; the latter stressed the consequences of a fall in production, the imminent spread of the epidemic to as yet unaffected areas, and the dangers of popular riots. Timashev undertook to discuss with the Council of Ministers the appointment of an individual with extraordinary powers to combat the epidemic.[25] The result was a resolution of the Council of Ministers, passed at its meeting of 20 July, asking the Red Cross to send medical "flying squads" to the stricken area and to appoint a field commander to be selected by agreement between the MVD and the executive of the Red Cross.[26] According to Rein, he was personally selected for the job by Stolypin himself and hastened to St. Petersburg from Volhynia, where he had received the telegram informing him of the appointment. True to form, he dispatched squads of physicians, student-medics, and Sisters of Mercy even as he himself prepared to travel south. He had the good sense to take with him the outstanding epidemiologist D. K. Zabolotnyi—unlike the MVD bureaucrats, Rein did believe in employing experts—and was shrewd enough to have a long conversation with Avdakov, presumably about how to handle the mineowners.[27]

Once there, Rein found his efforts hampered by the unwillingness of local authorities to take the initiative, the lack of trained personnel, the unequal allocation of resources, and the traditional preference of officials for piecemeal temporary measures. The situation was serious; more than 200,000 cases had been reported in four *gubernii* (Khar'kov, Ekaterinoslav, Kherson, and Tauride), as well as in the Don army *oblast'*; the fatality rate among those who contracted the disease was running at 45 percent.[28] Immediately on arriving in Khar'kov, Rein met with the mineowners and made it clear that his efforts would require both their cooperation and their financial support.[29] Then he met with representatives of the *guberniia* administration, zemstvos, municipal dumas, commercial interests, and railway officials. To his dismay, the meeting lasted almost twelve hours, most of which were spent in futile wrangling among the various groups as to whose responsibility it was to take emergency measures. Rein left the meeting convinced that he was bringing together agencies and groups that ordinarily had little to do with one another and that even in the face of danger found it almost impossible to cooperate.[30]

Having toured the mines, Rein found that many had completely inadequate sanitary arrangements; on his instructions the mineowners hired emergency sanitary personnel and opened an information office to communicate basic instructions about cleanliness to the people.[31] Some of the problems he had to face dramatized the difficulties occasioned by separate jurisdictions; although the zemstvo *guberniia* of Ekaterinoslav put up some 400,000 rubles for antiepidemic measures, the neighboring Don Army *oblast'*, under the jurisdiction of the War Ministry, allocated only a "few tens of thousands of rubles" despite the fact—as Rein noted bitterly—that it contained one of the wealthiest districts in the empire, Taganrog.[32] He dispatched six of his flying squads to the Don region, but even with his extraordinary powers he could not tell the Russian army what to do and was forced to petition the Military-Sanitary Administration to send more physicians and feldshers into the area. The Sanitary-Executive Commissions, in which the MVD had placed considerable faith, were, in Rein's judgment, "powerless"; according to published reports, they seem to have done nothing except order the closure of spirit shops and taverns.[33]

Before leaving South Russia in late September, Rein prophesied that cholera would again reach epidemic proportions in the spring; in Kiev and in Kherson he commented on the shortage of sanitary physicians at the *uezd* level and on the need for more laboratory facilities in the zemstvo provinces.[34] These concerns led him to insist that the various "temporary" measures that he had taken be carried over into the spring and summer of 1911; Stolypin later formally agreed to this extension.[35] Having done as much as he could and by now convinced of the need to establish one centralized agency to direct public health affairs, Rein returned to the capital to report on his efforts in South Russia to the tsar, the premier, and the Red Cross.

Taking advantage of an audience with Nicholas II on 12 October, Rein broached with the tsar his plan for the creation of a ministry of public health and advocated the creation of an interdepartmental commission to work out the detailed legislation. In a written report that he submitted to Nicholas II in person (and apparently without

Stolypin's knowledge), Rein, like von Anrep before him, argued that neither the local administrative agencies of the central government nor the zemstvos and municipalities could deal effectively with epidemics because of the absence of an agency capable of centralized planning and direction.[36] In phrases worthy of a seventeenth-century mercantilist, he played upon the relationship between health and national power: "Hundreds of thousands of people perish, enormous financial resources are wasted, the economic well-being of the populace is destroyed, the prestige of the state in other countries is diminished, the people's trust in their rulers is undermined."[37]

Elaborating on the potential for popular disorder, Rein went on to point out that

the people are not yet taking the entirely proper view that every death from [contagious] diseases . . . is, in essence, a kind of violent death, comparable to the perishing of individuals in the collapse of a building erected without the supervision of the authorities, or in a train crash as a result of improprieties on the railways. But the cholera discontents, which turned into the present disorders, demonstrate that even in the ignorant mass of the people there exists some sort of unconscious feeling of dissatisfaction with the existing arrangements for the protection of public health. It is time to put an end to these arrangements.[38]

Having argued that his proposal was both sound political economy and an inescapable moral obligation, Rein left the meeting convinced of the tsar's support. Two days later, one newspaper had already heard rumors that a ministry of public health would soon be established and that Rein would be its first head.[39]

THE KRYZHANOVSKII CONFERENCE

The tsar's support for Rein's scheme, coupled with his earlier instructions to the government regarding the prevention of epidemics, placed Stolypin in an awkward position. On the one hand, he was no more enthusiastic about the idea of a separate ministry of health than he had been when von Anrep proposed it but, on the other hand, he could not rule out the idea entirely, given the favorable attitude of his royal master. He therefore wrote quickly to Rein to say that, before anything else was done, all of Russia's antiquated medical legislation would have to be reviewed, a task he thought Rein could complete— or so he said—in two or three months. His letter also stressed the need to place restrictions on the growth of zemstvo medicine: "The zemstvos [he wrote] have deviated a long way from the limits of existing law. It is necessary to define strictly in law their rights and duties."[40] After cautioning Rein against the "precipitate action" of creating an interdepartmental commission and suggesting that he was saving Rein from "frequently unfair and malicious criticism," Stolypin announced his intention: "I propose at first to form our internal departmental commission [within the MVD] of competent persons; work out in that body the main fundamentals of reform, and only then place your project before the legislative institutions."[41]

Acting with all speed, no doubt to present Rein with a fait accompli and the tsar with evidence of his concern, Stolypin established a review committee in the MD within a fortnight of Rein's interview with the tsar. Presided over by Deputy Minister of the Interior S. E. Kryzhanovskii, the review committee soon became known as the Kryzhanovskii Conference, undoubtedly because of its unwieldly formal title, "the Special Conference to discuss shortcomings in the existing organization of medical-sanitary affairs in the empire and to work out the general bases for a restructuring of this organization."[42] In addition to Kryzhanovskii and Rein himself, Stolypin appointed three officials from the Main Administration for the Affairs of Local Economy and three from the Office of the Chief Medical Inspector; the Medical Council was permitted to elect its three representatives.[43] With such a composition the Kryzhanovskii Conference was almost certain to reach the same impasse that had thwarted von Anrep's early attempt at reform because the only real support for a separate ministry such as Rein desired came from the Medical Council itself.

Before the conference could hold its first meeting, there was a brief flurry of activity in the Duma, organized by the tireless von Anrep, who had not given up hope that a separate ministry might one day be created. With the assistance of P. V. Sinandino, the former mayor of Kishinev and a physician keenly interested in public health, von Anrep introduced a resolution on 27 October 1910, signed by eighty-three members of the Duma, which called for the establishment of a ministry of state health protection (*ministerstvo gosudarstvennogo zdravookhraneniia*).[44] The resolution began by contrasting the tsar's earlier appeal for a speedy reorganization of medical affairs with the grim death tolls from cholera, plague, scarlatina, typhus, and diphtheria in 1909 and 1910. Noting earlier unsuccessful efforts at reform by the Medical Council and the continuing proliferation of responsibilities both inside and outside the MVD, the resolution condemned inactivity and appealed for "decisive and radical measures."[45] Its authors took clear aim at the MVD, whose increasingly diffuse and complex responsibilities had little in common with the improvement of public health; the MVD, they argued, could give health reform neither the funds nor the radical initiatives that were required. Hence a new ministry was absolutely necessary, both "to bring a common system" to the existing chaos and to oversee "consistently and methodically" the introduction and enforcement of new laws.[46] After a brief debate in which left-wing deputies predictably berated the government for callous indifference to the health of the Russian people, the resolution was approved and sent to the Duma's Commission for Public Health, with instructions to draft an appropriate legislative proposal. In fact, however, the resolution had been buried; for all their rhetoric, the Duma deputies were no more enthusiastic for such a sweeping reform than was Stolypin himself. Liberals and radicals feared that the establishment of a strong ministry would seriously curb the autonomy of zemstvos, municipalities, and village communes, and many rightists were loath to do anything that might impair the effectiveness of the MVD as a police agency with unfettered powers. Stolypin was able to fob off the small group of deputies who were seriously interested in reform by pointing to the review committee that he had just set up within the MVD.

The fortnightly meetings held by the Kryzhanovskii Conference between November 1910 and May 1911 must have been a continual frustration for Rein. There was general agreement among the participants that the zemstvo institutions should be given more to do at the local level so as to keep them away from matters of state and that government and public (*obshchestvennye*) institutions ought to work together in new local councils of public health (*sovety po delam narodnogo zdraviia*, but beyond this point unanimity disintegrated.[47] In simple terms, it rapidly became clear that only the representatives of the Medical Council were seriously interested in sweeping reforms; Antsiferov and Vitte from the Main Administration for the Affairs of Local Economy resolutely defended the status quo because it gave them a large role, whereas the Chief Medical Inspector, L. N. Malinovskii, did his best to reverse the demotion that his office had suffered in 1904 and to put his office on a par with, or even above, that of his rivals Antsiferov and Vitte. Rein's high hopes that the conference would endorse his proposal for a separate ministry had run aground on the reefs and shoals of bureaucratic ambition, jealousy, and indifference.

Rein elaborated his position in a lengthy report that buttressed and extended the arguments that he had already made to Stolypin and the tsar.[48] He now maintained that the state's obligation to promote public health was equal to its role as protector and promoter of Orthodoxy, industry, trade, agriculture, and education. With appendices full of statistics, he continued to stress the economic costs of epidemics and poor health: "Disease results in the sickliness of the population, which is reflected in the productivity of the nation, in the physical constitution of the contingent of newly-married [people], and consequently in the army, weakening the might of the state and its international significance."[49]

While conceding that the zemstvos had done a good deal to improve medical care in rural areas, Rein pointed out that there were many zemstvo districts and provinces where medical assistance of any kind was virtually inaccessible to the population because of the distances involved, where trained midwives were the exception rather than the rule, and where little of the medical budget was spent on sanitary improvements. In any case, he noted, many epidemics entered Russia through its western, southern, and eastern frontier regions, where zemstvo institutions had not been introduced; some strong central agency was absolutely necessary to introduce reforms in these areas while coordinating zemstvo efforts in the thirty-four zemstvo provinces.[50]

The novel elements in Rein's 1911 proposal concerned the relationship of the new ministry to other departments of the government. He specified that, in matters of health and medicine, departments should be required to subordinate themselves to the new ministry, securing its permission before introducing bills into the Duma, asking its permission before undertaking large projects, sending it regular reports on medical matters, and subordinating themselves to its general laws.[51] If differences arose (as undoubtedly they would), they were to be settled in a new review body, to be called the Central Sanitary Council, which was to bring together the heads of existing medical departments, senior officials of the new ministry, and representatives of *guberniia* administrations, zemstvos, and municipalities. Citing the examples of the English Local Government Board and the German *Reichsgesundheitsamt*, Rein argued that wherever "authoritative, planned, systematic preventive work" was undertaken, low mortality from epidemic disease and a general improvement in the level of health were apparent. He was utterly convinced that a powerful central agency was essential to the success of health reform.

Antsiferov and Vitte took a very different view and attacked the very idea of a separate ministry. It would, they pointed out, lack competence over military medicine; it would be powerless to enforce its regulations without the cooperation of the police and the supervisory agencies in the MVD; even more tellingly, its ability to function as a ministry would be seriously impaired by the existence of the Zemstvo and Municipal Statutes because questions of their interpretation would be settled not by the new ministry but by the Senate or even by the Council of Ministers. If it were thought desirable to establish a supervisory agency for zemstvo and municipal medicine, then in their view this agency must be the existing Main Administration for Affairs of Local Economy. They even went so far as to suggest that such a step would "complete the reforms of 1904" because it would reaffirm that "medical questions cannot be settled apart from financial considerations."[52] Throwing out a carrot to Malinovskii, they conceded that it "might be acceptable to elevate the rights of the Chief Medical Inspector to those of a deputy minister," so long as their Main Administration retained complete control over the economic and legal aspects of public health.[53]

Malinovskii, however, had his own plans for the future. Like Antsiferov and Vitte, he thought that the absence of police power would render a new ministry ineffective and entirely dependent on the MVD. In his view, its establishment was "premature." Instead, he proposed that its functions should be exercised by a Main Medical-Sanitary Administration within the MVD, formed by upgrading the existing office of the Chief Medical Inspector into an agency equal in rank to the Main Administration for Affairs of Local Economy. Any differences between these two senior agencies could be settled, he claimed, by establishing an Imperial Sanitary Council representing both medical and economic interests and concerns.[54] Both Malinovskii's proposal and the position taken by Antsiferov and Vitte sidestepped a review of existing legislation in favor of a modest administrative reorganization.

Rein remained firmly committed to his proposal and indeed was convinced that he would triumph in the end because he had the tsar on his side. He reckoned, however, without the adroitness of Stolypin. Malinovskii finally secured the approval of Antsiferov and Vitte for his Main Medical-Sanitary Administration, provided "that it remain exclusively an organ of supervision and control, without economic or financial functions."[55] When Kryzhanovskii reported to Stolypin the various points of view which had emerged, the premier quickly opted for Malinovskii's proposal, although he told Rein that his decision was prompted by tactical considerations and that "in principle" he agreed with Rein's arguments for the separate ministry. With one move, Stolypin had easily outflanked Rein, rewarded Malinovskii, and produced tangible evidence of his concern for health reform which he could now present to the tsar. In June, he promised Rein that the legislation embodying Malinovskii's proposal would be sent to the Duma in the autumn. Whether or not such a draft was in preparation, the whole subject was thrown open once again by Stolypin's assassination in Kiev in September.

THE REIN COMMISSION, 1912–1914

Stolypin's death removed the chief obstacle that had blocked Rein's plans for reform. His successor as premier was the Minister of Finance, V. N. Kokovtsev, who had none of his predecessor's loyalty to the MVD. As Minister of the Interior, Stolypin was succeeded for a brief period by State Secretary A. A. Makarov, with whom Rein discussed the whole question shortly after his appointment. To his delight, he found Makarov far more sympathetic to his plans than Stolypin had been. Together they agreed that there was little point in proceeding with the legislation proposed by Malinovskii; the Duma was in the final year of its five-year term, was likely to be preoccupied with the political aspects of Stolypin's assassination, and had in any case shown little interest in pursuing von Anrep's proposal for medical reform. Instead, Makarov and Rein agreed that a complete review of medical and sanitary legislation ought to be carried out by an interdepartmental commission, which would produce finished legislative proposals that could be presented to the Fourth Duma to be convoked in the autumn of 1912.[56]

Makarov took the proposal for an interdepartmental commission to the Council of Ministers on 21 December 1911; securing a favorable response, he then presented the plan to Nicholas II during a formal audience. The scope of its inquiry, the details of its organizational structure, and its actual composition were approved by the tsar and the Council of Ministers on 16 February 1912.[57] Less than six months after Stolypin's death, Rein was finally poised to undertake the mission that he had set himself some four years earlier. In the belief that this was his great opportunity to save the empire from the ravages of disease and the monarchy from the machinations of the revolutionary movement, Rein enthusiastically set to work.

Despite the commission's unwieldy size and interdepartmental character, Rein's personal influence over it was enormous. He laid out the scope and direction of its work, chose most of its members, chaired all of its plenary sessions, and organized its subcommittees, retaining for himself control over the subcommittee on finance and organization. For his chief assistant he chose probably the only person in the empire who understood the legal complexities of the subject, N. G. Freiberg, author of the standard compilation of existing medical-sanitary law.[58] Malinovskii, no longer able to depend on Stolypin's protection, found himself chairing the subcommittee on sanitary measures, a position that made it clear that he was now playing second fiddle to Rein. As if to drive the point home, Rein chose as Malinovskii's deputy the distinguished bacteriologist N. F. Gamaleia; as editor of the respected fortnightly *Gigiena i Sanitariia*, Gamaleia had been campaigning for centralized planning of antiepidemic measures and for state-supported research in bacteriology and epidemiology.[59] Rein's colleagues on the Medical Council, themselves high-ranking medical officials and academics, chaired the other subcommittees: the Chief Medical Inspector of the Court, Professor N. A. Veliaminov, chaired the subcommittee on medical assistance and charity; the Director of the Medical Department of the Ministry of Public Instruction, Professor E. A. Neznamov, chaired the subcommittee on medical education; Ia. A. Pliushchevskii-Pliushchik, principal medical legal adviser to the MVD, chaired the subcommittee on forensic medicine. Besides representatives from no less than fifteen ministries, the Red Cross, and the Imperial Philanthropic Society, the commission also included several mayors and town councillors, members of various zemstvo boards, a few physicians from provinces lacking zemstvo institutions, and representatives of the Moscow Stock Exchange, the mining industry, and the Congress of Representatives of Industry and Trade.[60] With such a large and disparate membership, the real work was done in the subcommittees, not the plenary sessions.

Spokesmen for the community medical tradition were predictably outraged by the absence of formal representation from the Pirogov Society and by what appeared to be a random selection of zemstvo representatives.[61] Their immediate conclusion was that Rein was deliberately snubbing those best qualified to advise on the principles of medical and especially sanitary reform. To such accusations Rein remained impervious, and it is not difficult to understand why. Explicit participation by the Pirogov Society risked a reiteration of its earlier demands for constitutional reforms as a necessary preliminary to constructive activity; it would also have necessitated sending similar invitations to other medical societies, thus making the commission even larger than it already was. Co-opting individuals from zemstvos and municipalities was the normal means by which such commissions operated, and here Rein was simply following precedent. In any case he had no trouble finding individuals ready to serve. As far as expertise was concerned, the subcommittees either included or consulted with recognized medical authorities—whatever their politics—when drawing up specific legislative proposals. An outstanding example of this process was the participation of the distinguished epidemiologist and well-known radical D. K. Zabolotnyi in planning new leglslation to deal with epidemics. Rein was prepared to avail himself of scientific expertise, but he was determined not to make the commission a forum for the expression of political opposition to the regime. Suggestions were also made in the Pirogov Society's organ *Obshchestvennyi Vrach* that commercial and industrial interests would exercise a disproportionate and harmful influence upon the commission's work.[62] These charges seem to have stemmed from the almost hysterical anticapitalism typical of some zemstvo intellectuals. After his experience in south Russia in 1910, Rein appreciated that the cooperation of business and industry would be an important factor in the eventual success of his reforms. On the other hand, he had no reason to pander to commercial interests, and in fact the commission's recommendations in some areas went much further than representatives of trade and industry would have liked.[63]

The work of the Rein Commission extended over three years; the first full session was held in November 1912, the fifth and last in March

1914. The subcommittees were in almost constant session during this period. It resulted in the most extensive proposals for the reform of public health ever produced under the tsarist regime: over forty legislative proposals, twelve of them dealing with sanitation, four with medical assistance, eight with the training and obligations of medical personnel, four with forensic medicine, and fifteen with administrative reorganization at all levels.

The centerpiece of all its work was the proposal to establish a Main Administration for State Health Protection (*Glavnoe Upravlenie Gosudarstvennogo Zdravookhraneniia, GUGZ*). It was to undertake the overall direction and supervision of medicine, public health, and sanitation throughout the empire and to be responsible for seeing all of the other reforms through the legislative institutions. Although its jurisdiction was not to include military medicine (which would continue under the Naval and War Ministries), *GUGZ* was to assume almost complete control of the civil medical sector: only the medical administration of the Ministry of the Imperial Court was to be exempt from its control. All other ministries, including of course the MVD, were required to submit for its approval all measures that touched in any way on matters of public health.

The proposed structure of the new agency indicates the range of activities which it was expected to undertake.[64] Its Medical Department was to include four divisions: hospitals, medical assistance, pharmacology, and forensic medicine. This would be complemented by a Sanitary Department with three divisions: sanitation, epidemic disease, and chronic contagious and occupational diseases. A Department of General Affairs was to include the secretarial and accounting staff, as well as the inspectorate, which would take over the functions previously performed by the Administration of the Chief Medical Inspector in the MVD. This department was also assigned responsibility for the publication of a new journal (intended to replace the MVD's *Vestnik obshchestvennoi gigieny, sudebnoi i prakticheskoi meditsiny*) as well as weekly bulletins concerning epidemic disease. The Learned Branch (*uchebnyi otdel*) was to direct education in medicine, pharmacy, and veterinary science and was to administer those institutions attached directly to the ministry: initially, the Imperial Institute of Experimental Medicine and the St. Petersburg Orthopedic Institute. Also attached to *GUGZ* were a Statistical Section, a Technical-Structural Section, a *Jurisconsult* Section, the existing Veterinary Administration, and a new state laboratory.

This vast administrative structure was to be guided by three advisory bodies, two of which—the Medical Council and the Veterinary Committee—were to be transferred from the MVD to *GUGZ*. In addition, a new Main Sanitary Committee was to advise on sanitary measures of statewide significance and to coordinate relations between the central government and the zemstvos and municipalities. Unlike the Medical Council and the Veterinary Committee, which were small bodies composed exclusively of scientific experts, the Main Sanitary Committee was to be an enormous assembly of government officials and representatives of local government with a membership approaching two hundred. Though not as large as the MVD, *GUGZ* was obviously meant to be a substantial addition to the St. Petersburg bureaucracy. Several hundred new positions would have been required to bring it to full operation; the potential for interministerial conflict inherent in its broad jurisdiction would soon have demanded a host of additional personnel in the *Jurisconsult* Section alone.[65]

Naturally *GUGZ* was not intended to stand alone in St. Petersburg. Its authority was to be felt throughout the empire through the establishment of thirteen regional (*okrug*) medical-sanitary departments, eight of them in European Russia, two in Siberia, and one each in the Far East, Turkestan, and the Caucasus. The commission also proposed to establish medical-sanitary councils at the *guberniia* and *uezd* levels, each with their own inspectorates, and new *uezd*-level organizations for combating epidemics. *GUGZ*'s jurisdiction was to extend to provinces without zemstvo institutions and also to those parts of the empire under special forms of military authority, such as the Cossack areas. Had all these plans been carried to fruition, agents of *GUGZ* would doubtless have become as familiar—and probably as contentious—a part of the local scene as the existing agencies of the MVD and the Ministry of Finance, compounding the bureaucratic assault on the countryside.[66]

Given Rein's plans for *GUGZ*, it should come as no surprise that many of the commission's proposals were designed to increase substantially the authority of the state over physicians and other medical personnel. This reassertion of authority can be seen clearly in the commission's proposals for the reform of medical education.[67] These drew a sharp distinction between medicine as an academic discipline and medicine as a vocation, leaving the former under the control of medical faculties and placing the latter squarely under the control of the state. In place of the existing two-tiered degree structure in which both those who planned to teach and those intending to practice took the same initial degree (*lekar'*), the requirements for which were set by the medical faculties, the commission proposed two different paths. Those planning to teach would initially study for the new degree of candidate of medical science, pursuing a longer, broader, and more onerous program than that required for the *lekar'* degree; then they would proceed to the M.D., which was to become essentially a proof of ability in one particular specialty (e.g., internal medicine, surgery, ophthalmology, etc.). Faculties of medicine were to set the requirements for these degrees and to examine the candidates. Those intending to practice would follow a quite different program: they would work not towards a degree but towards receiving one of three titles (zvaniia)–that of physician (vrach), sanitary physician (sanitarnyi vrach), or forensic physician (sudebnyi vrach). Although these studies would be pursued within a medical faculty, the courses would be prescribed by the state (i.e., by the Learned Branch of GUGZ), and students would be examined by specially appointed State Examining Commissions. Henceforth, freedom of inquiry was to be permitted only to academic medicine; practitioners, especially those who might find employment as community physicians, were to be given a state-approved view of the social role of physicians.

The same trend towards greater state control is apparent in the commission's plan for the expansion of medical research, the collection of statistics, and the development of hygiene education. Besides taking over the Imperial Institute of Experimental Medicine, GUGZ was to establish and run a vaccination institute, an institute of tropical medicine, and (under the aegis of the Medical Council) a state laboratory for research in hygiene, pharmacy, physiological chemistry, forensic medicine, toxicology, and bacteriology. Elsewhere in the commission's proposals are plans for a network of regional forensic-medical research facilities and institutes for the study of sanitation. To be sure, the need for expanded research facilities had been a constant theme in the medical press, but their relatively small growth in the two decades after 1890 had been sponsored almost entirely by the zemstvos.[68] The commission was thus proposing a substantial shifting of the major responsibility for medical research from the local level to the central government. This is equally true of medical statistics, where for years the really significant work had emanated from zemstvo sanitary bureaus and from the Pirogov Society. True, the Main Administration of the Chief Medical Inspector published annual reports on public health and medical assistance, but these were of little use as a basis for planning. The statistical section of GUGZ was assigned a much larger role, involving the collection, digestion, and publication of information not only about Russia, but also about foreign states. It was to be concerned not only with morbidity and mortality, but also with antiepidemic measures and medical-sanitary legislation. Most important of all, it was given the power to prescribe the rules and forms for medical registration and reporting which, together with the supervisory duties of the inspectorate, meant that GUGZ could control the collection and publication of statistics by the sanitary bureaus of zemstvos and municipalities. Popular hygiene education, another area in which sanitary bureaus and the Pirogov Society had been active, was also accorded a high priority by the commission.[69] All three divisions of *GUGZ*'s Sanitary Department, as well as its Learned Branch, were assigned responsibility for publishing and disseminating information about the purity of water, the importance of diet, the evils of alcohol, and the prevention of epidemics.

Most revealing of all were the commission's recommendations on the professional activity of physicians. Whatever the differences that had divided Russian physicians, there is no doubt that most of them believed that a national professional organization was desirable, that such an organization ought to speak for all physicians, and that it ought to play an important role in the formulation of state policy concerning public health. That they had not been able to find the appropriate form in which to cast the organization does not mean that the idea had been entirely abandoned. Rein and his colleagues on the Medical Council, however, subscribed to a much narrower definition of professionalism, in which most physicians were purely and simply practitioners. As practitioners, their activity was important enough to warrant regulation through legislation and state supervision. Thus the commission understood professional activity to mean nothing more nor less than state regulation of the legal and ethical aspects of medical practice. The subcommittee to which this subject was entrusted concentrated on such matters as illegal practice, medical confidentiality, and the ethical aspects of surgery and anesthesia. Clearly the intention was to produce a code of ethics which could be enforced on all physicians in state or public service through the inspectorate of *GUGZ*.

But what of the private practitioners who made up approximately one-third of those in practice? How to enforce professional discipline on those outside state service was a serious problem. For advice on this problem as well as on the particulars of the code, the commission turned to several medical societies, although the Pirogov Society itself was once again ignored. At this point, supporters of a professional medical estate began to make their opinions heard again. The St. Petersburg Physicians' Mutual Assistance Society revived its earlier campaign for the creation of an autonomous medical corporation but did so in somewhat different terms. In 1902, it had taken the position that state action should follow, not precede, the growth of "estate consciousness" among physicians. In 1912, the society argued for immediate state action. Its current president, Dr. K. P. Sulima, the Medical Inspector of the City of St. Petersburg, urged the commission to recommend the establishment of an autonomous corporate organization modeled on the German and Austrian chambers of physicians.[70] His proposal envisioned chambers composed of all physicians, whether salaried or self-employed, practicing in a given area; they would regulate the professional activity of their members, defend their interests, and advise the government on the formulation of public health policy. This form of professional organization, while by no means acceptable to the community physicians who dominated the Pirogov Society, probably would have enjoyed considerable support among other salaried physicians in government and institutional service.

Not surprisingly, Sulima's proposal ran into heavy opposition in the Rein Commission, especially in the plenary sessions where ministerial representatives and provincial governors spoke out against the creation of an autonomous medical estate. Influenced no doubt by memories of 1905, the commission in the end flatly rejected Sulima's proposal on the grounds that "an organization of physicians with rights of jurisdiction, and with the right of raising questions of state significance . . . is, in the interests of the state, inadmissable."[71] Obviously the commission wanted to encourage physicians to confine their professional interests to such matters as salaries, pensions, trust funds, and refresher courses, leaving matters of high policy to *GUGZ*. If they insisted on trying to influence state policy, they would have to work through, or rise within, the new bureaucratic apparatus. If they wished to advance other professional interests, they would be forced to do so through medical societies organized under the 1906 laws for unions and associations and thus subject to the double scrutiny of *GUGZ* and the MVD. Rather shrewdly, the commission had drawn a sharp line between physicians' medical activities, which were so important that they demanded regulation, and their other professional activities, in which—allegedly—the state had no interest.

Nevertheless, the problem of disciplining private practitioners remained. To deal with it, the commission devised an ingenious solution based on a severely truncated version of the Sulima proposal. It recommended the creation of much smaller Councils of Physicians (*sovety vrachei*), the jurisdiction of which would be confined exclusively to private practice.[72] Councils would be created at the provincial, regional, and municipal levels, wherever there was a concentration of at least three hundred private practitioners. Chosen by a complicated two-tiered electoral system, the councils were empowered to make regulations concerning the ethics of private practice and to deal with infractions by individual practitioners. They could levy penalties against offenders, up to and including a one-year suspension from practice. To ensure overall state supervision of the councils, the commission proposed to establish a special disciplinary board under the

Medical Council to review and hear appeals against decisions of local councils. These councils were quite unlike the bodies proposed by Sulima: they did not represent all physicians, dealt only with private practice, and had no power to speak for the whole profession on broad issues of policy. Like the Councils of the Bar, the Councils of Physicians were designed primarily to ensure that practitioners operating outside the state service were still subject to state authority.

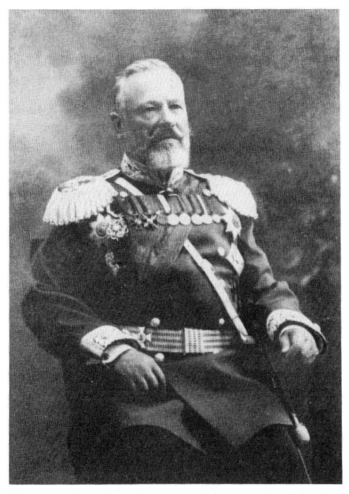

Fig. 9. G. E. Rein, medical reformer, loyal servant of the tsar, and nemesis of the community physicians, proudly posed for this official portrait just before his world collapsed in February 1917.

COMMUNITY MEDICINE OR STATE MEDICINE?

Rein and his commission received a predictably bad press from the organs of the Pirogov Society and were regularly denounced by its spokesmen. The tone was set by A. S. Durnovo, a regular columnist for *Obshchestvennyi Vrach*, who greeted the commission's formation by condemning the "opportunism" of St. Petersburg careerists, concerned only with "dead norms and regulations . . . the inventions of irresponsible chancery clerks."[73] On the opening day of the Twelfth Pirogov Congress in 1913, P. N. Diatroptov published a lengthy and telling critique of the assumptions on which the commission was operating, pointing out the dangers that its recommendations held for the future of community medicine.[74] Once again the Pirogov Congress had on its agenda the question of professional organization, the discussion of which took on a new urgency in view of the rumors that were circulating about the Rein Commission's refusal to sanction the creation of the broadly powerful chambers of physicians favored by the admirers of Germany. To be sure, the Pirogov Society had never favored such *soslovie* institutions anyway, so the congress gave Dr. Sulima a poor reception when he tried to rally support there for his proposal and instead reiterated its previous position that only the Pirogov Society could or should speak for Russian physicians as a profession.[75] The fact that Sulima's plans were rejected by the Rein Commission was not, of course, seen by the *pirogovtsy* as a reason for abandoning their hostility to its work; their position remained that the Rein proposals, if implemented, would destroy Russian community medicine.

The fears of the *pirogovtsy* were, in this instance, more than justified. To be sure, Rein claims in his memoirs that he was misunderstood; that his aim was not to destroy zemstvo medicine but to strengthen its effectiveness by providing a coordinated overall plan of activity. However, the student of his work during the years 1912 to 1914 will scarcely be persuaded by such a dubious argument, advanced by Rein during the difficult years of emigration and after a severe dressing-down by the Provisional Government's investigating commission for the cavalier attitude that he displayed towards the Duma in 1916 and early 1917. It is undeniably true that the proposals of the Rein Commission did not take matters of public health away from the zemstvos; indeed, by establishing in law that public health was an obligatory, rather than an optional, responsibility of local governments, they appeared to strengthen the position of zemstvo medicine. However, the greater state supervision that this change required would ensure that local autonomy was not increased. At the same time, the commission's proposals guaranteed nothing to the zemstvos by way of state revenues earmarked for medical purposes, nor did they even raise the matter of cost sharing between central and local governments. It is thus no exaggeration to say that the Rein proposals provided a means by which zemstvos and municipalities might easily bankrupt themselves and their taxpayers in the struggle to provide norms of medical care which would be set in St. Petersburg.[76]

In any case, the Rein proposals so changed the conditions under which zemstvo and municipal physicians would operate as to make it impossible for community medicine, as understood by the *pirogovtsy*, even to survive, let alone flourish. Greater state control over medical research, the collection of statistics, popular hygiene education, and epidemic prevention inevitably meant the emasculation of zemstvo and municipal sanitary services. Zemstvo sanitary physicians had prided themselves on being social critics and social reformers, but Rein's reorganization of medical education was obviously aimed at replacing them with obedient functionaries in an expanded system of state medical police. No longer would mere practitioners of medicine and sanitation be permitted to link the improvement of public health with the granting of civil and political rights; Rein's new sanitary physicians would function as technologists whose successes could be measured solely by falling morbidity and mortality rates. Their concerns would be pure water, better sewage systems, and the improvement of housing, all of these divorced from any larger social or political issues.

The political outlook that helped Rein to formulate his program was almost deceptively simple. Where liberal and radical health reformers saw the tsar's subjects as downtrodden but worthy potential citizens, Rein saw only so many hands to be employed, hands whose loyalty could be assured by fair treatment. Hence his determination to reduce mortality from epidemics. Like his seventeenth-century mercantilist predecessors, he was all in favor of larger, healthier populations that would work harder in civilian life and fight more effectively in the army. He saw no conflict whatever between the ideology of tsarism and the cause of *ozdorovlenie:* one had only to break the absurd connection that the *pirogovtsy* always insisted on making between sanitary improvement on the one hand and the extension of civil and political rights on the other.

Yet for all that Rein appears to be little more than a naive monarchist hoping to please his sovereign, he was in one respect singularly astute: he understood implicitly that tsarism was threatened not only by the radicalism of community medicine but also by the very idea of medical professionalism. Whatever the differences that separated physicians who sought a professional corporation from those who preferred a public-professional society or even an activist union, most Russian physicians did share certain fundamental attributes of professionalism. Chief among these was the assumption that physicians ought to control medical education and research, define their own legal and ethical obligations to society, act to improve the status of their occupation, and carry out their work free from interference by external authority. Rein did not share this outlook; his view was the traditional Russian one, in which the physician was regarded not as a professional providing a service to society but rather as a servant—or, better, servitor—of the state. Just as Witte recognized that zemstvo self-government was incompatible with the preservation of autocracy, so Rein understood that the state could not allow itself to be dictated to by an autonomous group of experts who claimed to have scientific truth on their side.

The proposals made by the Rein Commission, particularly those dealing with medical education and the professional activity of physicians, were in fact a deliberate counterattack on the ideals espoused by supporters of an autonomous profession. They restricted to a minimum the opportunities that physicians might take to act as a homogeneous social group. They reduced almost all physicians to the status of mere practitioners whose every move was to be supervised by agencies of the state. They prescribed the legal and ethical obligations of physicians and established a new institutional framework through which to police them. They made a concerted attempt to put the state, through its control of universities, in control of the development of medical knowledge. Rein led this counterattack not because he deplored expertise; on the contrary, he valued it enormously and wished to harness modern medical knowledge to make the country healthier and its people less barbaric and more productive. However, the only path that he could see that would permit the tsarist regime to accommodate medical expertise was the one proposed by his commission, in which the state would grant substantial power and autonomy only to the academic wing of the profession and then only on the implicit condition that it help the state to regulate the practitioners in its best interests.

It was Rein's misfortune to be overtaken by events. The commission finished its plenary sessions in the spring of 1914, and Rein decided to spend the summer overseeing the final version of his report and the publication of the commission's transactions. He was thus caught off guard by the outbreak of war in Europe in July. At first he saw no reason why the war should interrupt in any way the great work upon which he had been engaged for so long; indeed, in his view the danger from epidemics and the mismanagement associated with multiple jurisdictions argued for the speediest possible implementation of the commission's proposals. He was soon to discover, however, that the war would affect his plans and his career in ways that were as unexpected as they were unwelcome. Although he had far surpassed Botkin and von Anrep in preparing the way for a centralized ministry of health protection, his proposals still required legislative sanction and that, for a host of reasons unforeseen in the summer of 1914, was to prove enormously difficult to obtain.

5
WORLD WAR I
AND THE CONTROL
OF PUBLIC HEALTH

A centralizer such as Rein should have had everything to gain from the outbreak of war in August 1914. In tsarist Russia, however, the war did not increase the power of the civil government; instead, within months, its authority had almost ground to a halt. Effective power quickly devolved to the army at the front and to the so-called voluntary organizations—the Union of Zemstvos and the Union of Towns—in the rear. To Rein's dismay, he found himself virtually paralyzed by a war that continually provided more scope to the community physicians, who now grouped themselves round the Union of Zemstvos and the Union of Towns. Thanks to the unpreparedness of the army's medical corps, the duration of the war, and the tendency of corps commanders to rely on the assistance provided by the voluntary organizations, the community physicians enjoyed a windfall opportunity to reorganize and rejuvenate themselves. The Union of Zemstvos soon became, in the words of William Gleason, "one of the most important medical offices in Russia,"[1] and the Union of Towns was not far behind. Rein found himself an unwilling spectator as the community physicians used the medical bureaus of the two unions to revive and extend their involvement in public health matters throughout the country. This was the very development that Rein had wished to arrest, but he had reckoned without a war that outstripped the capacities of the regime.

Early in 1914, it seemed to be only a matter of time before the community physicians were tied to the apron strings of Rein's new ministry. The war reversed this situation, providing the professional intelligentsia as a whole and the community physicians in particular with fresh opportunities to extend their influence at the national and local levels. Thanks to the desperate plight of Russian field commanders, the medical staffs of the voluntary organizations quickly found themselves enjoying a freedom of action which, although not unrestricted, was far greater than they could have expected had Rein's ministry been established before the war broke out. The activities of the medical bureaus of the voluntary organizations must be seen against the background of these prewar conflicts over the control of public health administration. Many of the physicians who worked for the two unions had sympathized with the 1905 alliance between the Pirogov Society and the radical opposition. Having lived through the years of crisis, disarray, and despondency which characterized community medicine after 1905, they plunged into war work with the specter of the Rein Commission hanging over them. No more than Rein himself could they have foreseen the enormous role that the war would carve out for them. Indeed, for the first year they were almost wholly occupied with the day-to-day problems of caring for the sick and wounded. Nevertheless, once they began to realize the possibilities that the war had opened up, they were determined to make the most of them.

By the autumn of 1915 at the latest, it had dawned on those directing the medical work of the voluntary organizations that what was at stake was not only the provision of immediate assistance to the army, but the larger question of the inevitable postwar reorganization of medical and sanitary affairs. Would it be directed by conservative centralizers such as Rein or by the community physicians themselves? Using their connections with the Pirogov Society, which cast off its prewar doldrums and hurriedly organized a host of conferences, the medical staffs of the unions were able to draw up vast programs of vaccination, disinfection, and urban sanitary improvements. The local committees of the voluntary organizations drew up wider social participation than had the zemstvos and town dumas, so that the community physicians were able to use these bodies to enhance their position as professional experts, while at the same time pressing for a broadened zemstvo and municipal franchise. By the end of 1916, the unions' sanitary bureaus had worked out an extensive reform program for postwar Russia and had created much of the institutional framework through which it could be realized. Rein, recognizing what was afoot, continually urged the tsar to put him in control by creating a separate ministry but, by the time Nicholas II decided to act, both of them were caught in the torrent that swept away the old regime and its supporters. The events of February 1917 seemed to ensure that the long overdue reform of medicine and public health would be carried out by the community physicians, whose incontestable importance to the war effort gave them considerable leverage over the tsar's successors so long as the latter remained committed to fighting the war.

THE MEDICAL NEEDS OF THE ARMY

The first German shells fired against the Russians in August 1914 did even more damage in the rear than at the front. Within days of the opening salvos, it became apparent that the medical services available to the Russian army were completely inadequate for the tasks at hand. Russian patriots only days previously had greeted the tsar's declaration of war with unbounded optimism and gestures of support, but they suddenly found themselves faced with appalling evidence of the army's lack of planning. M. V. Rodzianko, President of the Fourth Duma, was one of the many who expressed shock when makeshift evacuation trains rolled into the railway stations of Moscow, disgorging their hideous cargo of wounded and maimed soldiers who had received no medical attention en route and for whose urgent needs absolutely no preparations had been made: "Chaos reigned supreme. Freight trains arrived in Moscow packed with wounded who lay on the floors of cars without straw litter, themselves often without clothes, with badly dressed wounds and having had no food for several days."[2] Scenes such as this, which soon became commonplace in most cities and towns with hospitals and rail connections to the front, provided grisly evidence that the army had been caught unprepared and spurred the formation of civilian agencies that would endeavor to stem the mounting chaos.

Why was the army's medical staff so unprepared? True to military form, they were prepared to fight the last war but not the next. In the wake of a less than distinguished performance in the Russo-Japanese War, the Military-Medical Administration was reformed between 1908 and 1910.[3] The chief lesson learned in the east, that sanitary needs required as much attention as medicine and surgery, became the central theme of the reform. All administrative positions from top to bottom were renamed from "military-medical" to military-sanitary." The duties of all personnel were rewritten to ensure that, for example, inspectors of army hospitals would now see to the sanitary state of the hospital and its surroundings and that regimental physicians would attend to the sanitary state of the troops in their charge. Although overdue by perhaps a quarter of a century, the reform was nevertheless a big step towards the modernization of any army that had for too long regarded the physician as "a mere dispenser of castor oil."[4] Having taken this step, however, the army medical staff rested on its laurels. True, the new structure of the Military-Sanitary Administration included a Personnel Section that was supposed to ensure that adequate personnel was available in the event of war, a Mobilization Section charged with planning and overseeing the transition to a wartime footing, and a Hospital Section that was responsible for arranging for the requisition of beds and services from the civil sector in the event that casualties exceeded the capacity of the military's own hospitals. As of May 1911, these sections were fully staffed by experienced and highly educated military physicians.[5] However, as the events of August 1914 were to reveal with such damning clarity, none of these planning bodies had any idea of the potential destructiveness of German firepower.[6]

Ignorance was compounded by complacency. Just as the war minister, V. A. Sukhomlinov, brooked no criticism of his administration by Duma politicians, so the chief military-sanitary inspector, A. Ia. Evdokimov, refused to countenance any suggestion from physicians that his department was not ready for war. Even after the unimaginable had become a reality, Evdokimov never admitted that he had been caught off guard; indeed, he continually maintained, in the face of mounting evidence to the contrary, that the army's medical staff could cope with all eventualities and resisted not only the services offered by newly created civilian organizations, but even in some cases the help of the Russian Red Cross.[7] Evdokimov deserved to be sacked in the first months of the war, not because he grossly underestimated the destructiveness of the German assault—after all, he had to work with the military intelligence at his disposal—but because he so stubbornly refused to cooperate with efforts to rescue the army from the situation in which it found itself. Yet he survived, and one is tempted to speculate that he was protected and perhaps even encouraged in his intransigence by Sukhomlinov, who treated the mildest criticism as evidence of disloyalty.

Nicholas II, whose personal anguish over the suffering of his troops is beyond doubt, could not but intervene. Where the government had failed, the dynasty would not. In the wake of the Romanov tercentenary in 1913, it was natural for him to look to a member of his own family to play the role of savior of the army, and his choice, not surprisingly, fell on his cousin, Prince Alexander Ol'denburg, head of the Russian Red Cross. Founder of the Imperial Institute of Experimental Medicine and patron of a score of philanthropies, the prince was, in Nicholas' opinion, admirably suited for the role. On 5 September, therefore, he was named Supreme Head (*Verkhovnyi nachal'nik*) of an entirely new military formation, the Sanitary and Evacuation Section; in this capacity he was to supervise "all organs, organizations, societies and personnel of the sanitary and evacuation service, both in the theater of military operations, and in the interior of the empire."[8]

That Ol'denburg was intended to have dictatorial powers is clear from his orders, which specified that all government and public institutions and personnel, and indeed the entire population, were subject to his authority. Even more significant is the fact that the prince was beyond the control of the war minister and hence of the Council of Ministers itself; he was responsible only to the commander in chief (Grand Duke Nikolai Nikolaevich, until he was supplanted by the tsar himself in August 1915) for his work at the front and only to the tsar personally for his work at the rear.[9] Dictatorial powers were clearly essential because the problems of administration and coordination which Ol'denburg faced were enormous. At the front, despite Evdokimov's attitude, there was a fairly good working relationship between the army medical staff and the Red Cross but, in the rear, Ol'denburg's duties meant potential conflicts with the Ministry of the Interior and its medical inspectorate, with the governors and provincial administrative institutions, and, above all, with the zemstvo and municipal medical and sanitary agencies.

Ol'denburg was required to work with the community physicians not only because he needed their personnel and hospital facilities but because the tsar had already recognized a special wartime role for the zemstvos and towns. Early in August, the Moscow provincial zemstvo had sought imperial sanction for the creation of an All-Russian Union of Zemstvos, which would provide medical and other assistance to the army; a group of mayors followed suit with a request concerning the formation of an All-Russian Union of Towns.[10] Thankful, no doubt, for such a display of patriotism from men who had more than once during his reign been in opposition to the regime, Nicholas replied with messages of gratitude and good wishes. Between them, the zemstvos and towns employed almost a quarter of all the physicians in the empire and controlled a substantial proportion of the hospital beds available in European Russia; hence they were of crucial importance in any effort to bolster the faltering abilities of the Military-Sanitary Administration.[11]

Although working with the voluntary organizations was a necessity, the prince had no intention of permitting them to take over functions that he believed rightly belonged to the army and to the Red Cross. In this attitude he was supported by his newly appointed deputy, V. K. von Anrep, who after his term as a Duma deputy had become a member of the executive board of the Red Cross. Even before receiving his appointment as Supreme Head, the prince had established a clear demarcation line (running from Moscow to Khar'kov) separating areas adjacent to the front, and hence under the jurisdiction of the army and the Red Cross, from areas east of this line and hence under the jurisdiction of the voluntary organizations.[12] It was not only the prince's institutional loyalty that led him to preserve a distinct sphere of operations for the Red Cross; the tsar's orders had specified that the voluntary organizations should work under its flag, and the prince's intention was to make their subordinate role indisputably plain. He may also have wished to put as much distance as possible between the hard-pressed front and the enthusiastic rear: help was welcome, but meddling was not.

The destruction wrought by the German guns soon made it impossible to maintain separate spheres, at least with regard to the evacua-

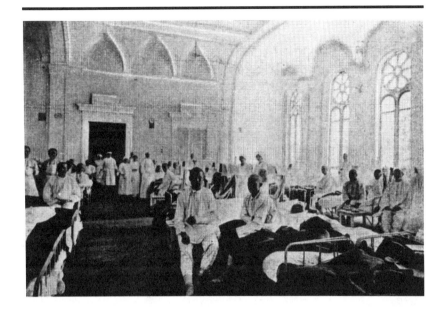

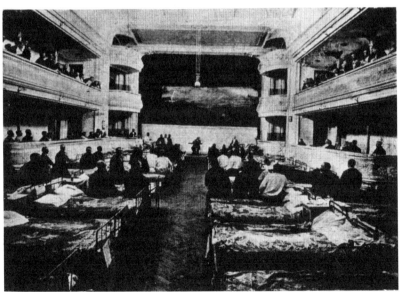

Fig. 10. The Union of Towns hastily converted to medical uses whatever buildings were available: in Kiev *(top)* a medical society building, and in Poltava *(bottom)* a theater.

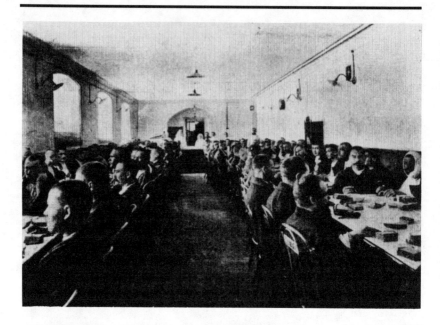

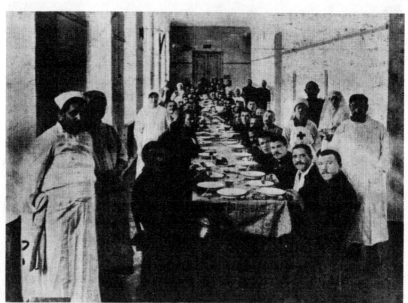

Fig. 11. Convalescing soldiers were fed in improvised dining halls such as these in Poltava *(top)* and Vladikavkaz *(bottom)*.

tion and hospitalization of wounded soldiers. Casualties were far too high for the army and the Red Cross to handle them alone, either at the front itself or in the areas adjacent to it. Physicians were in such short supply that, at first, line officers were detailed to organize sanitary measures and to run evacuation stations, a military and a medical absurdity when these jobs could have been done by medical personnel from the voluntary organizations.[13] Corps commanders themselves subverted Ol'denburg's instructions by appealing to the voluntary organizations to cross the line and help to stem the chaos at the front. With the encouragement of General Brusilov, the Zemstvo Union began in September to send medical teams and field hospitals into Galicia. The prince was outflanked; he could scarcely insist that officers let their men die to protect the pretensions of the Red Cross. In any case, the physicians who joined the two unions had little or no confidence in the military and civil bureaucracy and saw no reason why they should stay behind an artificial demarcation line. The more they did at the front, the more they were asked to do. The prince was soon forced to abandon his earlier policy and to countenance a steadily increasing role for the voluntary organizations. This was, however, a grudging concession; in areas other than evacuation and hospital care, such as the treatment of special groups (for example, maimed, tubercular, or mentally ill soldiers), the prince held to his original policy, enforcing his wishes by controlling the kinds of activities for which the unions received government subsidies.

Meanwhile, in St. Petersburg, Rein was anxious that the temporary demands of the war should not overshadow his grand plans for the reorganization of Russian medicine. Like everyone else, he expected the war to be over in six months and hence wished to get on with the implementation of his recommendations. His first concern was to secure the approval of the Council of Ministers, so that the legislation to establish *GUGZ* could be sent to the legislative institutions.[14] However, the new minister of the interior, N. A. Maklakov, was by no means sympathetic, and Rein had to seek the tsar's help to have his proposal discussed by the council in September 1914. Between those who, like Maklakov, opposed the creation of a new ministry and those who simply thought the measure untimely, support was neither unanimous nor enthusiastic. In the end, the council approved in principle the establishment of *GUGZ* but decided to postpone sending the legislation to the Duma until the war was over. After three years' work in the Interdepartmental Commission, this decision was a blow for Rein, but he treated it as a setback, rather than a defeat. Still confident of the tsar's support, he appealed to Nicholas to override the council; if necessary, he argued, *GUGZ* could be established by means of Article 87, which provided for the enactment of emergency measures when the

Duma was not in session. No constitutionalist, Nicholas might well have agreed but, when Prince Ol'denburg got wind of it, he was adamantly opposed. His task was difficult enough already, without having Rein established as a rival authority in those areas not under military jurisdiction. For the moment, at least, Rein was stymied; he could do nothing unless the tsar changed his mind and overrode the prince's opposition.

MEDICAL SERVICES ON THE HOME FRONT

The community physicians were far too busy to celebrate Rein's discomfiture. In the first months of the war, they were almost entirely occupied with evacuating soldiers from the front and providing hospital facilities for them in the rear. Within four months (September–December 1914), the medical staff of the Zemstvo Union made 150,000 hospital beds available for military use; some of these were existing beds diverted to wartime needs, but others were in new hospitals created wherever space was available.[15] Within six months, the Zemstvo Union had equipped and staffed 45 hospital trains that carried sick and wounded soldiers from all over the western front to relocation points and thence to hospitals in the interior.[16] Empty railway cars had to be completely outfitted with hospital beds, surgical facilities, medical instruments, kitchens, and all the paraphernalia that these demanded; physicians, nurses, and other medical personnel, as well as cooks and attendants, had to be hired. After Brusilov's appeal for help in Galicia, the Zemstvo Union also sent field detachments and several mobile surgical teams.

Rapid organization was easy for the Zemstvo Union, which was able to call upon the experience and expertise of local bodies (the zemstvo medical-sanitary bureaus), thus establishing the rapid exchange of information between the center and the regions that the situation demanded. The Union of Towns, however, was hampered by the absence of medical or sanitary organizations in many towns, by the shortage of medical personnel in urban areas, and by the lack of elementary urban sanitary facilities. A 1913 survey conducted for the Pirogov Society by D. N. Zhbankov disclosed that 43 percent of Russia's most populous towns had no civic medical organization, and 63 percent had no permanent sanitary organization whatsoever. During the early months of the war, the call-up of physicians hit the cities with particular severity, depleting a supply of medical personnel which was already inadequate. The same 1913 survey also showed that Russian towns were, from a sanitary point of view, extremely poorly served: only 219 had a piped water supply, canalization was a rarity, and baths, laundries, and disinfection facilities were sadly deficient. Thus in 1914 the Union of Towns was in no position to rival the Union of Zemstvos in providing for evacuation and hospital trains; the focus of its activity was rather on the towns of the interior where, in the words of its first medical officer, Dr. Nikolaevskii, "everything had to be created de novo."[17]

Towns, especially those located on the railway evacuation routes, had to move especially quickly because of the threat of infectious diseases. True to form, Evdokimov had blithely assumed that the Military-Sanitary Administration could cope with the problem of infectious disease among soldiers by using its own isolation hospitals in the interior military districts, ignoring the fact that many of the latter were located in epidemiological danger zones. In any case, the desperate haste that marked early efforts to evacuate the sick and wounded resulted in the indiscriminate dispatch of soldiers suffering from cholera, smallpox, and typhus into the very heart of the country. Neither the army nor the Red Cross were able to separate and control infectious diseases at the rudimentary front evacuation points, which had inadequate disinfection, bath, and laundry facilities. The medical staff of the Zemstvo Union, although aware of the problem, were forced to send on without treatment the infectious sick, at least during the first few weeks when their own facilities were still being created. Before the end of 1914, there were outbreaks of typhus, typhoid, and relapsing fever, which reached epidemic proportions in the provinces of Kaluga, Voronezh, Riazan, and the Povol'zhe.[18] Small wonder that the Union of Towns moved at a furious pace to create isolation hospitals and to remedy the most glaring deficiencies of urban sanitation.

Russian soldiers were not the only agents who spread infectious diseases in the interior. Indeed, if the War Ministry had embarked on a deliberate policy of promoting epidemics on the home front, it could scarcely have taken measures more calculated to achieve this result than those it adopted during the first year of the war. With the army's isolation hospitals already swamped and before adequate preparations had been made for facilities elsewhere, trainloads of prisoners-of-war and "unreliables" were transported from the fronts to central Russia, spreading disease as they went. Many of the Turkish prisoners of war had been captured in areas of the Caucasus where typhus had already broken out. The hygenist N. I. Teziakov witnessed the arrival of one such train in Balashov, en route from the Caucasus to Penza. When the wagon doors were opened, not only were there numerous cases of typhoid among the living, but many corpses had to be removed and disposed of.[19] Neither food nor water, let alone medical attention, was provided on these trains, nor were the physicians at their destinations alerted in advance. Many of the tsar's own subjects were treated no better. Jews, Germans, Latvians, and Poles in the west and Turks, Greeks, and Armenians in the Caucasus were liable to immediate deportation if declared "unreliable" by the War Ministry. They arrived without warning at evacuation points and thus became an additional complication for the organizers of evacuation and a further source of infection on the home front, either because they were already suffering from infectious diseases or because they contracted them during the evacuation itself. Prisoners and "unreliables" helped to fuel the typhus epidemic, which by January 1915 had spread to Tambov, Iaroslavl', and other areas. Thus serious epidemics began in Central Russia several months before the exodus of refugees which was instigated by the great retreats along the western front in July and August 1915.

As problems mounted on the home front, fewer physicians were available to deal with them. By 1915, 14,500 physicians (almost 44 percent of the available total of 33,000) had been drafted or called up from the reserves and militia.[20] Although precise figures about the pattern of impressment are not available, certain observations can be made with reasonable certainty. It was not the policy of the War Ministry to deplete the ranks of physicians in direct government service so long as others were available; as a result, such "essential" services as provincial medical administration, the police *gorodovoi* physicians, and prison physicians were left to get on with their work. The Russian state had always regarded community physicians and private practitioners as supernumerary state servitors who could be pressed into service as required, and hence a large number of those conscripted and called up came from their ranks. In the cities, the call-up most affected municipal physicians; civic, charity, and private hospital physicians; and self-employed practitioners. In the countryside, zemstvo medical and sanitary physicians at both the provincial and district levels were pressed into service.

Although the physician-patient ratio was ordinarily considerably better in the countryside than in the cities, the shortage of physicians and other consequences of the war played havoc with rural medical services.[21] The tireless Pirogov statistician, P. I. Kurkin, reported in 1915 the effects of the war on zemstvo medical services; he based his findings on questionnaires completed by more than 40 percent of the districts in forty of the zemstvo provinces of European Russia.[22] His first conclusion was that rural hospital services had not only stopped growing but had actually declined. The respondents indicated that, although nearly 1,500 new beds had been made available, 5,467 had been diverted for use by soldiers; hence, there was a 10 percent net reduction in beds available for the local population.[23] Second, he reported on the almost universal phenomenon of "deserted" medical districts (*pustovavshie uchastki*), caused by the military call-up of physicians. More than a quarter of the districts in these forty provinces had lost all their physicians, while another seventy-two reported that one-half to two-thirds of their physicians were gone. Although Kurkin had no figures for the provincial zemstvos, the situation there cannot have been much better, and he described the exodus as "a new crisis which has arisen in the sphere of Russian zemstvo medicine."[24] It was not simply the decline in services that disturbed him; even more worrying was "the intrusion of feldsherism into the sphere of zemstvo *uchastok* medicine."[25] Probably correctly, Kurkin concluded the feldshers were taking up the slack in "deserted" areas; some districts replied that neighboring physicians might look in or act as nominal administrators, but feldshers must have borne the brunt of coping with the rural population. In view of the traditional hostility of community physicians towards "independent feldsherism," it is significant that only 10 of the 187 districts which replied admitted that their services were being run by feldshers, and only 1 stated that its feldshers were being paid more for the extra work (although several mentioned increased salaries for physicians). Other makeshifts were also employed: the complete or partial closure of rural hospitals and even the impressing of medical students. Essential maintenance was not being carried out, while long-term plans to build new hospitals and to upgrade feldsher posts into medical stations had been shelved. Kurkin commented gloomily on the "profound and burdensome disorder" into which zemstvo medicine was being driven by the war. Comparably detailed studies covering the same period for municipal medical services do not exist but, if things were this bad in rural areas, they must have been far worse in towns, where there were almost three times fewer physicians per inhabitant.

THE MOUNTING THREAT OF EPIDEMICS

The second year of the war began in circumstances that suggested that it would be even more disastrous than the first. By July and August, Russian armies were forced to retreat from Poland and Galicia, setting off a human tidal wave that inundated central Russia with millions of uprooted, starving, and diseased unfortunates.[26] Refugees seeking to escape the war jammed evacuation points; as they awaited their chance to leave, camping out in the hot weather amid unsanitary conditions, cholera broke out, adding its toll to the suffering already caused by typhus. Soon epidemics of both diseases were raging in the provinces Volhynia, Minsk, Mogilev, and Grodno. Fear of cholera quickly became an additional motive for escape, and in the ensuing months some three million refugees fled by caravan, by railway, and on foot. One of the lines of escape went northward to the lakes and the Baltic provinces; another southward into the Ukraine and New Russia; yet another eastward into central Russia and even Siberia. Thus cholera and a host of gastrointestinal disorders, dysentery, typhoid fever, and paratyphoid spread throughout European Russia and beyond the Urals. Cholera was particularly virulent in August and September in the towns along the main refugee routes. Scarlet fever, measles, and diphtheria raged among the children. Trains stopped only long enough for corpses to be removed. With the coming of cold weather, cholera and the other hot-weather diseases abated, only to be replaced once again by typhus. By the end of 1915, according to the (probably incomplete) information compiled by the Zemstvo Union, thirty-nine provinces were affected by epidemic diseases, principally typhus, typhoid fever, and relapsing fever. Unless a coordinated plan was implemented quickly, Russia would surely be defeated not by Germans, Austrians, and Turks, but by lice, intestinal parasites, and impure water.

Given the immediacy and magnitude of the threat posed by epidemic disease, one might reasonably expect some initiative to have been taken by official Russia and its medical establishment. The historian looks in vain, however, for any sign that the threat was taken seriously in St. Petersburg. True, Rein continued to lobby the tsar to accept his proposals, which included new antiepidemic agencies at the *okrug* level, but his efforts were fruitless. Nothing was heard from the Council of Ministers, the MVD, the Medical Council, or the Anti-plague Commission. Nothing was heard from Prince Ol'denburg or from the Military-Sanitary Administration. Nothing was heard from the official centers of medical education and research at the Military-Medical Academy, the Institute of Experimental Medicine, or the Plague Fort at Kronstadt. Admittedly, the problems of public health were only one aspect of the crisis provoked by the government's evident inability to direct the war effort, a crisis that led to the fruitless negotiations between the tsar's ministers and the Duma's Progressive Bloc and to the tsar's decision to assume personal command of the armies at the front. Yet the general political crisis of August 1915 cannot by itself explain the utter lack of leadership which characterized all official bodies charged with the protection of public health.

Rein had been warning since 1909 of the dangers of divided responsibility, reliance on piecemeal temporary measures, and the absence of a central agency to plan and direct medical and sanitary affairs. He had been thwarted first by the civil bureaucracy, chiefly the MVD, and then by the military in the person of Prince Ol'denburg. Rein's opponents within the regime were dogs in the manger; in opposing him while taking no action themselves, they assured that leadership would come from elsewhere, as come it did. The paralysis of the regime in the face of the epidemics of 1914 and 1915 seemed to prove what the community physicians had been saying all along: that only they were capable of reforming medical and sanitary affairs on the basis of reason, science, and humanity. This is not to suggest that, if Rein had been put in charge of *GUGZ* at the outbreak of the war, he could singlehandedly have averted the disastrous epidemics of the following years. At best, with the cooperation of Prince Ol'denburg and of the MVD, he might have been able to strike a more just balance between the needs of the army and those of the rear; at worst, he might have so alienated the community physicians as to impair severely the assistance that they were rendering to the war effort. One thing is certain: the absence of effective leadership from St. Petersburg gave the community physicians an unexpected opportunity to demonstrate what they could do, in the face of almost insuperable obstacles, to save Russia from both the ravages of disease and the inadequacies of the tsarist regime.

The epidemics of 1914/15 changed the focus of the medical work of the two unions. So long as their primary concern was with the wounded, therapeutic measures—first aid, field surgery, evacuation, and hospital care—far outweighed preventive measures. However, as attention shifted to the importance of antiepidemic work, the initiative for conceiving and executing preventive programs came to lie not with the therapists and hospital physicians, but with the bacteriologists, epidemiologists, and hygienists. Half a dozen individuals who directed these activities stand out with particular clarity, men who had long participated in the struggle to consolidate and extend the frontiers of community medicine, who were veterans of many battles against the tsarist regime, and who by 1914 had close ties to radical politics. They were haunted by three spectres: bureaucratic interference, of which the Rein Commission was the most recent and dangerous manifestation; the zemstvo reaction of 1906/07, which had done such damage to the aspirations and morale of medical radicals; and popular ignorance, which continually menaced the activities and even the lives of those who believed in reason and science. Each of these specters exerted its particular influence on the physicians' relationship with the tsarist government, with the propertied elements who dominated the executives of the two unions, and with the common people, whether encountered as soldiers at the front or as peasants and workers in the rear. These same men, haunted by the same specters, were to play important roles in the medical political controversies of 1917, so it is doubly important that their experiences during the war be clearly understood.

Given the importance that antiepidemic measures would play during the war, the Zemstvo Union was fortunate in securing the services of L. A. Tarasevich, P. N. Diatroptov, and Z. P. Solov'ev. Tarasevich, it will be remembered, had been forced out of Novorossiisk University in the wake of the 1905 Revolution, only to be dismissed from Moscow University during the Kasso purge of 1911. When the war broke out, he was teaching at the Moscow Higher Womens' Courses; he immediately went to work for the Zemstvo Union and became head of its anti-epidemic bureau. Wooed by the Social Democrats in 1906, he had not joined the party, but he did give it money—a good deal of money, according to an appreciative friend.[27] A clue to Tarasevich's political attitude on the eve of the war is provided by Olga Mechnikova, whose eminent husband spent the summer of 1911 in Russia as leader of a scientific expedition financed by the Pasteur Institute.[28] Tarasevich met his old teacher in Moscow and there joined the expedition, which was making a study of tuberculosis among the Kalmuks. Although Mechnikov had hitherto been extremely skeptical of the Russian revolutionary movement, he returned from this trip revolted by the excesses of tsarism and by the influence wielded at court by the odious Rasputin. He was particularly incensed by the purge that Minister of Education L. A. Kasso had carried out against radical elements in the universities, by the pogroms against the Jews, by official encouragement of the right-wing Black Hundred gangs. "Henceforth," Mechnikova concludes, "M[echnikov] thought that the problem of Russian life would be solved by the intellectuals apart from the government and in opposition to it."[29] Such a fundamental alteration in Mechnikov's outlook could only have come from conversations with scientists whose work he respected; Tarasevich, who had by now achieved an international reputation as a bacteriologist, must have been his principal confidant on Russian affairs. Tarasevich, then, was no apolitical scientist driven into opposition by the spectacle of wartime mismanagement; already by 1911, he was convinced that progress meant opposition to tsarism and had personally supported the organized opposition by subsidizing the Social Democrats.

Diatroptov's career was similar. A leading physician-radical in 1905, he had lost his job in Odessa, been exiled, and eventually found his way to Moscow.[30] In 1914, he was teaching with Tarasevich at the Higher Women's Courses, and he joined his friend in the Zemstvo Union, becoming head of its Sanitary Bureau. Whether or not he had been a Social Democrat in Odessa in 1905, he did not join the party in Moscow. It was no secret, however, that he was sympathetic to the revolutionary cause.[31]

Solov'ev, on the other hand, was an active member of the Bolshevik underground.[32] He arrived in Moscow by a somewhat different route, having been exiled for his political activities while he was a zemstvo physician in Simbirsk and Saratov. An epidemiologist with a special interest in tuberculosis and occupational diseases, he had by 1914 become Secretary of the All-Russian League for Struggle with Tuberculosis. Forbidden to secure employment as a zemstvo or municipal physician, he gravitated naturally and enthusiastically into the Zemstvo Union, where he became Secretary of the bureau that was headed by Diatroptov. Moreover, all three men were associated through the Pirogov Society as members of the editorial board of the monthly *Community Physician* (*Obshchestvennyi Vrach*). Through the society and its journal, they worked closely with another Bolshevik physician, I. V. Rusakov, a specialist in pediatrics and child hygiene.

Rusakov's past also included radical politics and a term of exile.[33] He joined the student underground in 1899, supported the radical All-Russian Union of Medical Personnel in 1905, and was arrested for participating in the Moscow uprising. After three years' exile in Tobol'sk, he returned to Moscow, where he became secretary of the editorial board of *Community Physician*. A member of the Pirogov Society's board of directors, he regularly represented the society at meetings of the medical bureaus of the unions. He and Solov'ev, the two Bolsheviks, were also relatively young men. In 1914 Rusakov was 37 and Solov'ev 38; Tarasevich was 46, while Diatroptov, at 54, was almost a generation older.

The youngest of all the physicians in senior positions with the unions was A. N. Sysin, who headed the Antiepidemic Bureau of the Union of Towns.[34] As a medical student in Moscow in 1899, he had been arrested for participating in student disorders and had been sent back to his home province of Nizhegorod. Undeterred, he joined the local Social Democratic underground and in 1901 was arrested and exiled to Siberia, where he remained until released under the political amnesty that Nicholas II was forced to concede during the 1905 Revolution. Finishing his medical studies in 1908, Sysin enjoyed during the next eight years a remarkably speedy rise through the ranks of community medicine. Serving first as an *uchastok* physician in Vologda, he moved to Saratov as a santiary physician, and then in 1911 he became head of the *guberniia* sanitary bureau of Nizhegorod. In 1913, he had moved to the sanitary bureau of the city of Moscow and, when the war broke out in 1914, he became, at the age of 35, director of the city's war-time sanitary organization and director of antiepidemic measures for the Union of Towns.

Sysin's meteoric rise to such a responsible position deserves some explanation. Perhaps because of his youth—he was only 27 when he returned from Siberia in 1906—he retained a spirit of optimism that others, such as Diatroptov, seem to have lost in the wake of 1905. He was also imaginative and dynamic. While the protagonists in the "pen versus test tube" debate agonized over the future of zemstvo sanitary services, Sysin got on with his job in a way that was to demonstrate the sterility of the debate. In his day-to-day work as a sanitary physician, at Pirogov Congresses, and especially at the 1912 Conference of Bacteriologists and Epidemiologists, Sysin constantly built bridges between medicine and technology. His work demonstrated that sanitary physicians ought to stop feuding over whether they should be publicists or research scientists and tackle the real problems of rural and urban water supply, which had now been linked definitively to the spread of cholera. In drawing up his plans he collaborated with geologists, hydrologists, sanitary engineers, and agronomists. At the 1912 Conference of Bacteriologists, he argued for the creation of a new zemstvo collegial organization that would bring together sanitary physicians, hydrologists, and engineers, as well as agronomists and insurance personnel. A leading Soviet historian of medicine has argued that it was the enthusiastic response to his fresh approach that brought Sysin the offer of a position in Moscow.[35]

Sysin's emphasis on the role of technologists in sanitary reform undoubtedly found favor with members of the Moscow Sanitary Bureau, especially with L. B. Granovskii, another Social Democrat and physician-activist in 1905, who was one of its most influential members.[36] Like Sysin, Granovskii had been particularly interested in industrial hygiene and had come to believe that a partnership between physicians and sanitary engineers was crucial to furthering the cause of urban sanitary reform. Their shared interests were soon reflected in the significant role played by engineers and other technical specialists in the sanitary work of the Union of Towns. Strong support for this new approach came also from N. F. Nikolaevskii, head of the Sanitary Bureau of the Union of Towns. Unlike Sysin and Granovskii, Nikolaevskii seems to have had no links with Russian social democracy, but he could scarcely have worked so closely with them without sharing their outlook, particularly after the union's plans for antiepidemic measures received such a setback in the summer of 1915. Sysin and Granovskii were both active in the Pirogov Society and on the editorial board of *Community Physician;* they certainly, and Nikolaevskii probably, shared with their colleagues in the Zemstvo Union the conviction that the tsarist regime was an insuperable obstacle to the progress of Russian medicine.

That so many radical physicians should have found their way to positions of influence within organizations that professed purely patriotic motives is one of the ironies of Russian history. Yet given the haste with which the unions were created, it was almost inevitable that they would attract such men, professionals who had been victims of tsarist persecution and who consequently lacked a secure institutional base within which to pursue their commitment to community medicine. True, the unions were ad hoc creations that could offer only a temporary institutional foothold. Moreover, their central committees were composed of the propertied men who enjoyed the limited franchise permitted in local government, men of the same class and type as

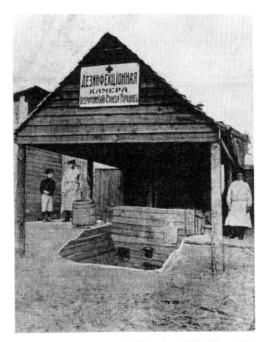

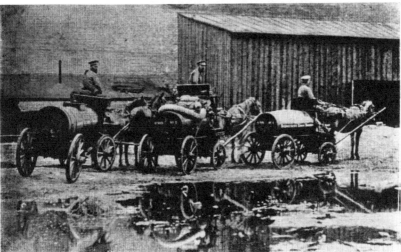

Fig. 12. Disinfection programs involved either bringing the men to a disinfecting chamber like this one at a railway station *(top)* or organizing convoys *(bottom)* to take the necessary chemicals to those encamped behind the front.

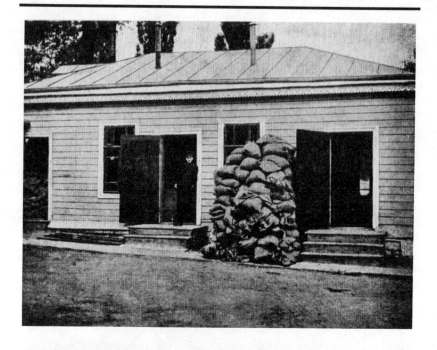

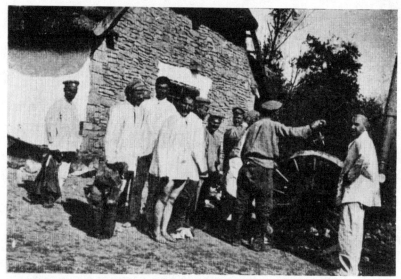

Fig. 13. With the right equipment almost any building, even a thatched cottage, could be turned into a disinfecting chamber or bathhouse.

those who had vented their rage over the events of 1905 upon community physicians and other third-element professionals. As they stood, the unions were less than congenial homes for politically minded professionals, but the very fact that they were ad hoc creations raised the possibility that they could be converted into instruments for change. They did at least provide an opportunity to transcend the restrictions on community medical activity which were inherent in the Zemstvo and Municipal Statutes, an opportunity that was bolstered by the urgent requirements of the army. They also held out the possibility that, through organizing at the local level to meet the wartime emergency, inroads could be made by the professional and technical intelligentsia upon the exclusive control of local, especially municipal, affairs by the propertied classes.[37]

Physicians were particularly fortunate in being able to wear their Pirogov hats one day and their union hats the next, thus enabling them to claim that what they were proposing as union employees and administrators smacked of no sectional or partisan interest but were rather measures demanded by an objective and rational medical science.[38] The Pirogov connection was to become the union physicians' trump card, played whenever it was necessary to outmaneuver the Red Cross or the Military-Sanitary Administration, whose physician-advisors could invoke no such prestigious support. Very quickly, what was to become an established pattern of relationships between the Pirogov Society and the unions became apparent. Plans were initially discussed within the medical bureaus of the unions; they were then revised by the directors of the Pirogov Society, who decided that they deserved fuller elaboration at a small conference or a larger congress; the resolutions passed at these meetings in the name of the Pirogov Society called upon the unions to do this and so; the unions' medical staff then sought the approval of their executives and funds from the government to carry out their plans. Between 1914 and the end of 1916, the Pirogov Society was the sole or joint sponsor of no less than seven such meetings, not to mention its Extraordinary Congress in 1916, which also discussed the role of the unions.[39] Among the topics discussed at special conferences were bacteriology, epidemic prevention, urban sanitation, tuberculosis, venereal disease, alcoholism, and mental illness. The full Pirogov Congress held in 1916 discussed many of the same questions and also devoted considerable attention to questions of housing, the food supply, and the reform of local government, indicating the extent to which the society's concerns mirrored those of the union physicians.

All this activity was a welcome fillip to the fortunes of the Pirogov Society, which had been sagging badly during the prewar years. The year 1914 had not, after all, brought Rein's comprehensive assault on community medicine and on the very idea of medical professionalization; instead it had brought the tempering experience of a war that not only arrested Rein's plans, but presented unforeseen opportunities to community physicians and the Pirogov Society to reassert their influence dramatically by organizing to meet the wartime emergency. Although the activities of the community physicians ranged over virtually every aspect of wartime medical work, from the supply of dressings to orthopedic care for the maimed, it would be inappropriate to review here a story that has been well told elsewhere.[40] Three aspects of their work do merit special attention, however: the campaign to organize antiepidemic measures because it revived the prewar conflicts between community medicine and the tsarist bureaucracy; the campaign to take over responsibility for the mentally ill because it revealed the continuing universalist aspirations of community medicine; and the effort of the Union of Towns to organize urban sanitary institutions because it demonstrated both the connection between medical and political reform and the gulf that was beginning to develop between zemstvo and municipal medicine.

THE ANTIEPIDEMIC CAMPAIGN

Tarasevich, Diatroptov, Solov'ev, and Sysin took the lead in organizing a concerted response to the epidemics that were quickly spreading from the front to the interior in late December 1914. Under the aegis of the Pirogov Society, a three-day conference brought together bacteriologists, epidemiologists, and representatives of the medical and sanitary bureaus of the unions, several provincial zemstvos, and major cities.[41] Immediate needs were as obvious as they were formidable. Isolation and disinfection facilities were required at the front, during evacuation, and in the rear. To be at all effective, they would have to reach not only Russian soldiers, but prisoners of war, "unreliables," refugees, and the civilian population along the evacuation routes and in the interior. Nowhere were there sufficient resources to do these jobs: not enough physicians or sanitary and disinfection personnel, not enough disinfection facilities, not enough hospital beds, not enough vaccines or laboratories in which to manufacture them. Nevertheless, at the Pirogov Congress the physicians set aside reality in favor of a declaration of optimum goals. Tarasevich spearheaded the passage of resolutions that called for preventive vaccination against typhoid, cholera, and dysentery and for the development of a multipurpose antiseptic vaccine that would prevent strep- and staphylococcus infections among the wounded.[42] His one concession to reality at this point was an admission that it was hopeless to expect that such vaccinations would be made mandatory by the military and civil authorities. Further resolutions called upon the government to provide the unions with special

funds earmarked for antiepidemic measures: the training of vacci-
nators, disinfectors, and other sanitary personnel; the construction
of baths, laundries, and disinfection chambers; the construction and
equipping of a network of isolation hospitals; sanitary improvements,
particularly to water supplies and sewage disposal in major towns and
cities. The only governmental action for which the physicians had
words of approval was the recent prohibition of the sale and consumption of alcohol. Although this measure was probably implemented to
prevent disorders during mobilization rather than for reasons of health,
medical evidence indicated that the physiological effects of alcohol
consumption greatly increased vulnerability to infectious diseases;
hence the congress applauded the ban as a useful temporary measure
and called for greater efforts to inform the people about the relationship between alcohol and disease.[43]

Armed with these resolutions, the physicians now put their union
hats on again and pressed the government all the harder for both the
money and the freedom of action necessary to implement them. More
detailed plans were formulated by a joint council of the medical and
sanitary personnel of both unions which began to meet in February
1915. These called for the erection of special isolation facilities in a
score of locations adjacent to the western and Caucasian fronts, administered either by the Union of Zemstvos or by the Union of Towns;
moreover, an additional 5 percent of all hospital beds elsewhere in the
empire were to be set aside for cases of infectious disease. In addition,
plans were made for vaccination programs and sanitary improvements in the interior towns and cities. Subsidies totaling 50 million
rubles were requested: 32 million for the Union of Zemstvos and the
balance for the Union of Towns.[44] Provided that official approval were
forthcoming in the early spring, the union physicians would have
their isolation facilities operating before the summer brought a recurrence of epidemic cholera and dysentery.

Predictably, the stumbling block was not the army but the civil government. In his first few months in office, Prince Ol'denburg had reluc-
tantly come to accept the necessity for cooperation with the unions to
deal with crises. The danger of infectious disease had already reached
crisis proportions. Accordingly, the special council he had established
to review requests for funds from the unions gave its approval to the
antiepidemic scheme and forwarded it to the Council of Ministers. It
was this body that dashed the hopes and plans of the union physicians by its outright and unexplained rejection of the whole scheme
on 1 March. Three months later, in May, the minister of the interior
announced that, because antiepidemic measures on the home front
were beyond the jurisdiction of the unions, the normal procedures
should be followed, that is, zemstvos and towns should individually

approach the ministry's Antiplague Commission for additional funds to cover specific projects within their jurisdictions.[45] Coming as it did in the early summer and on the eve of the retreats with their attendant exodus of refugees, Maklakov's statement virtually guaranteed an epidemiological disaster. He proposed to substitute amateurism for professionalism, localism for centralization, and piecemeal measures for planning. The union physicians, according to their temperaments, experienced despair, frustration, and rage. What joy was there in the eclipse of Rein if the alternative was Maklakov and his fumbling Antiplague Commission?

Once again, the army intervened, preventing a complete stalemate

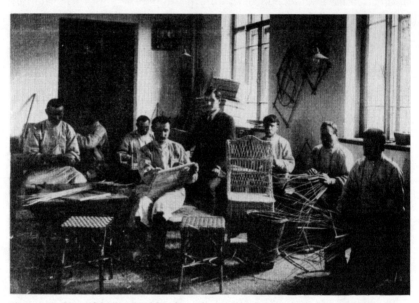

Fig. 14. Members of the imperial family preferred to support traditional charities, such as this wickerware workshop for blinded soldiers in Tsarskoe Selo.

between the government and the unions.[46] As July approached, the retreating soldiers and the refugees converged on the evacuation points, and the absence of medical facilities was felt more keenly than ever. Chief Military-Sanitary Inspector Evdokimov, anxious as ever to divert attention from the failure of his own department, joined in the chorus of criticism of the Antiplague Commission which emanated from the unions, the Pirogov Society, and the Duma. Evdokimov, Ol'denburg, and the commander in chief, Grand Duke Nikolai, must all have been under considerable pressure from field commanders to persuade the

Council of Ministers to reverse Maklakov's decision. A special meeting held in Petrograd on 14 August under orders from Evdokimov condemned the Antiplague Commission for failing to provide either coordinated leadership or sufficient funds to cope with the health problems occasioned by evacuation. Days later, probably even before Maklakov had had time to reconsider his decision, the newly created Special Council for Defense, the tsar's only significant concession to strident civilian criticism of the war effort, overrode Maklakov and ordered that the unions be granted 4 million rubles for antiepidemic work.[47] Thus, thanks to the army, which kept up the pressure for more funds for medical work. and to the mounting political crisis that the tsar could ignore no longer, union leaders and their friends and supporters in the Duma were able to secure some funds that could be given directly to the union physicians. Of course, the amount involved was a drop in the bucket compared to the 50 million rubles that had been sought; it did not begin to cover the extensive plans made in the spring and was quickly spent on extra hospital beds and on elementary sanitary improvements at or near the front.

Moreover, the army finally heeded the physician's advice about vaccination programs. In the spring of 1915, the union physicians had shifted from their earlier support for voluntary vaccination and instead began to insist on compulsory programs aimed, optimally, at both military and civilian personnel. In the late summer of 1915, Evdokimov finally conceded the necessity for vaccinations on the western front, initially against typhoid, and union physicians rapidly organized an extensive vaccination campaign, incurring in the process costs that were not covered by the subsidy given earlier. In the following year the vaccination and disinfection program was extended to the epidemiologically sensitive southwestern front and included efforts to prevent cholera and smallpox, as well as typhoid.[48]

The medical consequences of this activity are hard to determine, chiefly because of the absence of comprehensive statistics. Figures exist concerning morbidity and mortality from infectious disease in the second half of 1916. These indicate that, except in the case of cholera, where mortality was 36.8 percent, fewer deaths occurred than might have been expected: the overall mortality rate was 10.8 percent.[49] On the other hand, reasonably accurate figures are available only for soldiers and prisoners of war; among refugees and local inhabitants, actual mortality rates can only be guessed. What can be said is that, without the admittedly limited isolation facilities and sanitary improvements introduced during the summer, mortality rates, especially from cholera, would have been even higher. The vaccination and disinfection programs, useful though they were, came too late to prevent the spread of cholera, smallpox, and typhoid to the interior of the country and did nothing whatsoever to reduce the incidence of typhus and relapsing fever, both at the front and in the rear.[50]

For Russian medical politics, the consequences of the events of 1915 are considerably easier to assess. Among the union physicians and their colleagues working for zemstvos and towns, the old animosity towards the MVD was fueled afresh by Maklakov's rigid insistence that antiepidemic measures on the home front remain under the control of the Antiplague Commission. That Maklakov himself was dismissed from office brought little satisfaction; his successor, Prince Shcherbatov, made no change in MVD policy, and the Antiplague Commission, despite its brief humiliation, carried on as before. For the radicals who made up the medical leadership of the unions, the episode was one more forceful reminder of the gap that separated the tsarist regime from a modern, systematic approach to the problems of public health. Speaking at the April 1916 Pirogov Congress, Solov'ev described the Council of Ministers' refusal to support the antiepidemic campaign as "one of the clearest manifestations of opposition to the idea of the unification of public organizations to meet the pressing needs of the country in a planned way."[51] The intervention of the army and of the Special Council for Defense did make it possible for the community physicians to undertake a small part of their program, and this delayed opportunity to convert talk into action naturally spurred them to do even more. That they were confined to the fronts became a greater burden once they were permitted to do something rather than nothing. Frustration bred desire and determination, and both were reflected in the increasingly ambitious home front plans of the Union of Towns and in the growing impatience of physicians, not only at the government, but also at the executives of their own unions, because they appeared unable to fight for the physicians' program with sufficient force and professional expertise.

THE PROBLEM OF CARE OF THE MENTALLY ILL
The union physicians continually argued that tubercular, maimed, and mentally ill soldiers required special treatment and that the union physicians were best qualified to organize it. Here again they were faced with opposition from the Military-Sanitary Administration and the Red Cross and were even less successful in implementing their plans than they had been in mounting the antiepidemic campaign. Care for the mentally ill became an issue contested with particular bitterness, leaving a legacy of hostility between the unions and the Red Cross that even the February Revolution did not eliminate. In addition, the aspirations and activities of the union physicians raised the hackles of Russian psychiatrists, who were always distressed by the intrusion of somatic physicians into an area outside their expertise. Some atten-

tion at this point to the wartime conflicts will help to explain why, in 1917, the union physicians saw the Red Cross as an enemy, not an ally, in the cause of medical reform and also why psychiatrists who wanted reform did not regard the union physicians as the appropriate leaders of their cause.

Before the war, both community physicians and psychiatrists agreed that hospital and dispensary facilities for the mentally ill were inadequate and required improvement. One informed writer who reviewed the subject on the eve of the war estimated that there were about 500,000 mentally ill people in the empire, of whom at least one-third needed hospitalization, yet in January 1913 there were only 46,063 beds available in some 170 institutions.[52] Several Pirogov congresses passed resolutions calling for enlarged facilities, as did the conferences of the Russian Union of Psychiatrists. This apparent unanimity, however, masked a deep-seated hostility between the medical and psychiatric professions. For all their espousal of the cause of reform, Russia's community physicians were somatic physicians and no more disposed—perhaps even less—than their colleagues in government service or private practice to yield before the professional aspirations of psychiatrists. Julie Brown's recent work on the professionalization of Russian psychiatry gives much attention to the frustrations experienced by psychiatrists who found both the tsarist government and zemstvos significant obstacles to the fulfillment of their ambitions.[53] Although community physicians could always be relied upon to oppose control of their own work by nonspecialists, they largely abandoned this principle in their dealings with psychiatrists. The latter thus found their hospital and therapeutic work considered an appendage to the activities of somatic hospitals and their plans for preventive mental health disregarded by zemstvo and municipal sanitary bureaus. Brown concludes that, by 1914, psychiatrists as a profession were alienated not only from the tsarist state, but also from the zemstvos and municipalities, whose parsimonious attitudes jeopardized the very survival of the profession.[54]

These tensions and professional animosities recurred during the war and were compounded by the intransigence of the Red Cross and the suspicions of the Council of Ministers. At the beginning of hostilities, the Red Cross expected that mentally ill soldiers would be cared for exclusively in its lazarettos, staffed by Sisters of Mercy. Evdokimov, always the optimist, declared that these plans were entirely unnecessary because he already had at least 180 beds available in St. Petersburg and Khar'kov, a statement that reveals the extent of his grasp of the relationship between battlefield conditions and psychoneurosis.[55] Few psychiatrists would have agreed with his narrow definition of the mentally ill soldier as one "whose illness originates in traumatic depression."[56] In layman's terms, Evdokimov was trying to argue that special care was needed only for those whose illness was caused, not exacerbated, by the war, and caused specifically by the trauma of being under fire. German firepower alone made nonsense of the proposition that 180 beds would suffice, leaving aside those who contracted nervous disorders on account of the physical hardships involved or those with a history of neurosis or depression who found themselves again disoriented by the experience of military service. Evdokimov's refusal of assistance was soon shown to be absurd and, by the end of 1914, the lazarettos of the Red Cross were full of soldiers with spinal and brain injuries who needed more specialized care than could be provided by Sisters of Mercy whose training in nervous disorders was inadequate. Although some of the mentally ill did not require hospitalization, neither the army nor the Red Cross had appropriate dispensaries or outpatient facilities.[57]

The union organizations, already involved in evacuation and planning of antiepidemic measures, drew attention to the inadequacies of the Red Cross and offered to take over entirely the administration of care for the mentally ill. Perhaps because of the loss of face which it had already suffered, the Red Cross executive dug in its heels and categorically refused to permit the unions any role in the matter.[58] With criticism mounting, Prince Ol'denburg, anxious as ever to protect the Red Cross, asked Russia's most prominent psychiatrist, Professor V. M.Bekhterev, to work out a compromise. The only psychiatrist who was a member of the Medical Council of the MVD, Bekhterev was head of the Psycho-Neurological Institute in St. Petersburg and a former professor at the Military-Medical Academy.

Although he had close ties to the St. Petersburg bureaucracy at the turn of the century, Bekhterev had made himself somewhat more acceptable in community medical circles by his forthright defense of the liberty of the individual in 1905 and by his courageous intervention in the notorious Beilis case.[59] After consultation, Bekhterev recommended that the Red Cross remain in charge at the front and in charge of evacuation to all private hospitals in the interior; those who could not be accommodated therein would be sent to its lazarettos in Moscow, Petrograd, and Khar'kov. Bekhterev's report was also an indirect criticism of Evdokimov because it acknowledged the inadequacy of facilities for those suffering from trauma and called for a new specialized hospital in Petrograd as well as for special facilities in zemstvo and municipal hospitals.[60] Bekhterev's compromise left the Red Cross with more influence and the unions with less than the community physicians had hoped. Nevertheless both unions drew up plans for carrying out their role and submitted requests for additional funds from the government. These funds never arrived. As it had done when faced with the antiepidemic campaign, the Council of Ministers re-fused to authorize special subsidies, but in this case there was no spe-cial fund like that of the Antiplague Commission which could be drawn upon. The result was that the zemstvos and municipalities had to make shift, taking the patients that had been transferred to them by the Red Cross and somehow finding beds for them or arranging out-patient care without appropriate facilities or financial support.

The war provided Russian psychiatrists with few opportunities to advance their professional interests. Neither the Red Cross nor the zemstvo and municipal institutions appeared willing to recognize their claims to special expertise; the former continued to rely largely on charity administrators and nurses, while the latter too often placed the mentally ill and even psychiatrists under the jurisdiction of somatic physicians. Although the union physicians paid lip service to the idea of psychiatric expertise, their underlying assumptions were entirely char-acteristic: early in 1917, for example, a row developed when Diatroptov, evidently without consulting members of the Moscow Psychiatric Commission, persuaded the Union of Zemstvos to establish a psychi-atric subsection in its Medical Bureau. P. P. Kashchenko, a member of the commission and a leading Moscow psychiatrist who had been passed over for the appointment, complained bitterly that community psychiatrists were being ignored. His protests were dismissed and Diatroptov's action was upheld by the Joint Psychiatry Commission of the two unions, a body that was itself dominated by somatic physi-cians.[61] Such incidents confirmed psychiatrists in their view that com-munity physicians were unlikely to advance the professional interests of psychiatry as an autonomous medical specialty.

NEW DIRECTIONS
Throughout 1916, physicians working for both unions began to turn their thoughts towards the future, especially to the role that they and their organizations would play in postwar Russia. In part, this was a natural process of development: after all, they had built up super-visory staffs, field workers, and local committees, as well as material resources such as hospitals and laboratories. Those in charge were understandably concerned that all this should not vanish with the conclusion of hostilities. Doubtless the process was accelerated by the government's refusal to make additional subsidies available. The Union of Towns had hired extra personnel for its Sanitary Bureau in the ex-pectation that more vaccination campaigns and sanitary improve-ments would be funded and, when the money failed to materialize, the staff were set to other tasks.[62] One of these involved consideration of the medical problems that were expected to accompany demobi-lization, notably the threat of an epidemic of syphilis because of the

prevalence of venereal disease among the soldiers at the front. Physicians were also concerned that an end to wartime prohibition could produce waves of mass drunkenness and a dramatic increase in alcoholism. By the end of 1916, the two unions had established one joint working group to devise preventive measures against venereal disease and were planning another to find ways to arrest the spread of tuberculosis.[63] This last was the particular concern of Solov'ev, whose influence made it a high priority for the medical staff of the Zemstvo Union.

The medical concerns were real enough, but far more was at stake. There is clear evidence that physicians in both unions were increasingly bent on using their influence and resources to effect reforms in the structure of local government, reforms that would give themselves and other members of the professional and technical intelligentsia a larger role in local affairs than they had hitherto enjoyed.[64] Dependence on the whims and capabilities of the landowners and businessmen who dominated local government institutions had been a source of frustration for community physicians since the 1890s and especially during the conservative reaction of 1905–7; it was exacerbated during the war when physicians had to deal with men of the same stamp who ran the central committees of both unions as well as the local governments. Union physicians knew very well that it had not been the insistence of the union leadership but the intervention of the army that had produced the funds for the antiepidemic campaign and, when more money was not forthcoming, they privately blamed the leadership for not browbeating the Council of Ministers, pointing to their inability as laymen to explain in sound epidemiological terms why additional funds were necessary.[65] Many of the sanitary improvements so urgently undertaken by the Union of Towns would have been unnecessary if municipal dumas had paid attention to these matters during the prewar years, and an awareness of this fact was never far from the minds of those who had to do the work under duress in wartime. Finally, the predominantly left-wing political sympathies of the leading union physicians ensured that they would not stand aside from controversy simply because of the war, but rather would use the shortcomings of the existing structure as an argument for rapid and substantial change.

Solov'ev, who made no secret of his radicalism, took a particularly strong line on the need for local reform. His chief platform was the April 1916 Pirogov Congress in Petrograd, to which he reported on behalf of the Medical Council of the Central Committee of the Union of Zemstvos.[66] Acknowledging that many problems stemmed from the attitude of the government and the Red Cross, Solov'ev nevertheless reserved his main attack for the existing structure of local government.

The existing Zemstvo Statute, he argued, was an obstacle to both medical reform and the participation of physicians in local government. At a minimum, both the estate (*soslovnyi*) principle and the property qualifications for electors had to be abolished, as well as "the anomaly by which physicians are still regarded as 'serving' elements, without full rights of participation or of voting" when major decisions were made.[67] His carefully phrased call for "new, more suitable institutional forms in which to realize our objectives"[68] must have made it plain to his listeners that his personal preference was not for reforming, but rather for replacing both the zemstvos and the unions with more democratic and utilitarian institutions. The thrust of his speech was fully endorsed by Sysin, whose report on behalf of the physicians working for the Union of Towns ended with a demand for the immediate democratization of municipal government and a plea for the "deliverance" of Russian society from the influence and tutelage of the tsarist administration.[69]

After reports such as these to a congress presided over by Diatroptov, it is scarcely surprising that the final resolutions did not mince words. The most clearly political of these called for a complete democratization of all zemstvo and municipal institutions, as well as of the unions themselves, and for complete autonomy to set their own tasks and make their own decisions. In a thinly disguised attack on the Red Cross and Prince Ol'denburg's office, the congress called for an end to all "departmental monopolies and spheres of influence." All elements that made up local government, including "physicians and other specialists," should enjoy full rights of initiative and participation; hence, the resolution continued, many existing committees of both unions would have to be restructured to give physicians direct control over the organization of medical affairs. Finally, the congress called upon the unions to be guided by "the more democratic strata of the population" in cooperatives, professional societies, hospital funds, and other organizations.[70] In his closing speech, Diatroptov pointed to the similarity between the present circumstances and those that prevailed when the "Cholera" Congress met in 1905: the loss of autonomy, the stifling of public initiative, and the gulf that separated the government from the rest of society. Once again, he noted, physicians were performing both their professional and their civic duty in working for the complete democratization of state and society.[71]

The drive to reform local government involved more than passing high-flown resolutions. Something of its nature and direction can be seen also in the increasingly ambitious plans of physicians and other professionals working for the Union of Towns for reshaping the postwar Russian city. Lacking the local base of medical institutions possessed by the Union of Zemstvos, the Union of Towns had perforce to draw upon all the professional talent that it could find for its local committees. Given the shortage of physicians in urban areas and the nature of the improvements contemplated—disinfection, waste disposal, and water supply being the chief ones—it was natural that sanitary engineers and architects would play a significant role. Nikolaevskii, as head of the Sanitary Bureau, organized a small congress of physicians and technicians in November 1915, out of which came a plan to establish Sanitary-Technical Bureaus in major urban centers, beginning with Petrograd and Tiflis. A dozen more such bureaus were opened during 1916 in various regional centers. The Sanitary Bureau of the Central Committee worked with the regional bureaus, providing advice on water supply and purity and organizing drainage systems, filtration fields, and sewage farms. Laboratories in newly opened union hospitals were made available to the towns for bacteriological and sanitary work. To meet new needs a reorganization took place at the center, involving the creation in April 1916 of a Sanitary-Technical Consultation Department alongside the existing Sanitary Bureau. The new unit was composed of three sanitary physicians, two architects, and eight engineers and technicians. In their day-to-day work, in their visits to more than two dozen cities, and in their correspondence with more than 200 towns, the central staff tried, in Nikolaevskii's words "to ensure that our measures will not only meet present needs but also serve as a basis for the development of sanitary welfare (*blagoustroistvo*) after the war."[72]

This growing emphasis on the importance of technical expertise in postwar Russia blurred the limits between sanitary reforms per se and the whole field of municipal management and services. The idea of holding an All-Russian Congress on the Health of Towns was first discussed at the November 1915 meeting of physicians and technicians but, even before it could be realized, the Central Committee moved to create a Central Bureau for Municipal Affairs to provide information, advice, and assistance to cities and towns "in all matters and questions of municipal management,"[73] especially sanitation, technology, and financing. Members of the Sanitary-Technical Bureaus convened in mid-November 1916 and agreed to mount a thorough and systematic investigation of the sanitary state of all Russian towns;[74] the planning for this was undertaken by M. M. Kenigsberg, an experienced urban sanitary physician. The same conference also decided on the need for a new press organ in which the specialized concerns of sanitary physicians, architects, and engineers could be discussed more fully than in *Izvestiia Vserossiiskogo Soiuza Gorodov*. Prominent among the editors of the new journal, entitled *Vrachebno-Sanitarnyi Vestnik*, were A. N. Sysin and L. B. Granovskii. Their first issue (the appearance of which was delayed by the February Revolution) carried an editorial statement about the need for "worker-specialists in medical-sanitary and sanitary-technical affairs" to discuss "the prospect of peace and demobilization" and its relationship to the reform and rebuilding of Russian towns and cities.[75] How broadly they construed their mandate may be inferred from the fact that their first number carried two articles by A. K. Ensh, an expert on urban planning and the design and construction of garden cities.

The new directions taken by the physicians of the Union of Towns in 1916 and early 1917 had no counterpart in the Union of Zemstvos, although both groups agreed on the need to broaden and democratize local government. Where the municipal reformers, animated by a new vision of cities remade, stressed technical expertise, the physicians of the Zemstvo union assumed that they had already led the way down the road that others would naturally follow.[76] Their complacency and indifference towards the special needs of urban areas obviously irked Sysin and Granovskii; in the minutes of the Medical-Sanitary Council of the Union of Towns there are signs of an underlying hostility that made cooperative work between the two unions difficult and portended an imminent separation, if not a divorce, between the zemstvo and municipal wings of Russian community medicine.[77]

THE PYRRHIC VICTORY OF G. E. REIN

Whatever animosity the union physicians harbored towards Prince Ol'denburg on account of his hostile attitude to their work, they were forced to admit that he had, for the moment, saved them from the designs of G. E. Rein. If they were hoping that Rein's appointment to the State Council in 1915 would spell the end of his career as a would-be minister of health, they were reckoning without the vagaries of wartime politics. Indeed, there is some evidence to suggest that it was the very growth and unfolding aspirations of the unions' medical organizations that provoked second thoughts in St. Petersburg about the advisability of postponing reform until the end of the war. The result was that, despite the continued opposition of Prince Ol'denburg, the scales tipped in Rein's favor. Thus began, on the very eve of the February Revolution, the last bizarre skirmishes in the battle between Rein and the community physicians, a battle that had begun in South Russia in 1909.

Rein had spent the war years continuing to lobby for the establishment of a Main Administration for State Health Protection (GUGZ). Because opinion in the Council of Ministers had been divided when it first considered the matter, Rein never accepted the decision to postpone as final. Throughout 1915 and 1916 he made fresh attempts to persuade the council to reverse itself; the tsar wavered and eventually, in July 1916, he agreed to proceed with its establishment under Article

87 of the Fundamental Laws—a procedure theoretically reserved for the enactment of emergency measures during the prorogation of the legislative institutions, but one that was more frequently abused than used.[78] The tsar's order appointed Rein Main Administrator of State Health Protection (*Glavnoupravliaiushchii gosudarstvennogo zdravookhraneniia*) taking effect on 1 September 1916 and permitted him to proceed with creating the administrative council and learned advisory committee of *GUGZ*.[79] Prince Ol'denburg grudgingly consented, on the condition that he see every legislative proposal produced by Rein's new department before it went to the Duma.[80]

Rein's case for moving quickly, even by employing Article 87, was a strong one. He was convinced that it would take a long time—perhaps five years—to implement the whole program of the Interdepartmental Commission and therefore the sooner it was begun, the better. He saw no reason to scruple about the use of Article 87; after all, the Duma had had years in which to tackle the issue of medical reform and had done nothing. Moreover, there were literally hundreds of legislative proposals awaiting its approval; to put the *GUGZ* proposal into the normal legislative pipeline was to assure its eventual death from atrophy. The evident discomfort of the Council of Ministers at the seemingly uncontrolled growth of the wartime unions also played into Rein's hands.[81] As he pointed out to his interrogators in 1917, the establishment of *GUGZ* enabled the state to reassume control of medicine and public health during demobilization and the return to peacetime.[82] Prince Ol'denburg's powers were to cease automatically with the conclusion of hostilities; Rein was well aware of this and also assumed that the wartime unions should cease their activities. Whether he expected them to do so voluntarily or to be shut down by order of *GUGZ* is not clear, but he certainly did not envision their survival after the war was over. He pointed to the array of medical and sanitary facilities which had been created during the war—not only those administered by the unions, but also those created by the Red Cross and by semiofficial philanthropies such as the Empress's Supreme Council and the Tatiana Committee—and argued that only a central administrative agency could ensure that these facilities would be dispersed around Russia to the general benefit of all inhabitants. Because many of these facilities were in areas lacking zemstvo institutions (the western borders, Siberia), it was to his mind entirely appropriate that a state agency preside over their integration into the civil medical sector. Finally, Rein proved himself alert to the connection between demobilization and the spread of epidemics, arguing that only a statewide agency such as *GUGZ* could effectively control the spread of epidemics when discharged soldiers returned home.

Although Rein could not have known in detail what was afoot in the medical bureaus of the unions, he could not fail to be aware of the discussions that took place at the April 1916 Pirogov Congress. Even if he had only heard about the resolutions passed, he would have known that the union physicians, far from closing up shop when the war was over, were planning a large role for themselves in the reform of both medical affairs and local government. The rapid creation of GUGZ and the implementation of the recommendations of the Inter-departmental Commission—particularly those concerning the state and the medical profession—would serve not only to prevent the union physicians from falling heir to the extraordinary powers wielded by Prince Ol'denburg, but also to halt their plans to remake local government. The extent to which Rein employed such arguments in convincing the tsar to authorize his appointment must remain a matter for conjecture because of the absence of direct evidence. Nevertheless, in view of Rein's unwaveringly monarchist loyalties and his rigidly narrow approach to medical professionalization, there can be no doubt that he was fundamentally opposed to the directions in which the union physicians were moving in the summer of 1916. His claims in 1917 that he was ready to work with the community physicians, the zemstvos, and towns were not entirely disingenuous; he was prepared to do so, but on his terms, not theirs. As he indicated in a revealing comment to his interrogators, his plans for community representation on the advisory committees of GUGZ were modeled on the provisions that obtained for the council of the MVD's Main Administration for Local Economic Affairs.[83] Rein was always prepared to see representatives of community organizations *join* commissions and advisory committees, but he was completely opposed to allowing such people to *run* them.

Luckily for the union physicians, Rein's use of Article 87 ensured that the very Duma politicians who had paid so little attention to health matters would suddenly emerge as determined opponents of the establishment of GUGZ. Relations between the Fourth Duma and the government were at such a low ebb by this point that it was almost superfluous for the Pirogov executive to provide substantive arguments against GUGZ. Nevertheless they did furnish the Duma's hitherto somnolent Commission on Public Health with summaries of the same arguments that they had been using against Rein for almost a decade.[84] The commission duly recommended that the Duma refuse to grant the eventual ratification that was required by law for measures introduced by means of Article 87. Indifferent as ever to constitutional niceties, Rein withdrew the measure from the Duma's consideration but retained his position and carried on as if nothing had happened—

behavior that outraged the Duma deputies and for which he was severely berated when he appeared before the Extraordinary Investigation Committee in May 1917.

Rein barely had time to be fitted for the uniform appropriate to his new position when he was overtaken by events. His career as a minister of the tsar was reduced to a matter of days. Despite his sweeping plans, he found time during GUGZ's brief life to issue only one pronouncement, concerning the trade in saccharin. On 23 February, the very day when he had been due to appear before the Duma, disorders broke out in the streets of Petrograd. Four days later, leading Duma politicians hastily formed a Provisional Government headed by the president of the Union of Zemstvos, Prince G. E. L'vov. On March 1st, the tsar abdicated and Rein, in company with other ministers and high officials, found himself arrested by order of the Provisional Government. It was a spectacularly ignominious end to his grand design to save Russia and the monarchy.

6
THE CLEANSING HURRICANE: MEDICAL POLITICS IN THE 1917 REVOLUTION

For leaders of the Pirogov Society, such as D. N. Zhbankov, the February Revolution was welcome news indeed. The tsar's abdication, Rein's arrest, and the concomitant demise of the Main Administration for State Health Protection, Zhbankov assumed, would pave the way for the reorganization of Russian medicine upon the principles of decentralization and collegiality which he had for so long espoused. At the Pirogov Congress that met in early 1917, Zhbankov hailed the February Revolution as a "cleansing hurricane" (*ozdorovitel'nyi uragan'*) which once and for all swept away the specter of a ministry of public health run by St. Petersburg bureaucrats.[1] After decades spent criticizing the tsarist regime for mismanaging medicine and public health, it is scarcely surprising that Zhbankov and other leading *pirogovtsy* would consider themselves the logical persons to whom the new regime should look for guidance in reorganizing this aspect of Russian life.

The events of the next few days and weeks soon proved this assessment of the revolution to be both unduly complacent and strikingly short-sighted. For one thing, Rein's arrest—like those of the tsar's other ministers—was simply a security measure and revealed nothing about the Provisional Government's attitude to medical reform. *GUGZ* died with Rein's arrest because no commissar was appointed to take it over; the Duma politicians who allocated the ministerial offices among themselves apparently saw no need for a ministry of health as part of their democratic revolution. Moreover, the best medical talent among the senior Kadets (Constitutional Democrats) was employed elsewhere: the longtime *pirogovets*, A. I. Shingarev, became Minister of Agriculture, while N. Ia. Kishkin, also a physician by profession, was appointed commissar of the city of Moscow. Indeed, far from realizing Zhbankov's dreams, the Provisional Government's first steps suggested that the reform of civil medical affairs was not regarded as a matter of the slightest urgency.

Military medical affairs were, however, an altogether different business. It will be recalled that, initially, the Provisional Government was dominated by men such as Prince L'vov, head of the Union of Zemstvos, and A. I. Guchkov, head of the Central War Industries Committee, who had been working to shore up the Russian war effort and who regarded the February Revolution as an opportunity to purge the army of tsarist incompetence. Thus, although the Provisional Government committed itself in broad terms to the eventual reform of Russian society, in practice its leading members were interested primarily in reforms that would increase the fighting capacity of the army. Inevitably, this meant that Guchkov, as Minister of War, began to reorganize the entire relationship between the army and the rear, including of course military medicine and sanitation. Both his past involvement with the Red Cross and his fundamental political conservatism were reflected in the way in which he embarked on this reorganization.

On 7 March, less than a week after taking up his duties as Minister of War, Guchkov decreed the formation of a new Joint Sanitary Organization for Petrograd and the Northern Region excluding the front.[2] Although he apparently, and characteristically, acted without consulting the medical staff of either union, he intended to eliminate the isolation and rivalry of previous years by bringing together, in one coordinating body, representatives of the Military-Sanitary Administration, the Red Cross, the Petrograd municipal health organization, and the Petrograd committees of the two wartime unions. On the following day, Chief Military-Sanitary Inspector Evdokimov prudently offered his resignation for "reasons of health," and again Guchkov moved rapidly, appointing as his successor Professor N. N. Burdenko of Iurievsk University, hitherto director of the field hospitals that had been organized at the front by the Zemstvo Union.[3] No one knew better than the hard-pressed Burdenko the real cost of Prince Ol'denburg's attempt to maintain separate jurisdictions, and hence he was a good choice to promote coordination; by the same token, precisely because he had been so involved at the front in providing medical assistance to the wounded, he knew much less about the problems of the rear.

Within another week, the new regime had dismissed Prince Ol'denburg, a move that many interpreted as heralding the demise of the Sanitary and Evacuation Section.[4] Guchkov's Joint Organization had been assigned responsibility for the Northern Region, but the prince's departure raised the question of what agency would coordinate relations between the front and the interior of the country. While this news was being absorbed in Moscow by the Pirogov Society and the medical staffs of the unions, a sudden flurry of activity swept the senior levels of the Red Cross in Petrograd. On 13 March, the executive (*glavnoe upravlenie*) of the Red Cross met to discuss the implications of the collapse of the tsar's government. There were so many diehard monarchists on the executive that at first it seemed impossible to pass a declaration of loyalty to the Provisional Government. New elections were required before a "reformed" executive could pledge the full support of the Red Cross for the February Revolution.[5] The new leadership also speedily formulated a resolution that called upon the Provisional Government to entrust the Red Cross with the overall management of medical and sanitary affairs for the duration of the war.[6] In effect, the leaders of the Red Cross were playing upon Guchkov's lifelong association with their organization to ensure that they, and they alone, became the successors to Prince Ol'denburg's office and powers.

MOSCOW VERSUS PETROGRAD

While the Russian Red Cross was jockeying for position, the Provisional Government named a commissar to wind up the affairs of the Sanitary and Evacuation Section. The individual chosen was V. I. Almazov, a physician and Kadet deputy who had served on the Duma's Commission for Public Health. No stranger to the issue of medical reform, Almazov had once attended some of the meetings of the Rein Commission at the invitation of Rein himself, who was then still hoping to find allies in the Duma. Almazov was not converted to Rein's position, however; using arguments supplied to him by Zhbankov and the Pirogov executive, he joined in the battle against *GUGZ* in the Duma in late 1916 and early 1917.[7] Now he suddenly found himself entrusted with the task of replacing Prince Ol'denburg's office with some new agency that would unify and streamline the war relief work of the Red Cross and the voluntary organizations. Almazov began immediately to confer with the Joint Committee for the Northern Region, itself less than a week old. He also—perhaps because of his previous contacts with the Pirogov Society executive—sent an invitation to Moscow, asking that representatives of the medical bureaus of both unions come to Petrograd and assist in the work of planning the new agency. Even before they arrived, he was presented with one proposal worked out by the Joint Committee and another prepared by the durable tsarist bureaucrat, V. K. von Anrep, who obviously had no intention of vanishing into limbo just because his former master had abdicated. Both proposals addressed the immediate problem of improving medical assistance to the army. The arrival of the Muscovites, however, dramatically changed the focus of discussion.

The delegation from Moscow was led by Diatroptov and Tarasevich, accompanied by A. N. Merkulov, director of field hospitals for the Union of Towns.[8] From their behavior in Petrograd and their actions on returning to Moscow, it is clear that they were extremely upset to find that, even in its first days, the revolution was not living up to their expectations. Instead of waiting for direction from the unions' medical bureaus and the Pirogov Society in Moscow, Commisssar Almazov was already consorting with individuals and institutions unsympathetic to community medicine: the army and navy, the Red Cross, and even former Chief Medical Inspector von Anrep. The Muscovites took a very strong line, denouncing all proposals made to Almazov as unacceptable and insisting that the commissar create a temporary advisory committee on which representatives of both unions and of the city of Moscow would have equal standing with those of the army, the navy, the Red Cross, and the city of Petrograd. Furthermore, they specified that this committee should not confine itself merely to improving wartime medical services, but should work out a general proposal for the reform of all medical and sanitary affairs. After securing Almazov's agreement, the three returned to Moscow, where they quickly mobilized their colleagues to influence the direction that medical reform would take under the Provisional Government.

As luck would have it, the Pirogov Congress originally planned for November 1916 (for which the tsarist government refused permission) had been rescheduled for 4–8 April 1917. The Muscovites therefore had two weeks in which to produce an alternative proposal that could be approved by the Pirogov Congress and then presented to Almazov. Following what had become an established pattern, initial discussion took place in a joint meeting of the medical-sanitary bureaus of the two unions, to which Tarasevich, Diatroptov, and Merkulov reported immediately upon their return to Moscow. The upshot of this meeting was the appointment of a special committee of three—Z. P. Solov'ev, A. N. Sysin, and V. M. Bogutskii—to draft a new proposal "for central state organs of medical and sanitary affairs."[9] Working with all speed, these three produced a proposal that was discussed and approved on 23 March at a meeting of thirty-one community physicians employed by the two unions, by the city of Moscow, and by the Moscow *uezd* and *guberniia* zemstvo medical bureaus.[10] Sysin, speaking to the proposal, told his colleagues that it

envisions the formation of a council of representatives of central and local organizations, whose task will be to unify the medical-sanitary activity of all departments. This council should hold periodic meetings. As the executive and working organ of the council, the project envisions the organization of a temporary committee of eleven individuals in the office of the Commissar of the

Provisional Government. The business of the central organs will be not only to unify the so-called "Red Cross" work of the present moment, but also to unify all sanitary activity in general throughout the country with full autonomy for the public organizations."[11]

Sysin's explanation was rapidly overshadowed by an emotional speech from Diatroptov, who contrasted the "Moscow proposal" with those that, he claimed, were based on the bureaucratic decreeing of measures by *prikazi* in Petrograd. He appealed to his colleagues to support the Moscow proposal, "in order to remove the danger of disorder and of the usurpation of power which can be observed in some of the proposals which are being formulated *en masse* in Petrograd."[12] With one amendment (concerning representation for the front medical organizations), the proposal was approved, and the meeting broke up amid assurances that the proposal would be placed before the Pirogov Congress for discussion and approval.

Behind Diatroptov's exhortations to protect community medicine from interference by Petrograd lay a more powerful, but as yet unspoken imperative: the desire of the physicians employed by the two unions to secure an influential place for themselves in free Russia. By 1916, as we have seen, the concerns of the medical and sanitary bureaus of the unions had gone far beyond the organization of relief for the wounded; the unions' unique, extralegal status and the flow of subsidies had given these medical professionals the opportunity to organize and plan and the sense of exhilaration that came from being able, at long last, to carry out their plans, if only in a limited way. That they should wish to enhance and entrench their new-found authority in whatever political structure replaced the tsarist regime was understandable, but to do so required overcoming a number of significant obstacles, not the least of which was the historic opposition of Russian community physicians to any form of centralized direction of medical affairs.

Russian zemstvo and municipal physicians had always made local autonomy the central tenet of their faith in community medicine. In their vision of an ideal future, the free citizens of democratic Russia, acting in concert with local medical personnel, would organize and manage their own medical and sanitary services through *volost'* and *raion* duma assemblies. The local sanitary guardianship (*sanitarnoe popechitel'stvo*) would thus be both a school for and an embodiment of free citizenship in a democratic society. Centralized direction was anathema to those who accepted the mystique of zemstvo medicine. In the words of D. N. Zhbankov, administrator of the Pirogov Society, the centralized direction of medical and sanitary affairs was "in complete contradiction with the local and community medical sector." Centralization, he went on, meant "paralysis and inactivity," whereas local autonomy meant "growth and vitality."[13]

The experiences of physicians who had worked for the wartime unions were quite different: had not an abundance of "growth and vitality" occurred, thanks to centralized direction by the medical and sanitary bureaus of the two unions? Though none of them ever admitted it in so many words, the experience of planning and executing antiepidemic measures and sanitary improvements had converted these physicians to the need for unified, central direction. Moreover, the logic of the bacteriological revolution led directly to greater centralization, if only because of the costs of laboratory research and the possibilities for immunization. Now that more could be done to prevent disease, it was vital that it be done quickly and with a minimum of wastage and overlap. It is no accident that the moving spirits in the drive for reform in 1917 were all bacteriologists and epidemiologists: Diatroptov and Solov'ev of the Unions of Zemstvos, Tarasevich and Sysin of the Union of Towns. Zhbankov's populist vision of an autonomous *volost'* sanitary guardianship as the cornerstone of a new, healthy, democratic Russia had been made obsolete by the rise of bacteriology, immunology, and epidemiology.

If the traditions of the Pirogov Society were now an obstacle for the reformers to overcome, even more so were the political realities of the moment. Their institutional base lay in the unions, temporary creations occasioned by the demands of war, for which no provision had been made either in the Zemstvo or Municipal Statutes or in the idealized free Russia of Pirogov traditionalists.[14] Not only had the unions played no role in the events in the streets of Petrograd which brought down the tsarist regime; their leaders had in fact spent the war years putting military victory ahead of political reform. Now, in March 1917, with Soviet and soldier power already established features of the revolutionary landscape, the unions were becoming tainted by their connection with the inequities of prerevolutionary political society. They represented privileged Russia (*tsenzovaia Rossiia*). Should they, could they, continue to exist in a free Russia?

The unions were in danger of becoming a political liability for ambitious professionals such as Sysin and Diatroptov, who were anxious to further the cause of reform and to secure their place in the new Russia. After having spent more than a year elaborating plans for changing the face of postwar Russia, these men did not want to wait for *volost'* zemstvos and the constituent assembly to decide the nature of medical services in free Russia. The politically sensible course was rather to rid the unions of their tainted prerevolutionary lineage by supporting their immediate democratization, to reorganize their medical and sanitary bureaus so that their relevance to the new Russia would become even more obvious than their war relief work, and to create a new institutional base under the aegis of the Provisional Government from which to draw up firm plans for the reorganization of medical and sanitary affairs. This last objective was in fact an imperative: unless the Provisional Government could be shifted away from equating medical reform with improving aid to the wounded and unless the influence of the Red Cross and of military and civil bureaucrats in Petrograd could be reduced, there was no hope whatever that any real reform would occur in 1917. Hence the urgency with which the high-ranking physicians of the unions sought to mobilize support among the community physicians of Moscow; hence the alarmist emphasis on the specter of Petrograd *prikazi*; hence the delicacy with which the 1917 Pirogov Congress, heir to a tradition of four decades of opposition to centralization, was persuaded to endorse the creation of a new body that would liquidate remnants of the old regime, deal with immediate problems, and plan the reform of Russian medicine.

THE 1917 PIROGOV CONGRESS

Most of the physicians who approved the draft proposal for a Central Medical Sanitary Council at the Moscow meeting on 23 March were present at the Pirogov Congress, which opened on 4 April. Given the prominent place occupied by the subject of medical and sanitary reform on the congress agenda, it is noteworthy that this group stayed in the background for most of the discussion.[15] Not one of the four major speakers on the question of medical reform—Zhbankov, Uvarov, Tutyshkin, or Kanel'—had attended the Moscow meeting. Indeed, it seems that the text of the resolution adopted at the 23 March meeting was not put before the congress; instead, the congress approved a resolution that differed substantially from the one approved a fortnight previously, although it was presented by Diatroptov, who had chaired the earlier meeting. All of this suggests a certain unwillingness—prudent, perhaps, in the circumstances—on the part of those who had formulated the Moscow proposal to submit its text to full debate on the floor of the congress. Instead, K. I. Shidlovskii set the right tone for a reconsideration of old attitudes in his keynote address, which spoke of "the broad field for creative activity" that had been opened up by the revolution: "in the new state structure," he claimed, "the bases for hostility towards the creation of a central medical and sanitary organ no longer exist."[16]

First, however, came the settling of old scores. With enormous satisfaction, Zhbankov reviewed the society's opposition to the Rein project, praising the "cleansing hurricane" that had blown away both *GUGZ* and its author. As if to corroborate his words, the Provisional

Government on the following day announced that the Rein Commission had been disbanded.[17] In a second speech that was thoroughly in keeping with Pirogov tradition, Zhbankov demanded the destruction of all existing medical and administrative institutions from the Medical Council of the Ministry of the Interior (MVD) down to the *guberniia* medical agencies, the transfer of their functions to democratized institutions of local government, the outlawing of all private medical institutions, and "the broadest and most active participation of the population in the creation of the new order."[18] At the center, he would allow only an elected medical council composed of representatives of science, of community physicians, and of local governments, which "will preside over [*vedaet*] all the medical and sanitary affairs of the country, without breaking itself up or dividing into any departments or institutions whatever."[19] That such a body would have been unworkable probably explains Zhbankov's support for it; he had already made his hostility to central direction abundantly clear. Zhbankov had not attended the 23 March meeting in Moscow and, in view of his statements at the congress, it is unlikely that he would have supported the resolution that it passed. So great was Zhbankov's enthusiasm for the destruction of all vestiges of the old regime that he even proposed abolition of the Workers' Hospital Funds, on the grounds that representatives of community medicine had not been involved in drawing up the Hospital Insurance Law; on this issue, however, he stirred up a hornets' nest, because radicals were outraged by the suggestion that the nucleus of a separate factory medicine under workers' control should be dismantled.[20] The grand old man of Pirogov populism was beginning to discover that his assumptions were not shared by many of those attending the congress.

Zhbankov was followed to the rostrum by M. S. Uvarov, one of the few officials of the MVD who had maintained connections with the Pirogov Society in the decade before the revolution. Whatever Uvarov's personal views on the reform issue, there can be little doubt that senior MVD officials were hoping to regain the power that they had lost to the army and the voluntary organizations during the war years and were striving to ensure that the power to draw up reforms would be vested neither in some committee of advisors to Almazov nor in a council dominated by the physicians of the wartime unions, but in the MVD itself. The Chief Medical Inspector was already well aware of the aspirations of the Red Cross and the ambitions of the union physicians from Moscow. Therefore, it was necessary for the ministry to appear to bend before the tide of reform, while ensuring that the Office of the Chief Medical Inspector retained overall administrative power in the medical and sanitary sphere. When seen in this light, Uvarov's speech must be regarded as a tour de force. It elicited from the congress a resolution that congratulated the MVD on its "conversion" to the principles of community medicine, prompted no doubt by his opening remarks, in which he conceded that no "governing center" could interfere with the process of rebirth that was taking place, and lauded the importance of "free discussion at the local level." Yet his list of ten tasks in which a central organ could "participate," although beginning with such innocuous items as international conventions and conferences, went on to include several more controversial areas, among them legislation, financing, statistics, "the protection of all-state interests in the sphere of medical education" and "the realization of professional rights."[21] Uvarov was extremely careful in his choice of words, using ambiguous phrases such as "bringing necessary undertakings to completion" and "the speediest possible planned establishment of the new order." Rhetoric, it seemed, was of the essence for, when Rein had proposed to wield substantially the same powers through a central agency, he had brought down on his head the wrath of the Pirogov Society.

Uvarov's proposals for the immediate future were, in fact, a clear attempt to sidestep both the so-called Moscow proposal and the appointment of Almazov. He suggested the formation, *within the MVD*, of a committee representing public organizations, scientific circles, and appropriate government departments which could "put forward submissions" about the abolition of existing laws and their replacement by new temporary rules. This committee was also to undertake "preparatory work" for a future congress of elected representatives of local community organizations and of government departments, to "establish mutual relations . . . between the central medical and sanitary organ and local organs, and also the structure of the central organ, based on community principles."[22]

Uvarov's sincerity in proposing these measures cannot be questioned, but neither can it be doubted that he put them forward with the approval of MVD officials. After all, the MVD had been actively involved with proposals for medical and sanitary reform for more than a decade, and Uvarov's position was not in essence different from that taken by Stolypin and Malinovskii at the Kryzhanovskii Conference in 1909: while reforms were necessary, they must be carried out under the aegis of the MVD. Where Uvarov departed from previous MVD positions and also from that taken by Rein was in conceding participation by elected representatives of local community organizations and in stating that the new central organ would be based "on community principles." Yet the committee that he proposed would have no power except to "make submissions," presumably through the Office of the Chief Medical Inspector, to the MVD and thence to the Provisional Government, and it is by no means clear how far "community principles" would have survived this process. That Uvarov's speech represented a concession by the MVD in the face of new realities is clear; on the other hand, its magnitude should not be overestimated.

The two remaining reports on the general question of medical reform were given by well-known radicals—P. P. Tutyshkin and V. Ia. Kanel'—who indulged in lofty rhetoric about the democratization of the medical services to meet the needs of workers but contributed nothing to the immediate question of who should advise the Provisional Government and how such an advisory body should be constructed. The lengthy debate sparked by their reports also failed to come to grips with these issues; instead, a host of speakers rode their own hobbyhorses, defending the hospital funds, the eight-hour day, and workers' control of hospitals, praising the great traditions of zemstvo medicine, and warning against the possible spread of private practice and "feldsherism" in the countryside. Representatives of organizations of pharmacists and feldshers pleaded for an equal voice with physicians in determining the changes to be made, but among physicians there was more sentiment for including representatives of the Hospital Funds and the front medical organizations—presumably an implicit recognition that the February Revolution had been made by workers and soldiers, not by feldshers and pharmacists.[23]

The final day of the congress, 8 April, was devoted to the adoption of resolutions. Only at this point did the union physicians from Moscow begin to take an active part in the discussions; L. B. Granovskii, speaking for a so-called unifying group, produced a general proposal that called for the formation of a temporary central council to advise the Provisional Government, to be composed of representatives of "public organizations," including two members chosen by the Pirogov Congress and one each chosen by the hospital fund organizations of Petrograd and Moscow. Professor V. N. Sirotinin, President of the Society of Physicians of Petrograd and a former close associate of G. E. Rein, attempted to put an alternative motion that would have consigned the reform issue to a reorganized Medical Council within the MVD, but he was summarily ruled out of order. Attempts by feldshers, pharmacists, and veterinarians to secure representation for themselves were turned down because such amendments were deemed to conflict with the general motion and on the grounds that the council must be kept small and workable. Numerous other amendments were offered, but in the end only Granovskii's motion, redrafted by Diatroptov's organization committee, was put before the congress and approved.

Reduced to its essentials, the resolution authorized the existing allied public organizations to take over the management of medical and sanitary affairs, pending the creation of a new form of government by the Constituent Assembly, and it called for the creation of a Central

Council of representatives of public organizations. This new council was to coordinate the activities of democratized zemstvos and towns and of autonomous hospital funds, providing both direction and moneys for their work. It was also instructed to liquidate the Sanitary and Evacuation Section and other imperial institutions and to plan the construction of new central medical organs; finally, a crucial clause subordinated to the temporary Central Council both the personnel and functions of the Office of the Chief Medical Inspector and the medical departments of other ministries, thus blocking Uvarov's thinly disguised attempt to ensure that the MVD would retain control over the pace and direction of reform.

In what ways did the resolution approved by the Pirogov Congress differ from the Moscow proposal? First, the Pirogov resolution spoke only of a council of representatives of public organizations, whereas the Moscow proposal provided for both a larger council and a smaller executive committee and it included representation on both the council and the executive committee from three government departments: the Military-Sanitary Administration, the Fleet Sanitary Administration, and the Office of the Chief Medical Inspector. No doubt this was a concession to Almazov which recognized the difficulties of his position, but at the Pirogov Congress no hint had been given that existing bureaucratic agencies would be represented on the council. Second, the Moscow proposal was much more specific than the Pirogov resolution in listing the powers of the council and of its executive. Third, although the Pirogov resolution seemed to subordinate the center to local control, the Moscow proposal did nothing of the sort; not only did it ascribe to the council the power to "unify and coordinate the activity of all medical and sanitary departments, organizations, and establishments in the country," it also provided that the council could present its plans for reorganization directly to the Provisional Government. Instead of reaffirming the powers of zemstvos, municipalities, and hospital funds, the Moscow proposal called for the creation of local affiliates of the central council which would unify and coordinate activity at the local level. Thus both the composition of the temporary council and the general direction of reform endorsed at the Pirogov Congress was substantially different from that envisioned in the Moscow proposal. The point needs to be stressed if only because it has been assumed that the Central Medical Sanitary Council was virtually a creation of the Pirogov Society.[24]

THE PROVISIONAL GOVERNMENT AND THE MVD

The day after the Pirogov Congress ended, Almazov sent his proposal for a Central Medical Sanitary Council to the Provisional Government. Although he claimed in his covering memorandum that the wishes of the Pirogov Congress had been taken into account, there is little evidence of this in the proposal and, indeed, there was scarcely time for him to have done so. He made no mention of the primacy of local control, nor of a future congress to approve plans for reform, nor of direct representation on the council from the Pirogov Society. His proposal was, in fact, much closer to that approved at the Moscow meeting than to the resolution passed at the Pirogov Congress. On the other hand, he did not transmit the Moscow proposal verbatim; instead, he made several amendments, which presumably reflected discussions that had taken place in his advisory committee. Where the Moscow proposal had envisioned a broad council and a smaller executive committee, Almazov streamlined things a stage further: there would be a basic council of fifteen, which would do virtually all the work; only in "especially important circumstances" would its membership be extended to include a broader representation from local medical-sanitary councils.[25] This made the composition of the council especially important; here, Almazov deleted four of the community representatives in the Moscow proposal and replaced them with two bureaucrats and a representative of the Central War Industries Committee. The effect of this change was to give five of the fifteen seats on the council to representatives of existing government departments, while the voluntary organizations were given eight, and the Soviet one (the commissar himself was the fifteenth member). As Almazov stated, "The proposal aims at simplicity, unity, and co-ordination."[26] No doubt this was true, but it was a long way from what rank and file physicians at the Pirogov Congress thought they were approving. Indeed, the council that Almazov proposed looked remarkably like his temporary advisory committee; nine of its members were to be exactly the same, and only minor changes were made in the remainder of its composition.[27] Clearly, what Almazov wished to simplify, unify, and coordinate was the provision of medical services to the army in wartime. Where the Pirogov Congress resolution had suggested that the impetus for reform would proceed upwards from local zemstvos and sanitary councils, Almazov's proposal was for "top-down" planning, involving local agencies only where questions of evacuation and antiepidemic measures were to be discussed. Paradoxically, the union physicians now found themselves associated with a council that threatened to combine Prince Ol'denburg's emphasis on the primacy of military needs with G. E. Rein's penchant for centralized planning. If this paradox did not become immediately apparent, it was because the Provisional Government dragged its feet over accepting Almazov's proposal.

And what of the Ministry of the Interior? Senior offcials, who cannot have been pleased by the suggestion that the Chief Medical Inspector should be at the beck and call of the new council, must have been relieved that Almazov's proposal contained no such provision. Before the government took action, however, there was an opportunity, if not to scuttle the council, then at least severely to restrict its field of activity. On 15 April, the Deputy Minister of the Interior and the Chief Medical Inspector wrote to the Provisional Government, giving their views on Almazov's proposal.[28] Although they began by welcoming the establishment of such a council, they immediately proceeded to rehearse all of the problems that had been caused during the war by the establishment of Prince Ol'denburg's office, "staffed both at the center and at the local level by people unfamiliar with medical and sanitary affairs." Giving the Prince "the powers of an absolute monarch," they claimed, had an unfortunate consequence, in that "the activity of the permanent medical and sanitary organs [of the MVD] had been paralyzed." The message to the Provisional Government was clear: let us not make the same mistake again. "In arranging the terms of the council [their letter stated], it should be borne in mind that it is a temporary organ, created for the needs of the present moment, pending the reform of medical and sanitary affairs by the legislative order. This view is also shared by the resolution of the recent Pirogov Congress."[29]

The MVD officials were of course correct in suggesting that Almazov's proposal created a council somewhat too powerful for the tastes of the Pirogov Society, but it was bold indeed to cite the Pirogov Congress resolution in support of what was, after all, an attempt by the MVD to emasculate the council even before its formation. The authors went on to suggest several amendments, the intent of which was to eliminate its general leadership functions, to deprive it of the possibility of reorganizing the competence of existing departments, and to prevent it from standing between those departments and the Provisional Government. Their most important change concerned plans for the future: here they wished the council's role reduced to "preliminary review of legislative projects . . . which are presented to the Provisional Government by the departments under its authority."[30] From the MVD's point of view, the larger the council, the more likely that it would be ineffective; they therefore suggested six more members than Almazov had proposed.[31] This was a superb rearguard action by a couple of embattled but shrewd bureaucrats. Chief Medical Inspector Molodovskii had been in his job less than a year whe the tsar abdicated and evidently hoped that this unfortunate event would cause as little disruption to his career as possible. Deputy Minister Leont'ev seems to have been especially determined to keep Almazov and his advisers as far as possible from the MVD. When he heard that the commissar's temporary advisory committee had formed a subcommittee to review the operations of the Office of Chief Medical Inspector, he replied immediately that the MVD had already decided to carry out its own review and ended with a cool request that the commissar keep him better informed in future "in order to avoid parallel work on one and the same question."[32] The conduct of Leont'ev and Molodovskii surely calls into question facile generalizations about the melting away of the old regime. Nearly two months after the February Revolution, here were two bureaucrats doing their best to minimize its impact. One cannot help wondering how many others there were and how effective they were in delaying the first steps towards reform in the spring of 1917.

On 9 April, Almazov formally called upon the Provisional Government to establish the Central Medical Sanitary Council (CMSC). However, his superiors, apparently in no rush to do so, referred his proposal to the MVD, thus occasioning the response noted above. What happened after Leont'ev and Molodovskii penned their objections cannot be clearly established from the available sources. All that can be said with certainty is that the Provisional Government took no further action during April or May, while Almazov discussed the proposal again with his advisory committee. After that, it was submitted in an amended form to a four-day conference (20–24 May) of military and civil medical organizations which the commissar himself had called.[33] The so-called May Conference of Commissar Almazov is one of the ephemeral events of 1917; its transactions were never published and there are only fleeting glimpses of its proceedings in the sources. To it were invited representatives of *guberniia*, *oblast'*, and military medical and sanitary organizations (the latter including the front, the army rear, and the fleet). According to a brief published report, there were also representatives from Petrograd, Moscow, other large cities, and various organizations and societies; Almazov presided, assisted by Diatroptov, Tarasevich, and Igumnov.[34] A much broader range of interests and perspectives was thus represented at this meeting than at the Pirogov Congress: civil and military medical inspectors and administrators, rural and urban community physicians, the leaders of the medical bureaus of the unions, and representatives of various physicians' organizations. Almazov evidently called it to establish new provincial sanitary councils and to reorganize the antiepidemic campaign, sanitary technology, and psychiatric care for soldiers; the influence on this agenda of union physicians such as Diatroptov, Tarasevich, Sysin, and Kashchenko is apparent.

Why Almazov decided to have this conference discuss the CMSC proposal is unclear.[35] Possibly he felt a need to counter the maneuverings of MVD officials by appealing to a broad constituency that would put strong pressure on the government to act immediately; more probably Leont'ev's criticisms led the ministers to suggest that he rework the proposal before it was given final approval. Whatever the reason, the CMSC proposal that emerged from the May Conference was substantially different from that which Almazov had proposed on 9 April and vastly different from the original Moscow proposal of 23 March. Most important of all was the inclusion of a statement underlining the temporary nature of the council: it was to be established "pending the return of the army to a peacetime footing,"[36] a qualification that must have pleased Leont'ev and Molodovskii, who could still argue that this was a purely transitory body with no permanent jurisdiction. Furthermore, the composition of the council was altered yet again, this time to produce a larger body of twenty-seven. In addition to Ways and Communications, five other ministries were to be represented—Finance, Education, Labor, Welfare, and the Office of State Control. As if to offset this increase in the bureaucratic component, the number of zemstvo and municipal representatives was doubled from four to eight, and representatives of two medical societies—the Pirogov Society and the recently formed Union of Physicians of the Army and the Fleet—were also added. With these revisions, the conference approved the proposal and called on the Provisional Government to establish the CMSC as soon as possible.[37]

Before it dispersed, the May Conference took two further significant decisions. First, it resolved to shut down all remaining vestiges of prerevolutionary medical administration at the local level: the *guberniia* medical departments and the *uezd* and *gorodovoi* physicians; their functions were ordered transferred immediately to zemstvo and municipal governments where these existed and as soon as practicable in areas where such institutions had yet to be created. Second, it ordered the Office of the Chief Medical Inspector to cooperate fully with the CMSC in its efforts to reorganize medical administration. As a first step in this new role, the Chief Medical Inspector was instructed to prepare for the CMSC a detailed report on the mechanics of transferring the old *guberniia* medical departments to the zemstvos and municipalities.[38]

These final resolutions, aimed as they were at forcing the MVD to accept the reality and implications of the February Revolution, lend strength to the argument that Almazov called the May Conference to outmaneuver Leont'ev and Molodovskii. So does the fact that, in its wake, Molodovskii was replaced as Chief Medical Inspector by one of the leading Moscow zemstvo physicians, V. A. Kiriakov, who immediately began to prepare detailed proposals for the consideration of the CMSC.[39] Kiriakov had not been involved in the medical bureaus of the unions. His appointment is significant not only because it signaled the end of the MVD's attempt to use the confusion of March and April to recover some of its lost powers; it also indicates a revival of strength among those ordinary zemstvo and municipal medical personnel who had taken something of a back seat to the powerful bureaus of the wartime unions. Already at the 23 March meeting in Moscow, there were indications that some of the regular zemstvo physicians were dissatisfied with the influence being exerted by the unions and their staffs. Many rank and file zemstvo and municipal physicians, and perhaps not only physicians, must have begun to wonder whether the war and the abdication had not made the unions into the tail that would wag the dog. Kiriakov's appointment, coupled with substantial representation on the CMSC from the zemstvos and municipalities, offered hope that the enthusiasm of union physicians for creating a centralized administrative agency could be effectively restrained.

THE MOBILIZATION ISSUE

World War I was both a help and a hindrance to the aspirations of Russia's community physicians. On the one hand, through the unions, they had enjoyed unprecedented opportunities to organize and exert their influence at the national level; on the other hand, the army's insatiable need for medical personnel had played havoc with the provision of medical services to the civilian population. Zemstvo and municipal physicians, as well as those in government service and those in private practice, were eligible for the draft; only those employed by the Red Cross and the unions were exempt.[40] At every wartime medical conference, speakers complained that the army was mobilizing physicians without regard to the consequences in the rear. Moreover, it was said, the army constantly misused the abilities of those called up. Physicians were frequently assigned to perform tasks requiring no medical training or to do medical work wholly unrelated to their training and talents. Moreover, the Military-Sanitary Administration seems to have had no policy with regard to leave or rotation of duty, so that by 1917 some physicians had been serving in field hospitals at or near the front for more than a year without respite.

Inevitably, the frustrations engendered by these experiences found an outlet in the wake of the February Revolution. At the 1917 Pirogov Congress, discussion of the situation at the front was strongly influenced by the resolutions passed at a conference of army physicians which had met a few days previously.[41] The physicians asserted three general principles: that all military medical affairs must be controlled by physicians; that all military sanitary organizations must be reformed along collegial lines, with senior officers elected by their colleagues; and that physicians, whether in military service or employed by a civilian agency, ought to enjoy equal rights with officers. This conference also resolved that no physician should be required to do more than six months' service at the front. To release men for service at the front, it called for the mobilization of women physicians for service in the rear. Without waiting for official approval, army physicians had already begun to elect delegate congresses at the division, corps, army, and front levels and to introduce collegial principles of administration. The new Chief Military Sanitary Inspector, Burdenko, agreed to a general reform of the military medical corps, including the participation of Red Cross and union physicians in planning reforms that would satisfy immediate needs. All of these events were reported in detail to an enthusiastic Pirogov Congress.

The congress did much more than simply express its approval of these developments. At the urging of L. A. Tarasevich, President of the Medical-Sanitary Council of the Union of Towns and a member of Amazov's temporary advisory committee, it passed a resolution calling for "a speedy state mobilization of physicians of both sexes to meet the needs of the army and the country," entrusting its direction to "the central collegial organ in the Provisional Government."[42] Speaking in favor of the resolution and obviously choosing his words with great care, Tarasevich cautioned that "together with collegiality and local activity, it is necessary to observe the principle of the correct arrangement and economy of medical labor; that is, in certain circumstances, the centralization of technical and administrative forces—albeit elected and responsible—may be necessary."[43]

Here again, as in the case of the CMSC, the 1917 Pirogov Congress found itself approving the allocation of enormous powers to a central agency whose final composition and method of operation it was accepting on faith, largely at the urging of physicians who, like Tarasevich, were employed by the wartime unions. Truly this was an extraordinary Pirogov Congress. Such was the enthusiasm for defending the new order that only one of those present was courageous enough to call the mobilization extreme.[44] Nevertheless, his warning about its potential consequences throughout the country was ignored in the headlong rush to approve the resolution. Within a few months, such fears were to be amply justified.

Where did the idea of mobilizing all physicians originate? Once again, the paucity of sources impedes explanation. It is reasonable to assume that the subject was discussed in Almazov's advisory committee, probably in response to the resolutions passed by the army physicians. Was Tarasevich delegated to persuade the Pirogov Congress to lend its prestige to a measure that most community physicians would previously have found unpalatable? Mobilization of sorts, on a smaller scale, had already been practiced by the Medical-Sanitary Organization of the Union of Towns. To go from this to a full state mobilization was perhaps seen by union physicians as a fruitful extension of something already under way, rather than as a dangerous innovation. Certainly the pressures from front physicians for relief were real enough;

an exchange of physicians between front and rear had to be organized quickly by some central agency. In proposing a mobilization that would meet both military and civil needs, Tarasevich was evidently attempting to ensure that the new CMSC would become the supreme coordinating agency, replacing both the MVD and the Sanitary and Evacuation Section. Nevertheless, the other resolutions passed by the Pirogov Congress regarding the front—endorsing the army physicians' call for organizational unity, the exchange of physicians, and the internal reorganization of the Military-Sanitary Administration—opened the door to confusion because they encouraged the army physicians to proceed with substantial reforms immediately, without taking into account the needs of the civil sphere.

The problems soon became apparent. In the weeks after the Pirogov Congress, while the legislation to establish the CMSC was still awaiting action, front physicians forged ahead on their own. On 9 April, the Union of Physicians of the Army and Fleet was formed in Petrograd; from 11 to 16 April, it held a congress that, among other things, approved starting the exchange without delay. Whether by design or default, the Petrograd branch of this union, dominated by front physicians, began to set the scheme in motion, only to discover seemingly endless logistical problems.[45] Senior field medical officers and directors of field hospitals, despite their desire to leave the front, refused to take up jobs in the rear if they involved a drop in rank or professional status. For the exchange to work properly, therefore, senior physicians in the rear (many of whom were already advanced in years and fatigued from long service) had to be shifted to the front to create vacancies at a senior level. Many of them refused to go, pointing out that younger, healthier physicians could be sent in their places.[46] At Almazov's May Conference, participants discussed the situation and agreed that, if further disruptions were to be avoided, the exchange would have to be more carefully planned and more cautiously undertaken.[47]

MEDICAL REFORM IN THE ARMY

For Solov'ev, Sysin, and other union physicians who had expected the February Revolution to give them the opportunity to reshape the nature and direction of Russian medicine, the events of the spring and early summer were not entirely reassuring. The advent of change had been delayed by the stonewalling tactics of the MVD and by the indecision of the Provisional Government, whose failure to establish the CMSC after Almazov's May Conference was as frustrating as it was inexplicable.[48] The government stood by while the front physicians organized an exchange on terms that suited them, a development that made nonsense of the idea of employing medical personnel rationally and economically. Moreover, with plans for a summer offensive under way, the War Ministry was taking every possible step to improve both morale and efficiency in the army, including of course the Military-Sanitary Administration. Army physicians, urged on by the enthusiasm of their zemstvo colleagues for collective decision-making and caught up in the wave of revolutionary organizing which swept the army in the early spring, began to form elected sanitary councils at every level from the front down to the smallest evacuation point. Although the medical reformers sympathized with the desires of military physicians to make the army more democratic and more egalitarian, the new councils nevertheless presented difficulties. Chief among these was the fact that—following traditional tsarist military practice—they claimed responsibility for both military and civilian public health in the areas under their jurisdiction. Potentially, the new military sanitary councils could act at cross purposes with the plans of the reformers. However, the latter, who were still waiting for the establishment of the CMSC, could do nothing to stop the creation of the new councils, which were officially recognized by the War Minister on 22 June.[49]

The pace of change in the army threatened both to outrun developments in the civil sector and to disrupt the administration of military medicine. In an attempt to arrest and control it, Chief Military Sanitary Inspector Burdenko acted swiftly during June to restore and legitimize central authority and to build both personal and institutional bridges between the army and the home front. On 14 June, Tarasevich himself was appointed to the second most important medical post in the army, that of Chief Field Sanitary Inspector.[50] Only a fortnight later, the War Ministry announced the formation of two new coordinating bodies for military-sanitary affairs: the Main Military-Sanitary Council, which was to be the military counterpart of the (still uncreated) CMSC in the civil sector, and the Central Council of Fronts, which was to be created at Stavka to oversee the implementation of reform. Burdenko naturally became head of the Main Military-Sanitary Council (MMSC), while Tarasevich became head of the Central Council of Fronts (CCF). Both bodies were composed primarily of elected representatives of military physicians but also included representatives of the Red Cross and of the two unions.[51]

With Burdenko and Tarasevich—both of whom had come to the army directly from the unions—now presiding over the reform of military medicine, the union physicians had won a victory, albeit a limited one. They and not the Red Cross had finally emerged as the successors to Prince Ol'denburg and were now in a position to consolidate the role of the unions not only in the war zone but on the home front by drawing them more closely into the administration of the military districts. As long as the Provisional Government could retain the loyalty of the army—an increasingly dubious proposition—they had secured an institutional base from which to carry out some of their plans. Indeed, one could argue that, by the end of June, the reformers were making more progress in the army than in the civil sector, despite the fact that the latter was their stated priority. In the cities and throughout the countryside, it was not yet apparent that the February Revolution had produced any positive results, either in democratizing the structure of medical administration or in reversing the flow of personnel and material from civilian to military purposes. One well-known community physician, G. I. Dembo, sounded a warning that was to be heard increasingly during the summer of 1917: that physicians belong not to the military authorities, but to the Russian people, and that the Pirogov Congress had called for mobilization to meet the needs of the country, not militarization to meet those of the army.[52]

COMMUNITY MEDICINE OR DEMOCRATIC SOCIAL MEDICINE?

From the first, Almazov had included a representative of the Petrograd Soviet in his temporary advisory committee, and the various proposals for establishing the CMSC envisioned token representation from the Soviet. Such a limited role was bound to be unacceptable to Soviet radicals who wanted to introduce the principles of revolutionary democracy into all medical structures and institutions. The Soviet was committed to fight for immediate improvements in working conditions, the protection of labor, the expansion of hospital funds, and the elaboration of a scheme of social insurance. Its members also called for a definitive struggle against epidemic diseases, child mortality, and prostitution. Naturally enough, the Petrograd Soviet soon set up an agency to pursue its own priorities in the field of health reform.

By the early summer, the Central Executive Committee of the Petrograd Soviet had established a Medical and Sanitary Section that encouraged the reorganization of military medicine and propagated its own ideas about social medicine. The military subsection launched a program of support for the democratization of military medicine, demanding the inclusion of lower ranks and middle and lower medical personnel on the new military-sanitary councils. It also expressed concern about the struggle against venereal disease (which was expected to be a serious problem at the conclusion of hostilities) and announced its intention to ensure that demobilization, when it came, would be carried out in a proper "revolutionary-democratic spirit."[53] Precisely what this would mean for the demobilization of a syphilitic soldier was left tantalizingly vague. The subsection for social medicine quickly announced plans for a national congress that would "unify all democratic social-medical forces, elucidate the views of broad strata of the laboring population on these questions, coordinate these views with the demands of science, and debate the most urgent questions"[54] with a view to presenting draft legislative proposals to the appropriate government departments. It is significant that the Soviet planned to approach these departments directly; there was no mention of channeling their legislative proposals through the CMSC. It is also worth noting that the Pirogov Society was conspicuously absent from the lengthy list of organizations to be invited to the proposed congress on social medicine. In the minds of members of the Soviet, community medicine and democratic social medicine were very different things. The former was in their view inextricably entwined with political domination of the country by the narrow oligarchy that constituted *tsenzovaia Rossiia;* no amount of hastily arranged liberalization could make it acceptable in a revolutionary era.

By the summer, the Petrograd Soviet had more urgent matters to deal with than health reform: although agitation for the democratization of medical institutions continued, the proposed congress on social medicine was postponed. In Moscow, the city Soviet also became involved in medical issues when authorities at the (municipal) Golitsyn Hospital refused to introduce reforms in administrative practice, touching off serious disturbances among hospital workers. Although the Soviet deplored the reactionary attitude of senior hospital physicians, it also lectured the workers on the need for social responsibility as part of "revolutionary proletarian organization."[55] Meanwhile, at the (private) Sheremet'ev Hospital, the absolute refusal of its Guardian, Count S. D. Sheremet'ev, to countenance any reforms whatever, played into the hands of the Soviet by demonstrating the powerlessness of the "authorities"—in this case the Municipal Duma and the City Commissar—when faced with a diehard reactionary.[56]

With the Petrograd and Moscow Soviets already active in medical matters, it was only a matter of time before a national congress of Soviets established its own medical-sanitary bureau. If the CMSC did not soon meet and address itself to the issue of hospital reform, it would find itself overtaken by the Soviets, whose growing insistence upon the needs of workers, soldiers, and peasants suggested that they meant to take whole areas of health reform—especially social insurance, occupational health, and popular medical care—for their own territory. If this happened, the union physicians, the Pirogov Society, and the CMSC might all be pushed to the sidelines.

Soviet rhetoric about the socialization of medicine might have been less galling to many community physicians if real progress were being made towards introducing sweeping reforms. Instead, even the most basic measures were both slow in coming and disappointing in their significance. For example, both the Pirogov Congress and Almazov's

May Conference had called for an end to the MVD's archaic system of local medical administration.[57] Kiriakov's appointment as Chief Medical Inspector was meant to produce serious reform in the MVD, but the minimal changes he introduced fell far short of indicating the beginning of a new order.

On 28 June, Kiriakov published a circular on the reform of local medical administration.[58] Although he acknowledged that the traditional institutions "do not correspond to present needs," he argued that they must be retained "temporarily," pending new legislation, because they performed administrative functions of national significance which should not be interfered with. Certainly some lesser functions could be transferred to local governments, he went on, but even here zemstvos and towns would have to create new organs to perform them. Thus the existing institutions must retain broad powers in the areas of medical statistics, education, censorship, forensic-medical work, and the supervision of medical personnel. At this point, the only significant function of which they could be deprived was the supervision of zemstvo and municipal medical and sanitary work, including institutions and personnel. Where local governments were prepared to take on general sanitary supervision and the collection and publication of certain statistical information, these functions could also be transferred. However, these relatively small changes would apply only to areas where the zemstvo and municipal statutes were in force; elsewhere, local administration would continue largely as before. Although the circular spoke of all this as a new order, promising "full cooperation with the organs of local self-government," in the formation of new local medical and sanitary councils it is clear that more was left intact than altered. In essence, Kiriakov's June circular slightly expanded the jurisdiction of and granted full autonomy to the same local governments that had enjoyed qualified autonomy in this area since the 1860s. This was not a negligible change, but it fell far short of the Pirogov Congress' call for the transfer of all medical administrative functions to the local governments.

If some tsarist institutions seemed not to be changing quickly enough, the disappearance of others caused unforeseen problems. Before 1917, antiepidemic measures had been managed—or mismanaged, depending on one's point of view—by the Sanitary-Executive Commissions. Unlike the *guberniia* medical departments, they had no permanent existence but were temporary executive bodies that could be convened and dissolved by provincial governors in response to local outbreaks. Once convened, a Sanitary-Executive Commission could exercise virtually unlimited powers of medical police: it could demand information, publish and enforce rules and resolutions, close down public places, and requisition property. Community physicians had for years argued that these bodies abused their powers and mis-managed their tasks.[59] Along with Rein's GUGZ and the Antiplague Commission, the Sanitary-Executive Commissions were bade a joyous farewell by the reformers of 1917. Yet the need to exercise emergency powers did not go away, and it soon became apparent to those in-volved in antiepidemic work that they could not manage without such powers. No one realized the seriousness of the situation more clearly than A. N. Sysin, who was directing the antiepidemic programs of the Union of Towns. By August 1917, he was publicly lamenting "the present lack of responsible organs with juridical rights" and calling upon local governments to step in to fill the void. He even argued that new "com-missions for the struggle with epidemic disease" should include not only community physicians, but representatives of surviving govern-ment departments, particularly the provincial medical inspectors. Yet the legal vacuum continued, and by midsummer little had been ac-complished at the local level. Zemstvos and towns had rid themselves of interference by MVD bureaucrats, but they had neither assumed full control over local medical administration nor created appropriate new agencies to deal with those outbreaks of epidemic disease which the possibility of demobilization rendered more acute.

In mid-July, the Provisional Government finally authorized the cre-ation of the CMSC. The order was signed on 16 July, almost two months after Almazov's May Conference had called for its immediate introduc-tion.[60] In late July, its smaller Standing Council, consisting primarily of ministerial and organizational representatives, began to meet, and a full plenary session of the CMSC, including representatives from zemstvos and towns, was scheduled for 22 to 26 August in Petrograd.

The first concern of the Standing Council was with finances: having abolished the financial review agencies of the tsarist regime, it was necessary to create new procedures by which monies could be chan-neled from Petrograd to the rest of the country. The two unions and the Red Cross required continued funding for their medical assistance to sick and wounded soldiers; their representatives on the council not only drew up new financial arrangements, but also secured a declara-tion that they were the only public organizations legally entitled to re-ceive funds for this purpose.[61] It seems that the ministerial represen-tatives, like their tsarist predecessors, were concerned primarily with accountability in the expenditure of funds and hence did not want too many hands in the pot. Nor did the union representatives, who wished to keep firm control over the personnel, property, and equipment that the unions had built up in the course of the war. Another urgent matter was the provision of state funds to local governments for sani-tary and antiepidemic work, a process previously controlled by the Antiplague Commission. The new Chief Medical Inspector, Kiriakov, proposed arrangements by which zemstvos, towns, and other agencies of local government could obtain allowances and loans from the central government.[62] At Sysin's urging, the Standing Council also began to plan new agencies to replace the now defunct Sanitary-Executive Commissions. Indeed, the creation of a new financial-legal structure to replace the dismantled institutions of the tsarist regime occupied most of the council's attention and predictably elicited com-

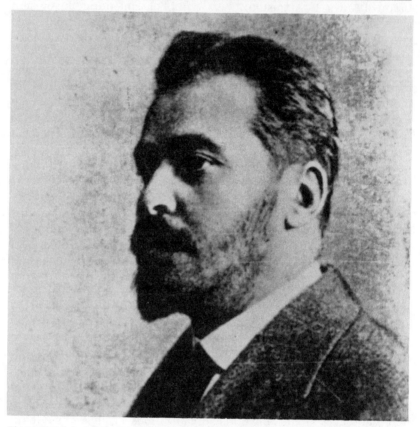

Fig. 15. Z. P. Solov'ev, leader of the left wing of Pirogov medical opinion in 1917. He immediately supported the Bolshevik regime and soon became the architect of the new Commissariat of Health Protection. Courtesy the Lenin Library.

plaints about its "bureaucratization" from more impatient reformers anxious for the advent of sweeping changes.

When the CMSC met at the end of August, it addressed itself to an agenda that harked back to the concerns expressed before and during the Pirogov Congress. Thus, in addition to approving Kiriakov's new funding rules (in so doing settling grievances that dated back to 1914), the CMSC discussed the creation of a new medical statistical agency, the formulation of new rules governing the professional activities of feldshers and midwives, and the reorganization of hospital administration and also announced plans for a congress on "health-resort medicine."[63] Of these, the reorganization of hospital administration was the most contentious: members of the CMSC were unable to agree on how much (or, better, how little) power should be conceded to hospital employees by physicians. Unable to swallow the extensive democratization proposed by the Soviet representative, Dr. Mandel'berg, the council decided to refer this issue for further discussion by new local medical-sanitary councils.[64] Many resolutions of the August plenary involved sending questions out for further discussion at the local level; the assumption was that the responses could be reworked by the Standing Council and then submitted to another plenary session of the CMSC before being sent to the government for legislative action. By this time, presumably, the constituent assembly would have created a new state structure.

This agenda for reform and the assumptions that underlay it had become glaringly inappropriate by the late summer of 1917. The revolution itself had created medical-political issues far more urgent than filling the vacuum left by the demise of the Antiplague Commission. Among these were the problems created by the continued mobilization of physicians and the mounting confusion at the local level, about which ample evidence was provided by local delegates to the August plenary.[65] While the army was denuding the country of physicians, local authority itself was breaking down. The revolution, it seemed, had only begun with the tsar's abdication and was not unfolding as many reformers had hoped. By the early summer, soldiers, workers, and peasants were assessing their own needs, formulating their own demands, and insisting on their satisfaction. One clear sign that the authority and assumptions of community physicians would be challenged was the formulation of the Soviet's program for the establishment of "democratic social medicine." Another was the announcement by the Workers' Hospital Funds of a forthcoming congress to plan a national scheme of social insurance.[66] Other, perhaps even more ominous, signs of ferment came from the countryside: as William Rosenberg has shown, peasants were no longer paying taxes; they were indifferent or even hostile to the *volost'* zemstvo elections; they distrusted village intellectuals, who were increasingly seen as outsiders, agents of an "alien" government that would neither end the war nor legitimize their seizure of the land.[67] By ignoring all this evidence that the revolution was far from over, the CMSC was to make itself a part of what Marc Ferro has called the "spectacular failure" of the February Revolution.[68]

The August plenary of the CMSC only served to demonstrate the gulf that now separated it from the new realities of power.[69] On 26 August, in a Petrograd teeming with rumors of an impending coup led by General Kornilov, the CMSC solemnly passed several resolutions aimed at bolstering its authority within the structure of the Provisional Government. The first enunciated the principle that the government should discuss no measure touching medical or sanitary affairs unless it had already been discussed by the CMSC; another called upon all ministries and departments to inform the CMSC of all legislative proposals that touched in any way on medical or sanitary affairs; a third asked whether the Council of Ministers would admit, as a full member, the President of the CMSC whenever measures proposed by it were under discussion. (Perhaps some members were now beginning to regret the speed with which Rein had been arrested and his ministerial status lost.) Taken together, these resolutions strongly suggest that members of the CMSC had little control over what the government did and that they were already being bypassed (as indeed they were) by ministries and departments bent on fulfilling their own ambitions.[70] They also suggest a striking lack of political realism. The government to which the CMSC was appealing for greater authority was itself in desperate straits, under assault from both left and right. It can scarcely have gone unnoticed by physicians whose sympathies were on the left that the CMSC refrained from denouncing the attempted coup that was taking place, as it were, before its very eyes. Moreover, the CMSC's declaration that only the unions and the Red Cross could legally assist the army was a challenge to both the soldiers' soviets and the front committees, while Kiriakov's complex rules for funding the medical work of local government agencies seemed to preclude any role for the sanitary bureaus of local soviets. Thus, wittingly or unwittingly, the CMSC appeared to tie its colors firmly to the masthead of an already foundering government and to set itself against any further leftward turn in the direction of the revolution.

RADICALIZATION AND MEDICAL POLITICS

A week before the convocation of the August plenary, the Pirogov Society began to publish a new medical weekly under the title *Medical Life* (*Vrachebnaia Zhizn'*). It was largely the creation of Z. P. Solov'ev, who, along with Bogutskii and Sysin, had drawn up the Moscow proposal in mid-March and who was known to be an open supporter of the Bolsheviks. Solov'ev had first proposed the new weekly publication to the Pirogov Executive in May; it was approved early in June but, reflecting the troubled times, did not begin publication until 15 August.[71] His rationale for starting a new publication in addition to the monthly *Community Physician (Obshchestvennyi Vrach)* was the need to provide a forum in which the big questions of medical politics—the organization of the profession, the reform of public health, the future of community medicine—could be debated in relationship to the rapidly changing world of revolutionary Russia. Whatever Solov'ev told the Pirogov Executive, however, his real aim was to save the great reforms envisioned in March by adapting to the new realities of the summer of 1917. Doing so, he soon came to believe, meant abandoning the Provisional Government, the CMSC, and the zemstvos, now identified irretrievably with the estate structure of the old order, and taking up instead the causes of the Soviets: immediate peace and recognition of the demands of soldiers, workers, and peasants.

Solov'ev's "new course," in which he was joined by I. V. Rusakov, A. N. Sysin, and F. D. Markuzon, has been portrayed by one recent historian as "a manifestation of the Bolshevik program of 'all power to the Soviets'," in effect, as an effort to Bolshevize Russian community medicine.[72] This argument rests on the rather slender evidence that both Solov'ev and Rusakov were members of the Bolshevik party. Yet there is no evidence that these two were acting in response to a decision of the party to "conquer" community medicine, nor even that they were responding to Lenin's April call for "All power to the Soviets," a slogan that he had in any case abandoned by August. In fact, the editorial line of *Medical Life* can be explained satisfactorily without resort to party intrigue by treating it in the context of Russian medical politics in 1917. Solov'ev, Sysin, and Rusakov had all been present at the March meeting that drew up the original Moscow proposal; all of them had subsequently witnessed the emasculation of their plans by the Provisional Government, the MVD, the army, and (it must be said) the CMSC itself, which it had taken too long to establish, which was too bureaucratic in its composition, and which was proving a poor weapon with which to fight for reform. Already disappointed and impatient, these three were also both perceptive enough to see that their hopes for reform were in danger of being destroyed by the failure of the February Revolution and bold enough to draw the logical conclusion. Since February, Russian community physicians had already reversed themselves on the central direction of public health administration and had approved a state mobilization of medical personnel. Was it unthinkable that physicians could be persuaded to abandon the Provisional Government and the zemstvos to find a place for community medicine in a revolutionary society?

The radicals' "new course" was heralded in the editorial that Solov'ev published to coincide with the meeting of the CMSC on 22 August. In it, he condemned the survival of "the spirit of old Petrograd" in the CMSC, warning that it might well become another tsarist interdepartmental commission. He also noted the proliferation of agencies involved in reform, such as the Medical-Sanitary Bureau of the Soviet, "whose tasks in many ways coincide with those of the council;" the Ministry of Labor, which had begun to review working conditions and factory medicine; and the Workers' Hospital Funds, which were beginning to plan their own medical insurance schemes. "Everything is going in all directions," wrote Solov'ev; the new council, he observed somewhat pessimistically, "will have to be pushed to deal with all these matters and to produce significant results."[73]

A week later, after the CMSC's disappointing plenary session was over, his tone was much more strident and his message unmistakable. Condemning the CMSC for doing so little to promote the democratization of public health administration at the local level, he pointed out that the local representatives who had attended the plenary were clearly dissatisfied by its inactivity and its failure to provide constructive leadership. The war, he claimed, was largely responsible: it commanded too much attention, consumed too many resources, and, as a result, local affairs were simply left to drift. But the war was only part of the problem: the CMSC itself appeared to be traveling "the old bureaucratic path of *ukazi* [edicts] and directives." Speaking directly to local activists, Solov'ev concluded:

No progress towards a real transformation can be made in this way. Only revolutionary initiative on the spot can put things on a direct path. It is necessary to collect for this [task] all the vital forces which are capable of creative work; to broaden the basis of the medical and sanitary structure, involving in it those democratic strata of the population who have hitherto stood on the sidelines. It is necessary that medical and sanitary affairs be treated not as the prerogative of a narrow circle of specialists, but as the immediate business of the organized people which understands and appreciates these matters.[74]

Coming on the heels of his comments about the CMSC, Solov'ev's references to vitality and creativity were plain: the future now lay with the soviets, not with the moribund institutions of the Provisional Government. In this regard, his choice of a title for the weekly took on new significance: *Medical Life* also became the symbol of medical vitality (*zhiznennost'*).

Solov'ev's decision to abandon the CMSC had personal as well as political implications: its president, Diatroptov, was an old associate in the Pirogov Society and also a colleague in the Union of Zemstvos. Other members of the CMSC's Standing Council, such as Vasilevskii,

MBs more left : not as tool
of Bolsh party but disengage from
Pirogov optim

Frenkel', and Durnovo, were also veterans of many Pirogov congresses and crusades on behalf of community medicine. Yet Solov'ev did not stand alone against these old associates: Sysin, Bogutskii, and Granovskii felt as strongly as did Solov'ev himself that the program of reform for which they had fought was in danger of being lost. Without attacking directly either the Pirogov Society or the achievements of community medicine, Solov'ev and his colleagues made the pages of *Medical Life* into a forum for those who sought to explore the continuing revolutionary possibilities of the idea of *ozdorovlenie*. Contributions were welcomed from Mandel'berg and other members of the Medical-Sanitary Bureau of the Soviet. This is not to suggest that the new publication became a forum for left-wing party ideologists; in a noteworthy contribution, I. V. Rusakov berated the socialist parties for not yet realizing that the time had come to abandon the "obsolete" zemstvo medical institutions and to create new, popular medical-sanitary institutions.[75]

In the wake of the August plenary, *Medical Life* became even sharper in its attacks on the War Ministry and, by implication, on the Provisional Government as a whole. Solov'ev's ammunition was provided by the continuing call-up of physicians—some 1,400 were added to the army's complement between June and early August—and by the exchange of front and rear physicians.[76] His editorial of 15 September was a spirited attack on the Military-Sanitary Administration for permitting the clerks who were running the call-up and the exchange to carry on "exactly in the old chancellery style," drafting those irreplaceable specialists most needed in the civil sphere and then squandering their talents at the front by posting bacteriologists as junior field surgeons and gynecologists as administrators of disinfection stations.[77] Worse was to come, however: according to Solov'ev's information, the army was considering a proposal to inscribe as military doctors all salaried physicians in the country, whether they worked for state, public, or private institutions; their regular employers were to pay their salaries to the army, which would then pay them out of the military budget.[78] Such a step would have put the army in command of all physicians and would effectively have reduced civilian medical care to the status of an appendage to the army and, in all probability, an unwelcome one as well. According to Solov'ev, the consequences of such a measure were too awful to be imagined. Harking back to the April Pirogov Congress and its call for the planned use of the medical resources of the country, he acidly inquired whether the present plan was the best that "our so-called reformed departments" could produce. For him, the choice was clear: wholehearted support for mobilizing medical resources to improve the health of the population; "decisive opposition" to militarizing the profession to meet the army's needs.[79] Within six months, the war had replaced the tsarist regime in his mind as the paramount obstacle to medical and social improvement.

Although the pages of *Medical Life* testify to the disillusionment of Solov'ev and Rusakov, they reveal little about the thinking of their more moderate colleagues in the unions and the Pirogov Society. How, for example, did Diatroptov and Tarasevich react to the events of July and August, 1917? By the time the CMSC held its first plenary meeting, in the wake of the July Days and the fall of Riga, St. Petersburg was rife with rumors of the collapse of Kerensky's government, of an impending coup by General Kornilov, and of the imminent evacuation of the city to escape the advancing Germans. Despite this atmosphere of turmoil, the CMSC did manage to meet, yet its records provide few clues to the thinking of the reformers who had hoped for so much only a few months previously. Their mute allegiance to the CMSC suggests that, whatever their dissatisfaction with the pace of reform under the Provisional Government, they were determined to cling to the existing order. Unlike Solov'ev, they believed that the soviets would not be able to make a fresh start, but rather would simply add to the confusion, ensuring that the revolution was destroyed by a German occupation. In these circumstances, their determination to cling to the CMSC and the Provisional Government was strengthened rather than weakened, not because they had so much to lose but because they still had so much to gain.[80] At the same time, their ties to the unions seemed more important than ever; in 1916 they had regarded them as the cornerstone upon which a new Russia might be built, but now they clung to them as the one hope for maintaining civil order and an organized war effort. It is only against this background that one can understand the hostility with which most of these men greeted the Bolshevik seizure of power on 23 and 24 October. Where Solov'ev and a handful of others were full of hope for the future, most of the physician-reformers of February were united in the belief that chaos was imminent.

7
SOVIET MEDICINE:
THE BOLSHEVIKS
AND MEDICAL REFORM

THE OCTOBER INSURRECTION

Armed rebellion is a dangerous enterprise. When the Bolsheviks planned their insurrection against the Provisional Government, they sensibly anticipated the need to provide medical care for those injured during the fighting. The soldiers, sailors, Red Guards, and militiamen who took up arms against the Provisional Government could expect no help from the doctors and hospitals of the Russian Red Cross or the Military-Sanitary Administration, both agencies that existed (it need hardly be said) to serve the needs of loyal troops. Rebels were, by definition, beyond the pale. Accordingly, on 25 October 1917 the Petrograd Military Revolutionary Committee (hereafter MRC) created a Medical-Sanitary Section to coordinate the work of several medical units that had been formed in factories and among rebel soldiers.[1] The MRC turned to the medical personnel of the Petrograd Soviet to find staff for the new agency but, as might have been expected, physicians who supported the Mensheviks or the Socialist Revolutionaries refused to participate.[2] Hence, M. I. Barsukov, a young Bolshevik military physician, was appointed commissar of the section; he was joined by several other Bolshevik physicians, among them A. N. Vinokurov, M. G. Vecheslov, V. M. Bonch-Bruevich, I. S. Veger, and S. I. Mitskevich, all of whom would soon play important roles in the new regime.[3] Mitskevich and Veger were medical radicals of long standing; the former had organized a radical discussion group among Moscow municipal physicians in 1905, and the latter's stormy career as a community physician had included many battles with conservative zemstvo boards and municipal *upravy.*[4]

In fact, the insurrection in Petrograd was carried out with remarkably few losses on either side, so that what might be called the first aid functions of the section were quickly fulfilled. In the streets, leadership was provided not so much by Barsukov's group as by a remarkable feldsher-midwife named T. A. Fortunatova, who organized women workers into a group of stretcher-bearers and medics soon to be known as the Proletarian Red Cross.[5] That access to medical facilities depended on politics and class background was underlined on the morning of 29 October, when cadets of the *junker* schools staged their abortive rebellion against the new regime. A first-aid station for wounded cadets was hastily organized by the Russian Red Cross, the Union of Zemstvos, and the Union of Towns. (It was directed by a lifelong *pirogovets*, M. M. Gran'.)[6] Not all union physicians opposed the October Revolution, however; in Moscow, the quick-witted Z. P. Solov'ev used his authority to obtain medical supplies for the rebels from the warehouses of the Union of Towns.[7]

Once resistance to the new regime had been quelled in Petrograd, Barsukov and his colleagues took up the other part of their original charge from the MRC, which was "to organize medical-sanitary affairs upon new principles,"[8] a task they interpreted as demanding the creation of a new, democratic social medicine—whatever that might mean. This first attempt at convening a meeting of medical officials and physicians in late October at Smolny—still the headquarters of the new regime—resulted in disappointment. Although representatives from the Military-Sanitary Administration, the Union of Zemstvos, and the Red Cross had been invited, none came; in fact, only three physicians and a few feldshers, dentists, pharmacists, and hospital orderlies turned up.[9] Fresh invitations to "comrades belonging to medical-sanitary professional organizations" produced a larger turnout on 5 November; the pro-Bolshevik feldshers, nurses, orderlies, and stretcher-bearers who attended—many of them probably from Fortunatova's Proletarian Red Cross—drew up a program of action which included the creation of an executive bureau, the reviewing of all new legislative proposals touching matters of health, and the extension of the authority of the *otdel* to military as well as civil medicine.[10] Inevitably, someone proposed that an All-Russian Congress of Medical Personnel be convened. In the ensuing weeks, Barsukov and his colleagues proceeded to widen their jurisdiction over both military and civil medical affairs, a strategy that worked well enough until it ran up against both the resistance of Lenin and—for quite different reasons—the opposition of the Pirogov Society.

Armed with this "revolutionary" program, the new agency did its best to assert its authority. A commissar was dispatched to take over military medical affairs at the Commissariat of Military Affairs (formerly the Ministry of War); one immediate result was the announcement on 8 November that the army's medical facilities were now open to Red Guards. At the same time, the informal first aid detachments of the Proletarian Red Cross received official recognition and support.[11]

Asserting the authority of the MRC's Medical-Sanitary Section beyond the hospitals and first-aid posts of Petrograd was made easier by the fact that, with the fall of the Provisional Government, most senior government officials had gone on strike. Mitskevich has left a graphic description of the scene at the empty offices of the Chief Medical Inspector in the Ministry of the Interior: "On the tables lay many unopened letters and telegrams which had recently arrived. The telegrams contained information from various locations about the severity of a typhus epidemic, and about cases of plague in Astrakhan *guberniia*. The identical scene took place at the medical offices of other government departments, and at the Red Cross." [12]

Barsukov's group were only too ready to fill the vacuum created by the striking civil servants. Choosing among themselves, they established three-person boards (*kollegia*) to run the medical departments of the principal ministries. Vinokurov, Veger, and Mitskevich took over at the all-important Commissariat for Internal Affairs (NKVD); similar boards were set up at the Commissariats of Ways and Communications, State Welfare, and Popular Enlightenment. [13]

LENIN AND THE PIROGOV SOCIETY
Riding the crest of the revolutionary wave, Barsukov and his colleagues went on to plan a Committee for the Protection of Public Health, a kind of revolutionary superboard that would completely reorganize Russian medicine. Having secured the support of a hastily convened meeting of "representatives of various medical organizations"—presumably the now familiar mixture of *rotnye* feldshers, Sisters of Mercy, hospital orderlies, and the Proletarian Red Cross—on 15 November, Barsukov, together with Vinokurov and Veger, put their plan before Lenin's government two days later. [14] This was a bold move indeed; had Lenin agreed, Barsukov and his colleagues would have been in a position to wield extensive powers, greater than those accorded the Central Medical Sanitary Council by the Provisional Government. That this initiative failed was due principally to Lenin himself.

Lenin had two good reasons for blocking Barsukov's plan. One—as yet unstated—was his growing conviction that the MRC and its agencies would soon have to yield before the government of people's commissars. The other, as he told Barsukov and Vinokurov, was his wish to prevent a head-on clash with the Pirogov Society. Almost certainly, Lenin was behind the reply that the Central Executive Committee of the Soviet (*VTsIK*) gave to Barsukov: a plea that he immediately convene meetings of left-wing physicians in Petrograd and Moscow. Barsukov replied that this was simply not feasible and again requested that the scheme be approved. On 20 November, *VTsIK* resolved that a special committee for the protection of public health should be created "in the event that convening such a conference of physicians is impossible,"[15] but, before any precipitate action could be taken, Lenin intervened. Both Vinokurov and Barsukov have testified that the Bolshevik leader cautioned them strongly against proceeding too quickly. Astute as always and surprisingly well informed about recent medical history, Lenin pointed out that this proposal for a superboard, reminiscent as it was of the plans of tsarist reformers, ran the risk of alienating the entire Pirogov Society; by taking a more modest course, the Bolsheviks might well attract and retain the support of left-wing *pirogovtsy*. Moreover, Lenin stressed, it was essential to create new local institutions that would be more representative of workers and peasants than the old zemstvos; it would take time to do so and still more time for these new bodies to appreciate the need for a coordinating central government agency.[16]

Barsukov's memoir account of this conversation not surprisingly depicts him as speechless with admiration for Lenin's brilliance, but in fact he may have been more than a little irritated by the leader's intervention. He and Vinokurov were two young turks; along with Veger, an old hothead, they had been ready to set Russian medicine on its ear; now, it seemed, they would have to restrain themselves. Their freedom of action was further curtailed when the Military Revolutionary Committee and its agencies were liquidated on 5 December by a government anxious to establish its undivided authority over the state apparatus.[17] With the MRC gone, Barsukov and his colleagues were now forced to work within the structure of the various commissariats. They were, however, as adaptable as they were ambitious and soon found ways to extend their influence.

Lenin's intervention, unknown outside the corridors of Smolny, did not prevent a public denunciation of the new regime by the Pirogov Society. Meeting in Moscow on 22 November, fifteen members of the society's executive condemned both "those forces which are destroying the country" and those physicians who were to be found "in the camp of the tyrants."[18] Was the passage of this resolution precipitated by recent events in Petrograd? If those who signed the declaration knew about Barsukov's planned superboard or about the *VTsIK* motion of 20 November, which seemed to give him the green light to proceed even without the support of physicians, then their hasty response and intemperate language are more than understandable. After all, they had not fought against the plans of tsarist reformers only to have a similar monstrosity foisted upon them by the left. Naturally, they could not know that Lenin himself was, almost at that very moment, reining in Barsukov's headlong quest for power. Regrettably, there is no evidence to prove or disprove these suggestions; all that can be said is that there was certainly time for news of Barsukov's plans to have reached Moscow and that the declaration reflects the manner in which most *pirogovtsy* could have been expected to respond.

In any case—and regardless of Barsukov's plans—most *pirogovtsy* did not welcome the new regime. Those who sympathized with the Socialist Revolutionaries or the Mensheviks were outraged by Lenin's actions, as indeed were the followers of Zinoviev and Kamenev among the Bolsheviks. Several of the radicals who signed the declaration fell into this category.[19] As for the others, many of whom considered themselves nonparty democrats, they undoubtedly shared—as Peter Krug has pointed out—the revulsion that was general among the intelligentsia at the actions of the Bolsheviks.[20] Community physicians were, after all, zemstvo professionals; as such, they were bound to be alarmed by the Bolsheviks' manifest hostility towards the political institutions of *tsenzovaia Rossiia* and by their apparent support for the crudest forms of egalitarianism. With the Bolsheviks seemingly bent on destroying the zemstvos and turning civil society upside down, many—perhaps most—*pirogovtsy* concluded that the achievements of decades could well be destroyed in a moment by radical ideologues and their ignorant supporters among the "lower depths" of Russian society. This prospect, if true, was dismal indeed.

P. N. Diatroptov, as President of the CMSC, was clearly beset by such fears. He not only signed the anti-Bolshevik declaration, but also called and chaired a meeting of thirty-five prominent physicians in Moscow a few days later; these included members of the CMSC, the medical bureaus of the unions, the Pirogov Society executive, and the medical department of the Moscow *guberniia* zemstvo. These physicians refused to recognize that the mandate of the CMSC had expired with the Provisional Government; instead, they accused the Bolsheviks of "interfering" in the work of the unions and in public health work at the local level. Members of the CMSC resolved to stay at their posts, making the argument that the current chaos made their presence and continued work all the more necessary.[21]

Not all *pirogovtsy* shared this view. Veger, though denounced in *Obshchestvennyi Vrach* for supporting the Bolsheviks, simply ignored the criticism and even continued to style himself a member of the Pirogov Society executive.[22] On 28 November, Solov'ev resigned from the executive, from the editorship of *Obshchestvennyi Vrach*, and from all Pirogov committees. His letter made it plain that he was in complete disagreement with the 22 November declaration. His fellow Bolshevik, I. V. Rusakov, also resigned all his Pirogov offices, claiming that he was proud to be a Bolshevik.[23] Both of these men were soon to make significant contributions to the creation of Soviet medicine, although that work had to await the transfer of government from Petrograd to Moscow. It is, however, worth noting that their resignations did not lead to anything like a mass desertion of the Pirogov Society by those left-wing physicians whose support Lenin had hoped to attract. At this point, only physicians who were also committed Bolsheviks were prepared to support the new regime.

Paradoxically, there was little similarity between the nightmare visions of Pirogov alarmists and the realities of Bolshevik efforts at reform. In the wake of Lenin's intervention, Barsukov and his colleagues slowed down their headlong rush to reorganize everything and set about trying to build support for the creation of a new Soviet medicine. Among ancillary medical personnel there was little difficulty: in Petrograd, Barsukov and Fortunatova organized a group of pro-Soviet pharmacists, feldshers, orderlies, and nurses into the grandly titled Pan-Russian Federated Union of Medical Workers, but this was really the same group that had been the backbone of the Proletarian Red Cross.[24] The new union attracted virtually no support among the physicians of Petrograd, so Barsukov left it discussing the "sovietization" of the Red Cross while he tried other ways to attract the support of physicians. On 2 December, members of the medical boards in the various commissariats met to discuss the reorganization of civil medicine; according to Barsukov, several feldshers and pharmacists and a few sympathetic physicians also attended. This meeting produced an appeal—which was quickly published—to all categories of medical personnel throughout the country to rally around the new government so as to reduce morbidity and mortality and improve sanitary conditions for the masses. The text of this remarkable document is worthy of reproduction in its entirety:

From the Colleges for the Administration of Medical Otdely in the Peoples' Commissariats of Internal Affairs, Ways and Communications, and State Welfare

The war, economic dislocation, and the waste of population and other consequences associated with them have placed before the Workers' and Peasants' government the question of struggling on a state-wide scale with morbidity, mortality, and the unsanitary living conditions of the broad masses of the population.

Comprehensive sanitary legislation is required regarding water supply, rational canalization, and sanitary supervision over commercial-industrial enterprises and residential housing; regarding the organization of a sanitary inspectorate, elected by the population, for the struggle with morbidity and mortality and, in particular, with child mortality, tuberculosis, syphilis, etc.; for the struggle with contagious diseases, and to provide the population with sanitary, salubrious resorts, etc. It is necessary to take pharmacies out of private hands and transfer them to public institutions of self-government (obshchestvennoe samoupravlenie). Resolution of pressing legal questions concerning assistant physicians is also necessary. Measures connected with demobilization need to be drawn up. It is also necessary to make an appropriate arrangement for [medical] statistical affairs.

It is possible to fulfil all these tasks if the broadest strata of the population are attracted to the work. To this end, the medical-sanitary organizations of public self-government, the *guberniia* and *uezd* sanitary councils, and also the Central Medical Sanitary Council should be employed on a broad scale.

In their present structure, these organizations are elected organs of zemstvo and municipal self-government, but broad strata of the local population, workers' and peasants' organizations, are insufficiently represented in them.

Full democratization of these medical-sanitary organizations is necessary, with broad representation from the local population. A congress of representatives of medical personnel who stand for the Soviet position is required in order finally to work out pressing medical questions.

In proceeding to realize the foregoing program, the Colleges for the Administration of Medical *otdely* in the Peoples' Commissariats of Internal Affairs, Ways and Communications, and State Welfare call upon all categories of medical personnel—physicians, feldshers, *feldsheritsy*, and pharmacists—who support the platform of the Central Executive Committee of the Soviet of Workers' and Peasants' Deputies, to rally round the peasants' and workers' government to carry out appropriate work in the interests of the laboring masses of the population.

(Signed) I. Veger, A. Vinokurov, M. Barsukov, M. Golovinskii, and M. Vecheslov.[25]

This document—the first official Bolshevik pronouncement on medical affairs—is remarkable most of all for its moderation. There is nothing in it to suggest that the Bolsheviks anticipated shutting down zemstvo medical services or dissolving the CMSC. Indeed, the existing institutions of community medicine are specifically called upon to join in achieving the desired reforms. The program outlined in the second paragraph is one that had been broadly espoused by every progressive community physician since the turn of the century. Even the tsarist reformer G. E. Rein would have agreed with much of the proposed sanitary legislation, as well as with the statist tone of the appeal. Especially noteworthy is the guarded statement concerning the legal rights of feldshers; here one finds none of the crude, inflammatory egalitarianism preferred by the *rotnye* feldshers who so readily supported the Bolsheviks. Taken all in all, the appeal was a deliberate attempt to rally as much support as possible from physicians by affirming the new regime's dedication to the cause of progressive medical reform. Nevertheless, there was also a clear political message: accept the October Revolution and its implications and demonstrate this acceptance by reconstituting existing agencies to include heavy representation from workers and peasants. Among those *pirogovtsy* who had already announced their unwillingness to cooperate with the new regime, this political message outweighed all other considerations and obscured the Bolshevik program for medical reform. The next issue of *Obshchestvennyi Vrach* passed over the 2 December appeal in silence; instead, it reported on support among physicians for the anti-Bolshevik declaration of the Pirogov executive and described at length the continuing chaos in local public health administration. Naturally many—though by no means all—of these disruptions antedated October, but all were now ascribed to the Bolshevik seizure of power. It seems that events at the local level—harassment of physicians by Red Guards, disruption of hospitals by self-important "commissars"—carried much more weight with most community physicians than did official statements from the new government. Therefore, Barsukov's appeal failed to achieve its desired result.

Meanwhile, in Petrograd, the Bolshevik physicians reorganized the medical bureaucracy. At the NKVD, the trio of Veger, Vinokurov, and Mitskevich replaced the old office of the Chief Medical Inspector with a new Administration of the Medical Sector, which was empowered to direct medical affairs throughout the Russian republic.[26] The old Administration for Local Economic Affairs, created during Plehve's reforms, was transferred from the NKVD to the new (and short-lived) Commissariat for Local Self-Government.[27] Despite efforts to promote change at the Military-Sanitary Administration, little had been accomplished, so Barsukov and his colleagues decided to force the issue by raising it in *VTsIK*. As a result, the government decreed on 5 December that the Military-Sanitary Administration would henceforth be run by a Council of Medical Boards (*Sovet Meditsinskikh Kollegii* or *SMK*) composed of members of the existing medical boards.[28] Once *SMK* had been created, its leading members, particularly Barsukov and Vinokurov, moved quickly to formalize its powers and status. On 22 December, at their first meeting, members of *SMK* decided that henceforth this body not only would run the Military-Sanitary Administration, but also would coordinate the work of all medical boards and departments throughout the government and would review all legislative proposals touching matters of health and medicine. They also elected Vinokurov their President and agreed that he should attend meetings of the government and speak to all medical issues.[29] One month later—24 January 1918—*VTsIK* approved a decree that formally recognized *SMK* as the highest medical authority in the land; its representative was accorded an advisory voice whenever medical matters were under discussion.[30]

Thanks in part to the obstinacy of the Military-Sanitary Administration, the Bolshevik physicians were able to create, by this somewhat circuitous route, a central body not unlike the superboard to which Lenin had objected in November. Why did Lenin find acceptable in

January what he thought premature in November? For one thing, the *SMK* derived its authority not from the Military Revolutionary Committee but from the government itself. Moreover, Lenin had begun to realize that little was to be gained by waiting: the events of December and January—to be described below—made it plain that most of the *pirogovtsy* were not ready to abandon their opposition to the new regime. In the circumstances, one might as well proceed with creating the nucleus of a future commissariat of health.

SKIRMISHES ON THE MEDICAL FRONT

From its creation, *SMK* became a base from which the Bolshevik physicians launched assaults against institutions that were controlled by their declared enemies. Vinokurov invited members of the CMSC to bring to a meeting on 30 December proposals for their own "reorganization upon democratic principles." Meanwhile, a little pressure was applied. *SMK* drew up a draft decree that dissolved the Union of Zemstvos; its property and assets were transferred to the state, and its existing Central Committee was dissolved and replaced by a new one appointed to liquidate the union.[31] This decree was approved by *VTsIK* on 29 December, the very eve of the meeting with members of the CMSC. If its intent was to teach Diatroptov and his colleagues that the Bolsheviks meant business, it must be considered a failure; no one from the CMSC turned up for the meeting with Vinokurov. During the next month, two further attempts were made to establish contact with the CMSC but, in the wake of the Bolsheviks' ruthless dissolution of the Constituent Assembly on 6 January, members of the CMSC were all the more determined to refuse contact with the new regime. More pressure was applied in early January when decrees were published nationalizing the assets of both the Russian Red Cross and the Union of Towns.[32] Unlike the Union of Zemstvos, these organizations were to be reorganized, not dissolved: Barsukov already had ideas about how the Red Cross could be "sovietized," and Mitskevich, sent to Moscow to investigate the unions, had reported that certain left-wing physicians, among them A. N. Sysin and N. A. Semashko, had shown interest in reorganizing the Union of Towns.[33] The Bolsheviks finally received an indirect answer from the CMSC later in the month. Several of its members, having held an unofficial meeting in Petrograd on 15–16 January, decided not to meet with *SMK*, but instead to travel to Moscow where, on the 24th, they met with members of the Pirogov Society executive. Here they decided, first, that a full meeting of the CMSC would convene in Moscow on 4 March to discuss urgent questions and, second, that an extraordinary Pirogov Congress should be held within two or three months to discuss both medical affairs and the formation of a national union of physicians.[34] In Petrograd, the Bolshevik physicians quickly decided that enough was enough and that, if the CMSC would not recognize the new regime, it would have to be abolished. Vinokurov reported on the situation to a meeting of Sovnarkom (as *VTsIK* was now called) on 15 February. On the following day, the government published a decree stating that the CMSC, a creation of the Kerensky government and composed of representatives of medical organizations that had refused to endorse the October Revolution, had lost its raison d'etre because of the creation of *SMK* and was therefore abolished. The decree also promised the creation of a new advisory council composed of representatives of the medical-sanitary *otdely* of soviets and of zemstvos that had adopted the Soviet platform.[35] The *SMK* had already (27 January) called upon all local soviets to form medical *otdely* and had announced that a congress of their representatives would be held in the near future.

Having dissolved the CMSC, the Bolsheviks made no move to stop the extraordinary Pirogov Congress that met in Moscow from 13 to 15 March. This was immediately followed by the conference on professional unity, at which was founded the All-Russian Alliance of Professional Associations of Physicians (*Vserossiiskii soiuz professional'nykh obedinenii vrachei* or *VSPOV*). Both the resolutions passed by the *pirogovtsy* and the founding of *VSPOV* occasioned much comment in the pro-Bolshevik press, the more so because of the opportunity to contrast the allegedly counterrevolutionary aims of these organizations with the staunchly pro-Bolshevik Congress of Medical Workers that Rusakov had cleverly fixed to meet at the same time. To be sure, the behavior of most Russian physicians gave Bolshevik commentators plenty of ammunition. Having quarreled about the creation of a professional association for three decades under the tsars, physicians had somehow managed to bury their differences and form such a body less than five months after the October Revolution. It required no great skill to see that soviets were regarded as a much more serious threat than the tsarist regime. Rusakov was to hammer this point home repeatedly in speeches and writings during the spring of 1918.

The general tone of the Pirogov Congress was negative. Some wanted to ignore political issues, and a small group (the membership of which is unknown) wanted to support the new regime—perhaps they had read the 2 December appeal?—but the vast majority lined up solidly behind a series of anti-Bolshevik resolutions. The new government was accused of "destroying the basic foundations of cultural life, trampling on the rights of man and citizen, plundering the state and national property, urging on the dark masses against the intelligentsia" and of being unable to solve "the serious crisis which has been created in all areas of Russian life."[36] The congress also called upon the government to reconvene the Constituent Assembly, stop interfering with the work of zemstvos and municipalities, and bring back the CMSC—demands that echoed those already made in the pages of *Vrachebnaia Gazeta*, the editors of which were also the senior officers of the recently founded Union of Physicians of the Army and the Fleet.[37] One would like to know whether, among the 500 participants at the 1918 Pirogov Congress, military physicians formed a significant group; unfortunately, the paucity of records of the congress makes such an inquiry impossible.

Having denounced the Bolsheviks in no uncertain terms, participants engaged in a two-day litany of complaints about what was happening to community medicine throughout Russia. Apparently forgotten were previous discussions that had lamented the impact of the war on civilian medical services or those at the August 1917 meetings of the CMSC which had focused on the increasing paralysis of local public health organizations as a result of the lack of leadership from Petrograd and the shortage of funds. Now the "catastrophic status"[38] of medical affairs could be ascribed to one source alone—the Bolshevik regime. It was the Bolsheviks who were said to be destroying everything by putting ignorant people in charge of public affairs, including local medical and public health services. Physicians had lost their dominant position on local sanitary councils. Hospitals had been taken over, said the old *narodnik* D. Ia. Dorf, by "the autocracy of craftsmen, orderlies, and sick nurses."[39] One of the congress resolutions lectured the government as follows: "The democratization of public medicine does not consist of passing its governance to incompetent organs, dominated by people poorly acquainted with questions of public health."[40] All this ringing rhetoric neglected one crucial fact: that most of the people who were well acquainted with public health matters had refused to recognize the October Revolution or to work with local soviets.

The 1918 Pirogov Congress has elicited the contempt of pro-Soviet writers.[41] The first and perhaps most devastating attack came from I. V. Rusakov, who on 15 March 1918 addressed a meeting of the Moscow Union of Medical Workers. His theme was the hypocrisy of the *pirogovtsy*, who had for decades trumpeted their allegiance to the idea of popular sovereignty but who deserted the popular cause during the revolutionary months of 1917. They had revealed their true colors, he claimed, in resorting to a strike: "This weapon, unsuitable for the struggle with the autocracy, was appropriate for the struggle with the proletariat."[42] Barsukov, in his magnum opus on the building of Soviet medicine, has pursued a similar theme; in his opinion, most *pirogovtsy* believed not in popular sovereignty but in limited popular participation in public affairs.[43] Hence their constant preference for the growth of sanitary guardianships, institutions that purported to involve the people in deciding their own affairs but that were really agencies through which the people could be kept under continuous medical tutelage. In the ideal world of the *pirogovtsy*, physicians would decide what needed doing, would convince the populace through the sanitary guardianship, and would then secure funds and approval from the local zemstvo or *raion duma*. After October 1917, this dream was shattered; now local soviets claimed the right to decide what needed doing, established medical *otdely* to work out the details, and expected physicians to cooperate, using their special expertise. According to Barsukov, "This is why not one physician-democrat can express himself in principle against the direction of activity by Soviet organs [of local government], even though physicians are in a minority within them."[44]

To what extent is this evaluation correct? It could, of course, be argued that Barsukov has made the highly questionable assumption that the soviets of 1918 were genuinely popular, democratic institutions, whereas in many cases they were unrepresentative frauds organized by the Bolsheviks. On this reckoning, it would appear that the *pirogovtsy* were correct to insist on autonomy. Yet this argument implies that the *pirogovtsy* would have abandoned their insistence on professional autonomy if only the soviets had been "genuinely democratic" institutions. Is this a reasonable assumption? What if a "genuinely democratic" *volost'* zemstvo, for example, had decided to dispense with physicians altogether and hire only feldshers? One can imagine the outraged reaction of the *pirogovtsy*. So it was not the authenticity of popular government, but rather its direction, that mattered. If these "unrepresentative" soviets had begun to give physicians *more* power rather than less, they would have been praised for their good sense, not condemned for "destroying the basic foundations of cultural life." There is, then, more than a grain of truth in Barsukov's criticism of the *pirogovtsy*.

Two other contemporary comments on the 1918 Pirogov Congress are worth noting because they shed light on the differing reactions of physicians, as members of the intelligentsia, to the new regime. For many, the question was, "Now that the barbarians are within the gates, what should cultured people (*kulturniki*) do?" Some argued for mass resignations. Undoubtedly, this tactic was discussed in the corridors and on the floor of the congress, but it was rejected on the grounds that the people would suffer. As one *pirogovets* put it, "It is not permissible to extinguish the last sources of light, which are still capable of illuminating the path."[45] But this meant only remaining at one's post, not cooperating with the new regime, lest it gain thereby an undeserved legitimacy. This posture drew scathing criticism from a nonparty physician who supported the regime:

It is impossible to be obsessed only with "the Bolshevik issue" and not take an active part in the positive structure of life—which is impossible at the present time without contact with the Soviet power—because of the fear that this participation could strengthen this power. Believe me, [the author is here addressing those *pirogovtsy* who held to this view] it [Soviet power] does not depend on you and it will not be swept aside by you. And it will not be swept aside at all so long as the people are the basis of it.[46]

Nevertheless, for the time being at least, most *pirogovtsy* seemed determined to keep their distance from the regime. More than 300 of them attended the founding meetings of *VSPOV*, where they agreed to contribute 1 percent of their incomes to create a fund to be used to fight for the improvement of their economic and legal situation.[47] One of the toughest anti-Bolshevik *pirogovtsy*, Ia. Iu. Kats, was chosen President of *VSPOV*. Only a few blocks away—ironically, in the former Hall of the Moscow City Duma—Rusakov attracted some two thousand medical workers (mostly feldshers, dentists, nurses, and orderlies) to the founding meeting of the Union of Medical Workers Acknowledging Soviet Power (*Soiuz meditsinskogo personala na platforme priznaniia vlasti sovetov*). Undeterred by the fact that he had as recently as 1916 argued for a professional association composed exclusively of physicians, Rusakov explained that times had changed and now the primary requirement was to mobilize medical personnel behind the new regime.[48]

THE BEGINNINGS OF COLLABORATION

While these congresses were going on, the government was completing its move from Petrograd to Moscow. The transfer of power, necessitated by the German offensive in late February, was not halted by the peace treaty signed at Brest-Litovsk in early March. By the end of the month, members of *SMK* had arrived in Moscow, and changes followed quickly in both cities. To fill the vacuum left in Petrograd by the departure of *SMK*, the Petrograd Soviet on 24 March appointed E. P. Pervukhin to direct a Commissariat of Public Health for the city and the surrounding region; despite vocal opposition from the Petrograd Union of Physicians, Pervukhin set about taking control over all aspects of medical and sanitary affairs.[49] The state of medicine in Moscow was reviewed by members of *SMK* as soon as they arrived; as a result, three members—Barsukov, Vecheslov, and Golovinskii—plus a local Bolshevik physician, N. A. Semashko, were delegated to organize a medical department for the city soviet, a task they completed in May.[50] Semashko, one of the exiles who had returned to Russia with Lenin in the famous sealed train, had headed the *uprava* in Piatnitskii *raion* during the October Revolution and had gone on to direct medical affairs for the soviet of *raion* dumas that had taken over municipal administration from the (now dissolved) city duma.[51] The most important result of the government's move to Moscow, however, was that both Z. P. Solov'ev and A. N. Sysin began to take a significant part in the determination of Bolshevik health policy.

When the October Revolution came, Solov'ev abandoned journalism for direct political activity, organizing medical assistance for insurgents in the Khamovniki district of Moscow, where he was president of the *raion uprava*.[52] After his editorial attacks on the Provisional Government and the CMSC during the summer, his support for Lenin can have surprised no one. As noted above, he swiftly resigned his Pirogov Society positions after the 22 November declaration. Along with Semashko, B. S. Veisbrod, and A. P. Golubkov, Solov'ev joined the medical college of the NKVD when it was reorganized after the move to Moscow. On 29 March, he was elected its president; he also became head of the reorganized Administration of the Medical Sector and, from 16 April, a member of the advisory college of the NKVD itself.[53] Over the next few months, he would become the key figure in the new government's medical apparatus, just as Barsukov had been the key figure while the government remained in Petrograd.

Sysin was not a Bolshevik like Solov'ev or Rusakov, but he had protested, if belatedly, against the 22 November declaration by resigning from the editorial board of *Obshchestvennyi Vrach*. Nevertheless, he did not sever all connections with the Pirogov Society and, indeed, attended the March 1918 congress. Perhaps the congress's only positive action was to establish a Commission on Epidemics; Sysin, who had already been calling for the establishment of new antiepidemic agencies in the summer of 1917, became its head. At the commission's first meeting on 2 April, members decided to circulate to local public health bodies a questionnaire on antiepidemic measures and to consider the results at another meeting in Moscow in early June.[54] The specter of a cholera epidemic during the summer months was already looming, and the Bolsheviks were just as worried by it as were the *pirogovtsy*. At a meeting of the SMK on 25 April, Vecheslov's proposal to establish a commission on sanitary education was discussed.[55] Somehow—the Soviet historians are silent on this point—Sysin was invited to spend a week (8–15 May) with members of the NKVD medical college, discussing how the government might cope with the expected epidemic. Presumably Solov'ev, who had worked closely with Sysin in the wartime medical bureaus, knew that the latter was prepared to work with the government despite his Pirogov connections; Sysin's mastery of the subject made it essential for the government to seek his views. Sysin's advice was that the NKVD go beyond Vecheslov's original proposal and create a department composed of three sections: sanitary technology and social welfare; epidemiological research and statistics; and sanitary education.[56] Shortly after these discussions, Sysin was appointed to head the new sanitary-epidemiological *otdel* established by the NKVD medical college.[57]

Sysin was not the first eminent non-Bolshevik physician to work with the new government, but his example was soon followed by many others. Once again, as so often in the recent past, it was bacteriologists and epidemiologists who played a leading role. Whether they had tired of the negativism of recent months, realized the pointlessness of standing aside or swallowed their principles because of the threat of cholera cannot now be determined with precision; what can be said is that, although the anti-Bolshevik declaration was never rescinded, leading *pirogovtsy* soon began to join Sysin in working with the new government. For their part, the Bolshevik physicians put aside rhetorical attacks against "bourgeois saboteurs" and worked with the existing personnel of the Pirogov Commission and the medical bureaus of the unions (still apparently functional despite the decrees passed in December and January).

On 23 May, thanks presumably to the persuasive powers of Sysin, four members of the Pirogov Commission on Epidemics—Zabolotnyi, Tarasevich, Diatroptov, and E. I. Martsinovskii—attended a meeting called by Solov'ev and Sysin at the NKVD.[58] Also present were members of various commissariats and departments, the Moscow Soviet, and (according to the Soviet historian Nesterenko) representatives of the two unions.[59] This meeting drew up a program of antiepidemic measures and planned their implementation; a few days later, a meeting of bacteriologists chaired by Tarasevich agreed that the preparation of vaccines would be carried out and controlled in the laboratories of the Women's Medical Institute in Petrograd and the Zemstvo Union in Moscow.[60] As summer arrived, typhus and cholera deaths began to mount; famine, a serious problem in several regions, increased mortality by reducing resistance. Solov'ev prepared a report for Sovnarkom which asked the government to provide more than 11 million rubles for antiepidemic measures.[61] By the time the Pirogov Commission on epidemics met (2–4 June), many of its members had already had significant dealings with the government, and its proceedings were soon to be overshadowed by the Congress of Soviet Medical Departments which *SMK* had called for mid-June. Nevertheless, old hostilities remained: at the urging of Ia. Iu. Kats, the commission passed a motion deploring the fact that the upcoming congress was not to be "a non-party (*bespartiinyi*) affair, so that the fight against epidemics would not be disrupted by party differences between center and localities."[62] Not surprisingly, the government had stipulated that only local health departments that had accepted the October Revolution could be represented at the congress. Like the tsar's Antiplague Commission and indeed the CMSC itself, the Bolshevik government was not about to place large sums in the hands of its potential opponents when there were more reliable ways to ensure that these sums were spent appropriately.

This collaboration between the new regime and leading bacteriologists and epidemiologists naturally raised the whole question of how such learned medical advice could be institutionalized. Even before the government moved to Moscow, the Bolsheviks had dissolved the old tsarist Medical Council; Zabolotnyi's suggestion that it be replaced by the staff of the Institute of Experimental Medicine, though interesting, was no longer feasible once the government had left Petrograd.[63] On 23 April, *SMK* agreed that any future learned advisory body ought to conform to certain guidelines: its membership should consist of individual scholars, not of representatives elected by public bodies; it should not be permitted to raise "organizational questions"; its conclusions and recommendations should not be transmitted to Sovnarkom unless approved by *SMK*.[64] A month later, in fact the day before the 23 May meeting discussed above, Veger and Vinokurov discussed these guidelines with a group of scholars from Petrograd and Moscow, most of them also members of the Pirigov Commission on Epidemics.[65] Evidently the proposed guidelines aroused a good deal of controversy; several of the scholars (who, it should be remembered, also had ties to the Pirogov Society, the CMSC, and the unions) raised objections to its proposed composition and jurisdiction. According to Solov'ev, who reported on the subject to *SMK* on 30 May, the scholars wanted a completely autonomous body—attached to Sovnarkom not *SMK*—which would include representatives of the Pirogov Society and elected representatives of the public organizations of Petrograd and Moscow. (Whatever the meaning of this last phrase in May 1918, it clearly was not meant to include the soviets.)[66] *SMK* agreed with Solov'ev that these proposals were unacceptable but did accept in principle appointed representation from universities and scientific institutions. Solov'ev was commissioned to prepare a final report on the subject, which was approved by *SMK* and sent to Sovnarkom on 24 June. His only concession to the scholars was to permit them to discuss "organizational questions," but all of their recommendations had to be approved by *SMK*.[67] Diatroptov and his colleagues may have come to the meeting believing that they could extract major concessions from the Bolsheviks as the price of their advice; if so, they were quickly disabused of such ideas. Having thrown the CMSC into the historical dustbin, the Bolsheviks were not about to welcome another such institution in through the front door.

SOLOV'EV AND THE CREATION OF THE COMMISSARIAT OF HEALTH PROTECTION

Now that Sysin had managed to involve the appropriate experts in the struggle against epidemics, Solov'ev could devote himself to organizing a new institutional structure for Soviet medicine. Soon after joining *SMK*, Solov'ev headed a small subcommittee that was asked to draft the legislation necessary for the establishment of a separate commissariat of public health. Barsukov and Vinokurov had always been in favor of the idea and, once the March Pirogov Congress made it plain that further delay by the regime was pointless, the plan was revived again. Solov'ev took charge, with the help of Semashko, Rusakov, and V. M. Bonch-Bruevich, who kept Lenin apprised of these developments.[68] In addition, Solov'ev was the moving force behind the Congress of Soviet Medical Departments which *SMK* organized in mid-June. He proposed the basis of representation: two representatives each from *oblast'* and *guberniia* soviets and from Petrograd and Moscow; one each from other cities and *uezdy*; all delegates must support "the platform of Soviet power."[69] He also prepared the program for the congress. Finally, drawing upon his experience as a medical journalist, Solov'ev became (with Rusakov and Vecheslov) principal editor of *SMK*'s new fortnightly publication, *Izvestiia sovetskoi meditsiny*, the first number of which appeared in mid-May. A vital adjunct to his organizing efforts, the new journal was full of articles about the need for a central state health agency, about how to organize local soviet medical departments, and about the importance of the forthcoming congress. Solov'ev also used the paper to print highly critical comments on the March Pirogov Congress.[70]

Legislative draftsman, congress organizer, and tireless publicist, Solov'ev was the dynamo that powered Bolshevik efforts to reform the relationship between medicine and society. His wartime experience with the Union of Zemstvos and the Antituberculosis League had convinced him that Russia needed a separate, powerful commissariat of public health which would bring under its jurisdiction the medical administrations of all government departments, the military included. World War I had taught him—and not only him—that rigid separation of military and civil medical administration could be harmful to the former and disastrous for the latter. It also taught him—as it had the tsar's ministers in 1915—that the state ought not to tolerate quasi-official agencies beyond its control, such as the zemstvo and municipal unions and the Red Cross. Accordingly, unification became the leitmotif of all Solov'ev's planning efforts at the national level, and it was also reflected in his design for the organization of local health departments. Solov'ev understood—with the clarity of one who had

been both an active *pirogovets* and a revolutionary at the barricades—
the imperative necessity to make a decisive break with the old local
institutional structure of zemstvo medicine. In his first editorial for the
new journal, he put his finger on the central issue: the position of the
pirogovtsy, he wrote, has always been that physicians, and only physicians, should play the leading role in medical-sanitary affairs, while
the people should only assist in this endeavor. Now that the people
themselves are leading, he went on, they expect assistance from physicians, but they are not receiving it.[71] The new Soviet medicine, he implied, would involve a permanent alteration in the relationship between physicians and the citizenry.

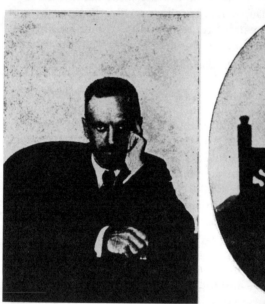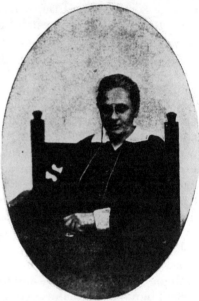

Fig. 16. N. A. Semashko *(left)* became Commissar of Health Protection at Lenin's insistence in July 1918. V. M. Bonch-Bruevich *(right)*, who acted as a channel of communication between Lenin and the leading Bolshevik physicians, was the first woman physician
to play a leading role in the formulation of health policy in Soviet Russia. Courtesy the
Lenin Library.

Solov'ev, Sysin, Rusakov, and Semashko all played important parts
at the Congress of Soviet Medical Departments which convened in
Moscow on 16 June. Sixty delegates were present at the opening and
an additional fifteen arrived during the next three days. This was by no
means purely a gathering of Bolshevik physicians. Forty-five of the
sixty were physicians, but only twenty-eight of them were Bolsheviks

(unfortunately it it not known how many of the physicians were Bolsheviks). Nesterenko gives the following figures for occupation: 45 physicians, 7 pharmacists, 4 medical students, 1 nurse, 14 feldshers, and 4 "without a medical title"; for party affiliation, 28 Bolsheviks, 7 Left Socialist Revolutionaries, 3 Menshevik Internationalists, 2 anarchists, 1 "Unity" group, 31 *bespartiinye*, and 3 unknown.[72] No minutes of the proceedings of this congress have survived, although the resolutions that it adopted were published in *Izvestiia sovetskoi meditsiny*, along with summaries of the principal reports.[73] In large measure the resolutions of the congress simply approved the proposals put to the delegates by members of *SMK*; it is difficult to estimate how much real debate took place. Nesterenko hints that some delegates found the proposals too vague, particularly regarding the financing of local services and improvements.[74] Certainly no challenges to Bolshevik domination were permitted; the president of an organization of feldshers, invited as a guest, clashed with Solov'ev and was immediately deprived of his status and excluded from the hall.[75] Presumably a lively debate took place on the subject of whether insurance medicine would survive as a separate field of activity or be integrated into the structure of Soviet medicine; Mensheviks would have supported its survival, but the congress, following Rusakov, voted for full integration.[76]

Solov'ev got from the congress what he wanted most—"grass-roots" approval for the creation of a Commissariat of Health Protection (*Narodnyi Kommissariat Zdravookhraneniia or NKZ*). On the very eve of the congress, *SMK* reviewed Solov'ev's draft legislative proposal, which called for the centralization and integration of all government medical departments under *NKZ*. Another proposal, apparently favored by Pervukhin and Bonch-Bruevich, would have allowed departments transferred to *NKZ* from other commissariats to function as discrete units run by specialists in the field.[77] Both variants were introduced and discussed at the congress, but Solov'ev's more radical approach was the one endorsed by delegates.

Nevertheless, approval of the *NKZ* project by the congress did not ensure clear sailing through the final stages of consideration by the government. For reasons not yet apparent, Veger tried to derail further consideration of the project, and Vecheslov and Artemenko voted against sending it to Sovnarkom at the *SMK* meeting on 25 June. Perhaps they preferred the Pervukhin proposal; Tsvetaev, now head of the Military-Sanitary Administration, attended the meeting and stated firmly that the total unification of medicine under *NKZ* was impossible under existing conditions.[78] Despite his opposition, a second meeting the following day voted to send the Solov'ev version to Sovnarkom, accompanied by a note that asked the government, whether or not it immediately centralized all medical affairs under the *NKZ*, to declare

NKZ the supreme directing medical body in the country.[79] Then members of *SMK* proceeded to nominate administrators for the new commissariat: Vinokurov was to run it with Pervukhin as his deputy, in consultation with a nine-person college, including Solov'ev, Rusakov, and Semashko.[80] On 30 June, Veger and Vecheslov sent a minority opinion to Sovnarkom; they were invited to attend a future meeting and Vinokurov was instructed to discuss the proposal with all other interested commissariats. It seemed for a moment as if all of Solov'ev's plans might come unstuck, but not so. On 9 July, the draft proposal appeared in *Izvestiia*, along with a list (prepared by Pervukhin) of eminent medical figures who were already working with the regime. Before the Sovnarkom meeting on 11 July, Lenin told Semashko that he wished him, and no one else, to be commissar; Semashko claims he demurred, but that Lenin was adamant. At the meeting itself, which Semashko apparently attended, Vecheslov, Veger, and Tsvetaev argued strongly against the proposal as an unworkable bureaucratic nightmare; someone even accused Semashko of "Rein-like belching." Nevertheless, Lenin was solidly in favor, and eventually the decree was approved.[81] Semashko was appointed Commissar, Solov'ev his deputy; Pervukhin, Bonch-Bruevich, Golubkov, and Dauge made up the college. Sovnarkom had stipulated that *NKZ* was to take over all of the medical institutions and other property that had belonged to the Zemstvo and Municipal Unions. The new administrators of *NKZ* were given one week in which to draw up operating rules, a plan for the orderly transfer of all other government medical departments to *NKZ* jurisdiction, and decrees taking over the two unions and the Red Cross.[82]

On 18 June, Semashko brought to Sovnarkom the final text of the *NKZ* Statute. Rein himself could not have described its areas of responsibility more broadly: the preparation of legislative norms; supervision and control over their implementation; the publication of obligatory sanitary rules for institutions and citizens; assistance to all institutions in the republic in fulfilling medical-sanitary tasks; the organization and administration of central medical-sanitary institutions, both scientific and practical; financial control over and assistance to central and local institutions; unification and coordination of the medical-sanitary activity of soviets.[83] The administrators of *NKZ* were to receive advice from three sources: (1) a learned medical committee, (2) an advisory council of representatives of workers' organizations, and (3) periodic congresses of Soviet medical departments. The only surprise had to do with administrative structure; although *NKZ* was to take over all other medical jurisdictions, there would be separate *otdely* for military medicine (hitherto under the army and the fleet); insurance medicine (hitherto under the Commissariat of Labor); school sanitation (hitherto under the Commissariat of Enlightenment); and railways and waterways (hitherto under the Commissariat of Ways and Communications). This initial structure represented a retreat by Solov'ev in the direction of the Pervukhin plan; perhaps because of the controversy already generated, Semashko may have thought it prudent to throw a sop to critics of this new "bureaucratic utopia."

The battle against cholera also played a part in the Sovnarkom decision to establish *NKZ*. The new commissariat was assigned 25 million rubles for antiepidemic measures and was instructed to send immediate aid to Tsaritsyn and Petrograd.[84] Semashko was ordered to make twice-weekly reports to Sovnarkom regarding the struggle with cholera. The very first meeting of the college of *NKZ* on the night of 12 June was devoted to organizing the anticholera campaign; presumably this was largely a matter of setting in motion the plans that had been drawn up in recent weeks in conjunction with members of the Pirogov Commission on Epidemics. Within a month, the medical bureaus of the unions, as well as their hospitals, laboratories, and warehouses, were transferred to the jurisdiction of *NKZ*. As a result, the new commissariat fell heir to a ready-made institutional structure, complete with material resources and a passably functional network of local committees which could be mobilized for antiepidemic work. Given the overlap in personnel, it is perhaps no exaggeration to describe *NKZ* as the unions' medical bureaus under new management.

While epidemic cholera was being fought in various parts of European Russia, Semashko and Solov'ev went on creating the new bureaucratic empire of *NKZ*—a process that the Soviet historian Nesterenko has called "the unification and gathering-in (*sobranie*) of medicine."[85] Some of the tasks involved were much easier than others. Tarasevich agreed to become head of the Learned Medical Committee, the membership of which was announced on 23 July.[86] Vinokurov, passed over by Sovnarkom in favor of Semashko, became Commissar of Social Welfare; in this capacity he speedily and happily transferred to *NKZ* all of the hospitals and medical equipment of the former Medical Department of the Charities of Empress Marie.[87] Taking over the workers' hospital funds was a more complicated business, which took more than six months.[88] Not surprisingly, the greatest resistance to *NKZ* came from the military medical administration. Tsvetaev remained adamantly opposed to the new commissariat; neither he nor senior officials in the Commissariat of Military Affairs would even attend meetings to discuss matters with *NKZ*. Finally, in late August 1918, Sovnarkom had to issue specific orders for the transfer of the Military-Sanitary Administration to the jurisdiction of *NKZ*; Tsvetaev, who still refused to cooperate, was dismissed from his position in September.[89] Even so, the fleet held out against *NKZ* for almost another year; not until 13 June 1919 was its medical-sanitary administration finally put under *NKZ*.[90] As in tsarist times, those who ran military medical affairs were the most stubborn opponents of efforts to bring military and civil medicine under a common jurisdiction. Even Rein had been forced to give way before the cherished independence of the army and the fleet but, where he had failed, Solov'ev ultimately succeeded. When the Red Army was formed in the course of the Civil War, its medical administration was also under *NKZ* jurisdiction.

Solov'ev's victory is a useful reminder that, where matters of substance are concerned, it was the October Revolution that really acted as a "cleansing hurricane." Despite Zhbankov's paean to the downfall of tsarism, the February Revolution did not lead to the decisive changes that the most enthusiastic reformers had sought. Sysin, for example, was able in all conscience to hail the changes wrought by the October Revolution because they made possible what had previously been impossible. In an important article in *Izvestiia sovetskoi meditsiny*, summarizing his reports to *SMK*, Sysin argued that the October Revolution had cleared away all of the principal obstacles to effective antiepidemic measures. At the national level, it had destroyed all of those various departments and committees—holdovers from tsarist days—that had always stood in the way of creating a strong central agency to run public health affairs. At the local level, it had wiped out the separation of administrative and public (*obshchestvennye*) functions that had characterized tsarism and was replacing the old zemstvo and municipal organs, some of which had not demonstrated a great commitment to sanitary improvements.[91] In the early summer of 1917, Sysin had pointed out the urgent need for new local bodies that would have the power to fight epidemics effectively; the CMSC had not moved quickly enough, but the new leaders of *NKZ* understood what Sysin was talking about and acted speedily to minimize the damage. To be sure, Sysin was one of the first non-Bolshevik physicians to support the new regime, but the point he made can scarcely have been overlooked by others: regardless of the distasteful bullyboy tactics of various local commissars, Red Guards, and Bolshevik enthusiasts, the fact was that October had done far more than February to make possible a sweeping reform of the relationship between medicine and society.

The Bolsheviks' first reforming steps went in an entirely different direction from that predicted by the frightened and confused physicians who attended the 1918 Pirogov Congress. Far from turning rural medicine over to feldshers and other inferior practitioners, the Bolsheviks decided to phase out feldsher schools, encourage trained feldshers to go to university medical schools, and persuade the army to stop relying on *rotnye* feldshers.[92] Nor did the Bolsheviks take hospital administration out of the hands of physicians and give it, as Dorf had claimed, to "craftsmen, orderlies, and sick-nurses."[93] In its resolution on hospital administration, the June Congress of Soviet Medical Departments called for hospitals to

achieve a harmonious combination of specialized medical competence and democratic administration. The college of physicians should be given the right to evaluate, from a medical-sanitary point of view, every measure concerning [the running of] the hospital, because even purely economic or administrative regulations may influence the internal life of the hospital and consequently affect [the welfare of] the sick.[94]

Despite the pretensions of hospital workers, encouraged at least in the short run by the Commissariat of Labor, the victory of Semashko and Solov'ev was also a victory for physicians, who now had *NKZ* behind them in any further dealings with middle and lower medical personnel.

Finally, despite fears that private practitioners might be singled out and punished as bourgeois entrepreneurs, the initial Bolshevik attitude towards private medical practice was perhaps more tolerant than that of Pirogov traditionalists such as Zhbankov. *SMK* made no statement at all on private practice. In a report to the June Congress of Soviet Medical Departments, Golovinskii suggested in passing that Soviet *medotdely* ought to keep private practitioners "under observation" while proceeding to organize socialized medicine for the whole population.[95] This approach echoes that of V. A. Levitskii at the 1917 Pirogov Congress, when he argued against Zhbankov's proposal that private practice should be outlawed forthwith. In fact the Bolsheviks in 1918 had no clear idea what they would do with private practitioners; their attention was directed elsewhere, particularly at pharmacies, which they moved speedily to nationalize in December. Pharmacists—not pharmacy owners—had a long history of involvement in radical politics, and this decree was a predictable consequence of the triumph of Bolshevism.[96]

Taken all in all, what was remarkable about the new regime was not its alleged radicalism, but rather its determination to build a strong centralized agency capable of realizing the program of reforms which progressive physicians—especially those in the unions' medical bureaus—had hoped the revolution would achieve. The hand at the helm may have been Solov'ev's (under the watchful eye of Lenin), but Rein had certainly had a hand in designing the vessel and Sysin in charting its course.

CONCLUSION

Tsarist Russia entered the twentieth century with a political and social structure unlike that of any other European state, and this uniqueness was reflected in the assumptions and limitations that governed the administration of public health. In matters of medicine and sanitation—as in so much else—the army and the fleet were laws unto themselves. Civil medical administration suffered from its subordinate status in the Ministry of the Interior, from its almost total preoccupation with routine clerical and forensic medical work, and from the jurisdictional confusion and overlap that characterized so much of tsarist government. The zemstvo and municipal institutions had done much to improve the medical care available to many inhabitants of European Russia, but both its quantity and its quality were uneven, and large parts of the empire, especially the frontier areas, remained untouched by these improvements. In any case, the ability of these relatively new institutions to take bold initiatives was considerably limited, not least by their dependence on the central government for a good deal of financial support as well as policing and law enforcement.

Although the Russian medical profession had matured considerably during the second half of the nineteenth century, its members still found themselves legally subject to the authority of a state that controlled licensing and discipline and that treated all physicians, no matter what the form of their employment, as servants whose persons and skills were the state's to command whenever it so chose. Eminent members of the profession holding academic, court, and senior administrative positions in St. Petersburg made up a medical establishment that operated under an informal accommodation with the tsarist regime. Naturally physicians whose medical interests were primarily theoretical and experimental were more welcome in this charmed circle than those who sought out the environmental causes of disease

197

or advocated social change as an effective means of prevention; the latter found a much more congenial home in the zemstvo medical organizations, especially in Moscow and the provinces of central Russia. One bizarre result of this disposition of interests was that reformers who believed Russia ought to create a powerful ministry of health found themselves opposed both by officials in the MVD who feared such an innovation and by community physicians in the provinces who resented interference in local autonomy.

Between 1900 and 1905 the autocracy came under attack. Physicians—especially the community physicians who dominated the Pirogov Society—joined the increasingly strong and vocal opposition to the tsarist regime. At the same time, the St. Petersburg medical establishment found its dominance over the profession challenged by those who claimed that knowledge, not official position, ought to be the only legitimate source of authority. Enthusiasts for "collegiality" defied the authority of government-appointed *nachal'niki;* zemstvo medical boards denounced the government agencies responsible for anti-epidemic measures; organizers of a radical medical union broke with the gentility and gradualism that had characterized previous attempts to organize Russian physicians into a national association. Bacteriologists, who had been especially provoked by the regime's intransigent defense of institutions such as the Antiplague Commission, soon led their Pirogov Society colleagues in approving resolutions that embodied the principal demands of the political opposition to the autocracy. Fed up with a regime that called upon them to fight cholera epidemics while making it as difficult as possible to do so, the community physicians looked forward to the creation of a new and better Russia that would follow the collapse of the autocracy and asserted their collective obligation to the Russian people to help bring this great day closer. The Pirogov Society's "Cholera" Congress in March 1905 marked the culmination of this spirit of militant radicalism among physicians.

Even after it became clear that the tsarist regime would survive the Revolution of 1905, the partisans of *obshchestvennost'* still believed that Stolypin's proposed reform of local government, particularly the establishment of *volost'* zemstvo institutions, would allow the professional intelligentsia to play a significant role in the future development of Russia. This optimism ignored the influence that the propertied classes still exercised over so much of Russian public life. As a consequence, the premier's change of course in the summer of 1907 led members of the liberal and radical intelligentsia to engage in a profound reconsideration of the assumptions upon which they had based their work. The medical counterpart of this reappraisal was the debate over the future of zemstvo medicine, a debate that raged in the medi-

cal periodical press until the outbreak of war in 1914. For the traditionalists who looked back to the impressive achievements of zemstvo
medicine, the difficulties of the moment could easily have been tran-
scended if only community physicians would abandon the tempta-
tions of bacteriology and laboratory research and the seductions of
private practice to recapture the high ideals, social commitment, and
moral purity of their forefathers. The fact is, however, that both Russian society and western medicine had changed a great deal since the
days of Molleson and Erismann, and the essentially populist ideology
of community medicine had not kept pace with these changes. As
many of the contributors to this debate pointed out, zemstvo medical
services could be faulted for weaknesses in both patient care and epidemic prevention, not to mention the clearly obsolete prejudice of traditionalists against laboratory research. The universalist aspirations of
zemstvo medicine and of the Pirogov Society were under attack in this
new age of medical specialization and innovation. One sees the discomfort of the traditionalists most clearly in their inability to welcome
the growth of industrial hygiene and occupational medicine, the establishment of workers' hospital funds, and the application of advanced technology to the problems of urban sanitation. If most of the
traditions of community medicine took a buffeting in this debate, one
article of faith remained surprisingly strong; as late as 1913, community
physicians showed themselves unwilling to reconsider their increasingly questionable assumption that the state had no significant role to
play in the promotion of improved public health.

With community medicine in such evident disarray, it is scarcely
surprising that the academics and bureaucrats in St. Petersburg attempted to reassert state control over both the medical profession and
the future development of Russian medicine. Stolypin, who found
himself caught between the tsar's desire for decisive action and his
own compulsion to protect the integrity of the MVD, managed to stave
off the challenges mounted first by von Anrep and then by Rein. Not
until Stolypin's assassination in 1911 did the centralizing reformers
have a clear opportunity to elaborate their program for greater state
control over all aspects of medical life: education, practice, research,
popular hygiene education, epidemic prevention, the collection of statistics, and even physicians' professional activities. Under Rein's leadership, the Interdepartmental Commission worked out a set of legislative
proposals designed to harness medical professionals to the service of
the tsarist state and to cut once and for all the ties between medical
professionalization and political radicalism. What made this reform
program particularly significant was the fact that it emanated from individuals such as Rein and Gamaleia, whose position at the forefront
of modern medicine could not be questioned. Following English and

German precedents, the reformers sought to create a strong central agency that would, among other things, take direct charge of the fight against epidemics in the frontier regions, while at the same time coordinating the efforts of the community physicians in the zemstvo provinces. Had the war not intervened, there is little doubt that Rein would have worked very hard to make the Main Administration for Health Protection a force to be reckoned with in Russian life.

The Great War decisively altered the fortunes of both Rein, the would-be reformer, and his opponents, the community physicians. The first few months of war proved repeatedly that Rein had been entirely correct to warn of the potentially disastrous consequences of the failure to create a central agency to plan and direct the administration of public health. In addition to the army's sudden need for many more physicians and hospital beds than its staff had expected and the concomitant decline in services available to the civilian population, Russia also faced a grave threat of epidemic disease not only among soldiers but throughout the country, thanks to the movement of prisoners of war, so-called "unreliables," and refugees. The tsar's decision to entrust the solution of all these problems to Prince Ol'denburg and his Sanitary-Evacuation Branch virtually sidelined Rein for the duration of the war. More importantly, the dependence of Ol'denburg and army field commanders on the personnel and material resources of the zemstvos and municipalities, coupled with the lack of effective leadership from St. Petersburg, meant that the community physicians soon found themselves with far more actual and potential influence than they had enjoyed in many years.

Many of the bacteriologists and epidemiologists who had been in the forefront of the opposition in 1905 and who retained their conviction that the tsarist regime was the chief obstacle to the creation of a healthier Russia now joined the medical staffs of the voluntary organizations. Buttressing their authority with the prestige attached to the Pirogov name, these physicians organized technical branches, the aims and guiding assumptions of which were far more radical than the allegedly patriotic motives that had brought their parent organizations into being. Conflicts over the organization of antiepidemic measures and over care for the mentally ill revived and exacerbated the prewar hostility between the community physicians on the one hand and the Council of Ministers and the Antiplague Commission on the other. In the plans that these physicians elaborated for the improvement of sanitation and health in postwar Russia, one can see members of the professional and technical intelligentsia trying once again to create that larger role for themselves which they had been denied by the outcome of the Revolution of 1905. In their calls for the democratization of zemstvo and municipal institutions and in their desire to broaden participation in the technical agencies of the unions, one can discern yet another attempt to diminish the control of local government by the propertied classes. The special importance of sanitary-technical expertise in the medical bureau of the Union of Towns reveals the extent to which those concerned with the development of urban management and services in postwar Russia had left the traditional assumptions of zemstvo medicine far behind.

Not surprisingly, the collapse of the tsarist regime resolved none of the larger issues and opened the door to intense jockeying for position and influence. The inclination of the Provisional Government—like its tsarist predecessor—was to put wartime medical relief work far ahead of general questions of health reform. Fearful that this opportunity to profit from the revolution might be lost, the union physicians pressed both the Pirogov Congress and the Provisional Government to create a new institutional base from which they could ensure that neither the Russian Red Cross nor the MVD would be able to block the sweeping reforms that they planned to introduce. However, it was May before the commissar appointed by the Provisional Government was able to beat off the clever rearguard action waged by tsarist appointees in the MVD who had done their best to treat the February Revolution as an event of minimal consequence.

The Central Medical Sanitary Council never became the effective reforming agency that the union physicians had sought. It could control neither the pace nor the direction of reform in the army, it was slow to find substitutes for the tsarist medical institutions that the revolutionaries had been so quick to abolish, and it had no answer to the challenge of "democratic social medicine" mounted by the Soviet. By the late summer of 1917, opinion among the reformers was divided. Many of those who had been ardent reformers in February now feared for the future in a Russia where hostility to intellectuals, zemstvos, and other tsarist "leftovers" seemed to be growing every day; their inclination was to cling to the existing order in the hope that the country would not be plunged into further chaos. However, a small group of radicals led by Solov'ev, appalled by the failure of their erstwhile colleagues to distance themselves from Kornilov's uprising, sought to find a place within the new revolutionary society for the old vision of *ozdorovlenie Rossii.*

In the wake of the October Revolution, most of the *pirogovtsy* behaved just as the MVD officials had done earlier in the year, when they acted as if unpalatable events could be reversed simply by ignoring their implications. The anti-Bolshevik declaration of the Pirogov Society's executive and Diatroptov's adamant refusal to respond to various initiatives from Lenin and the Bolshevik physicians seemed to validate the charge that most community physicians were simply unwilling to accept the October Revolution. The Bolsheviks, for their part, failed to appreciate that most of the *pirogovtsy*, who feared the rule of the mob and the devaluation of professional expertise, had little or no faith in the ability of the new government to implement a program of progressive medical and social reform. Physicians who claimed that the Bolsheviks were responsible for all the deficiencies in medical services in the year after the October Revolution were clearly exaggerating; against these claims must be set the fact that local soviets were curbing rather than augmenting the power and influence of physicians and medical boards.

The Commissariat of Health Protection owed much more to Russian precedent and tradition than to Bolshevik ideology. Faced in the summer of 1918 with the prospect of a cholera epidemic, the Soviet government did what Botkin, von Anrep, and Rein had called upon the tsarist regime to do; it established a strong centralized agency to direct medical and sanitary affairs and to coordinate antiepidemic measures. Solov'ev, who designed the new structure, had been persuaded by his experience before and during the war that departmental monopolies and overlapping jurisdictions were not only indefensible but positively evil; hence he was every bit as determined a centralizer as Rein had been and insisted on the creation of a "unified Soviet medicine" under one commissariat. Sysin, who planned the antiepidemic campaign, was similarly a product of his experience in the recent past. Like Rein, he was an early enthusiast for technological innovation; the war had given him the opportunity to design and implement preventive programs and sanitary undertakings on an ever larger scale, and the creation of the Commissariat of Health Protection promised him the chance to build upon the resources and structure of the wartime unions in carrying out new and (it was hoped) more effective antiepidemic measures. Clearly, the initial Soviet solutions to public health problems owed little to Marxism and much to the thinking of prerevolutionary health reformers.

In setting out to create what would subsequently be hailed as "the new Soviet medicine," the Bolsheviks were able to draw upon a number of exceptionally favorable circumstances. One was the traditionally large role that the state had always played in Russian medical life, a role that would have become even larger if Rein had had his way. Another was the legacy of service to the people which had become part of the ethos of Russian physicians, thanks to the influence community physicians had exerted upon the development of Russian medicine. Well before 1917, however, many community physicians had rejected the exclusively populist framework within which the Pirogov traditionalists had tried to confine the idea of community service. Hence, when the Bolsheviks attempted a new definition of the social obligations of physicians in a society that they were determined to make more urban and more industrial, they soon found willing allies among Russia's community physicians. Despite some initial misunderstandings and hostility, those who believed that the revolution was meant to play the role of a cleansing hurricane had much to gain and little to lose by making a speedy accommodation with a regime that, despite its rhetoric, appeared far more ready than the tsarist government to uphold the importance of modern technology and professional expertise.

NOTES

1: MEDICAL RUSSIA AT THE DAWN OF THE TWENTIETH CENTURY

1. According to the 1897 census, 92.6 percent of the population of the empire lived in its European part and only 7.4 percent lived in the Asiatic part. For a stimulating analysis of urban population growth before 1914, see Hans Rogger, *Russia in the Age of Modernisation and Revolution 1881–1917*, (London: Longman, 1983), 125–127.

2. The text of this memorandum remained unpublished for a decade; it finally appeared under the title "Zapiska o preobrazovanii tsentral'nogo upravleniia grazhdanskoi meditsinskoi chast'iu, sostavlennaia po porucheniiu G. Ministra Vnutrennikh Del', Egermeistera D. S. Sipiagina" in *Zhurnal Russkogo Obshchestva Okhraneniia Narodnogo Zdraviia*, no. 2 (1911): 73–78; no. 3: 72–74; no. 4: 72–75 (hereafter cited as *Zhurnal ROONZ*).

3. Ibid., no. 2: 73–74.

4. On the origins of the Medical Council, see A. I. Moiseev, *Meditsinskii Sovet M.V.D.: Kratkii istoricheskii ocherk* (St. Petersburg, 1913), 1–3.

5. *Zhurnal ROONZ*, no. 2 (1911): 74.

6. On the state of public health in the Imperial capital at the beginning of the twentieth century, see J. H. Bater, *St. Petersburg: Industrialization and Change* (London: McGill-Queen's University Press, 1976), and his more recent article, "Modernization and Public Health in St. Petersburg, 1890–1914," *Forschungen zur osteuropäischen Geshichte* 37 (1985): 357–372.

7. On the St. Petersburg bureaucracy and its difficulties, see George L. Yaney, *The Systematization of Russian Government: Social Evolution in the Domestic Administration of Imperial Russia, 1711–1905* (Urbana: University of Illinois Press, 1973); Walter M. Pintner and Don Karl Rowney, eds., *Russian Officialdom from the Seventeenth to the Twentieth Century* (Chapel Hill: University of North Carolina Press, 1980).

8. The growth of zemstvo medicine is the subject of an outstanding monograph by Nancy Mandelker Frieden, *Russian Physicians in an Era of Reform and Revolution, 1856–1905* (Princeton: Princeton University Press, 1981) (hereafter cited as Frieden 1981).

9. On the famine and its consequences, see Richard G. Robbins, Jr., *Famine in Russia, 1891–1892: The Imperial Government Responds to a Crisis* (New York: Columbia University Press, 1975), and Nancy M. Frieden, "The Russian Cholera Epidemic and Medical Professionalization," *Journal of Social History* 10, no. 4 (1977): 538–559.

10. Frieden 1981, 179. For her discussion of the proposed hospital statute and the campaign against it, see 161–177.

11. Article 386 of the statute governing the Ministry of the Interior, quoted by Veliaminov in *Zhurnal ROONZ*, no. 2 (1911): 76.

12. This was the *Vestnik Obshchestvennoi Gigieny, Sudebnoi i Prakticheskoi Meditsiny*, published by the MVD from 1889 to 1915 and edited by V. O. Gubert and M. S. Uvarov (hereafter cited as *VOG*).

13. *Zhurnal ROONZ*, no. 2 (1911): 77.

14. See above, note 11.

15. For the transactions of the Botkin Commission, see *Mezhdunarodnaia Klinika*, no. 5 (1886) and no. 6 (1887); for comment on its deliberations, see Frieden 1981, 138, 165.

16. *Zhurnal ROONZ*, no. 2 (1911): 76.

17. The activities of the Antiplague Commission and the crisis that they provoked among community physicians are discussed in Frieden 1981, 291–295. For its role in alienating bacteriologists from the Russian state, see John F. Hutchinson, "Tsarist Russia and the Bacteriological Revolution," *Journal of the History of Medicine and Allied Sciences* 40 (1985): 420–439.

18. *Trudy vtorogo s"ezda russkikh vrachei v Moskve* (Moscow, 1887) I: 14–19.

19. Eberman's paper, entitled "Concerning the Establishment of a Ministry of Public Health," was summarized in *Dnevnik shestogo s"ezda russkikh vrachei* (Kiev, 1896), no. 5: 12–14.

20. Ibid., no. 6: 25.

21. *Zhurnal Obschestva Russkikh Vrachei v pam. N. I. Pirogova* (hereafter cited as *Zhurnal ORVP*), no. 1 (1899): 18.

22. For his contribution to the campaign to form a physicians' protective and benevolent society, see John F. Hutchinson, "Society, Corporation or Union? Russian Physicians and the Struggle for Professional Unity (1890–1913)," *Jahrbücher für Geschichte Osteuropas* 30, Heft 1 (1982): 40–41.

23. *Zhurnal ORVP*, no. 1 (1899): 15–16.

24. "Programma doklada o neobkhodimosti uchrezhdeniia v Rossii ministerstva okhraneniia narodnogo zdraviia," *Zhurnal ORVP*, no. 3 (1893): 18–20.

25. Among the principal contributions to this controversy were L. G. Karchagin, "Ministerstvo obshchestvennogo zdorov'ia," *Vrach*, nos. 34 and 35 (1897); "N. Ch.," "O ministerstve narodnogo zdraviia," *Novoe Vremia*, no. 7925 (1898); G. M. Gertsenshtein, "Nuzhno-li nam ministerstvo narodogo zdraviia?" *Ezhenedel'nik Zhurnala Prakticheskaia Meditsina*, nos. 17–18 (1898); A. V. Pogozhev, "Mechty o ministerstve narodnogo zdraviia," *Novoe Vremia*, nos. 8088 and 8092 (1898).

26. K. I. Shidlovskii, "Materialy po voprosu o ministerstve narodnogo zdraviia: II. Literaturnye spravki," *Zhurnal ORVP* (1899): 23–24.

27. *Dnevnik sed'mogo s"ezda russkikh vrachei* (Kazan, 1899), 593–621.

28. See above, note 2.

29. A main administration [*glavnoe upravlenie*] was a government agency whose status was greater than a department but not quite that of a ministry. It was usually headed by a *nachal'nik* whose status was equal to that of a deputy minister.

30. *Zhurnal ROONZ*, no. 4 (1911): 75.

31. *Zhurnal ROONZ*, no. 3 (1911): 73. V. V. Pashutin, whose death had left the Presidency of the Medical Council vacant, was a pathologist; Veliaminov was a surgeon.

32. *Zhurnal ROONZ*, no. 2 (1911): 76.

33. For a sketch of Sipiagin as Minister of the Interior, see V. I. Gurko, *Features and Figures of the Past: Government and Opinion in the Reign of Nicholas II* (Stanford: Stanford University Press, 1939), 82–86.

34. These "bureaucrats with special commissions" were the MVD's roving troubleshooters; some of its most able functionaries had served in this capacity before promotion to department-level responsibilities. The most reliable guide to the inner workings of the MVD is Daniel T. Orlovsky, *The Limits of Reform: The Ministry of Internal Affairs in Imperial Russia, 1802–1881* (Cambridge: Harvard University Press, 1981).

35. These suggestions were very similar to proposals that had been advanced in 1898 by a subcommittee of the Medical Council; for details, see Moiseev, *Meditsinskii Sovet M.V.D.*, 19.

36. His six specialists were as follows: a representative of scientific and experimental medicine, a chemist, an expert in forensic medicine, a hygienist, an experienced hospital doctor or clinician-administrator, and a technical expert (either a civil engineer or an architect). *Zhurnal ROONZ*, no. 4 (1911): 72.

37 Gurko, *Features and Figures*, 84.

38. On Plehve's program for the reform of local administration, see Neil B. Weissman, *Reform in Tsarist Russia: The State Bureaucracy and Local Government, 1900–1914* (New Brunswick, N.J.: Rutgers University Press, 1981), 40–60, and Edward H. Judge, *Plehve: Repression and Reform in Imperial Russia, 1902–1904* (Syracuse: Syracuse University Press, 1983), 75, 85.

39. The text of the MVD circular of 6 April 1902 was reprinted in *Zhurnal ORVP*, no. 14 (1902): 255–257; for the outraged reaction of the Pirogov Society, see Ibid., 257–259. The incident is discussed in Frieden 1981, 289.

40. Frieden 1981, 289, has pointed out that Ragozin had attacked the Economic Department in no uncertain terms in 1899.

41. Ragozin was appointed President of the Medical Council on 6 July 1902, three months after Plehve became Minister.

42. For von Anrep's service record, see *Spisok vysshikh chinov tsentral'nikh i mestnykh ustanovlenii Ministerstva Vnutrennikh Del'. Chast' I* (St. Petersburg: Tipografiia Ministerstva Vnutrennikh Del', 1905), 95. His career after 1905 is discussed in chapter IV.

43. This account of the committee's work follows Moiseev, *Meditsinskii Sovet M.V.D.*, 28.

44. The text of the revised *polozhenie* appears in Moiseev, *Meditsinskii Sovet M.V.D.*, 21–26.

45. On these innovations and their significance, see Weissman, *Reform in Tsarist Russia*, 81–82; Judge, *Plehve*, 177; Frieden 1981, 259–290.

46. For the text of the *polozhenie* that established the Main Administration of the Chief Medical Inspector, see *Zhurnal ROONZ*, no. 3 (1904): 245–247.

47. *Zhurnal ROONZ*, no. 1–2 (1904): 113–114.

48. Ibid., 114–115.

49. The Pirogov Society's *Journal* quoted with obvious approval from an editorial in *Russkii Vrach* that made this point. See *Zhurnal ROONZ*, no. 1–2 (1904): 115.

50. Judge, *Plehve*, 72.

51. Six main areas of responsibility were assigned to the *guberniia* medical departments: the care of public health; supervision over fresh food, over physicians practicing or in service within the *guberniia*, over pharmacies and the trade in medications, and over civil hospitals; and forensic medical and legal matters. See L. I. Dembo, *Vrachebnoe pravo: Vypusk 1-yi. Sanitarno-sotsialnoe zakonodatel'stvo* (St. Petersburg, P. P. Soikin, 1914), 47–48.

52. Physicians had both a professional and a personal stake in reducing popular ignorance; many had been assaulted and a few murdered by outraged mobs during the "cholera riots" that accompanied major epidemics. On the riots and their aftermath, see Frieden 1981, 143–153.

53. Dembo, *Vrachebnoe pravo*, 50.

54. Ibid., 51.

55. This is a theme that recurs in many of the contributions to *The Zemstvo in Russia: An Experiment in Local Self-Government*, ed. Terence Emmons and W. S. Vucinich, (Cambridge: Cambridge University Press, 1982).

56. N. P. Iur'ev, *K voprosu o material'nom polozhenii vrachei, sluzhashchikh po vedomstvu Ministerstva Vnutrennikh Del' v guberniiakh i oblastiakh Rossii* (St. Petersburg, Tipografiia Ministerstva Vnutrennikh Del', 1904), 4–5.

57. L. Valerianov, *Prava i Obiazannosti Vrachei* (St. Petersburg, Vrachebnaia Gazeta, 1913), 29.

58. Iur'ev, *K voprosu o material'nom polozhenii vrachei*, 3, 7–11.

59. *Vrachebnaia Gazeta*, no. 39 (1907): 1099.

60. Ibid.

61. Ibid.

62. Iur'ev, *K voprosu o material'nom polozhenii vrachei*, 12–15.

63. Ibid., 14–20.

64. For an illuminating discussion of the aims, methods, and consequences of medical-police surveillance over brothels and street prostitutes, see Laurie Bernstein, "Sonia's Daughters: Prostitution and Society in Russia," Ph.D. diss., University of California, Berkeley, 1987.

65. Iur'ev, *K voprosu o material'nom polozhenii vrachei*, 24–25.

66. Levitskii, "Sel'skaia meditsina v ne-zemskikh guberniiakh," 790.

67. *Vrachebnaia Gazeta*, no. 39 (1907): 1099.

68. Iur'ev, *K voprosu o material'nom polozhenii vrachei*, 26–27.

69. In 1903, there were 3,528 physicians in the army, as well as 238 pharmacists and 9,798 feldshers and other lower medical personnel. See *Stoletie Voennogo Ministerstva, 1802–1902 gg*. VIII, Part 4, *Ocherk razvitiia i deiatel'nosti voennomeditsinskogo vedomstva* (St. Petersburg: M. O. Vol'f, 1911), 314.

70. For his service record to 1903, see *Spisok grazhdanskim chinam voennogo vedomstva pervykh shesti klassov po starshinstvu* (St. Petersburg, Voennaia Tipografiia 1904), 64. (He appeared in this list in his capacity as a professor at the Imperial Military-Medical Academy.)

71. The medical section of the Empress Marie Institutions included supervisory responsibility for the Clinical Institute of Grand Duchess Elena Pavlovna and the Imperial Clinical Institute of Midwifery.

72. The salaries and honors of Veliaminov and Pavlov may be compared, ironically on facing pages, in *Spisok grazhdanskim chinam voennogo vedomstva*, 64–65.

73. For biographical details about Pashutin's career, I have drawn on his autobiographical fragment, "Avtobiografiia," *Zhurnal ROONZ*, no. 3–4 (1901): 190–206.

74. V. V. Pashutin, *Lektsii obshchei patologii (patologicheskoi fiziologii), chitannyia studentam Imperatorskogo Kazanskogo Universiteta* (Kazan, 1878).

75. *Zhurnal ROONZ*, no. 3–4 (1901): 203.

76. S. [M.] Lukianov, "Pamiati V. V. Pashutina," *Zhurnal ROONZ*, no. 3–4 (1901): 185.

77. Ibid., 185–186.

78. On Erismann's role in the development of zemstvo medicine, see Frieden 1981, 99–104.

79. The whole story of this appointment is told with remarkable candor in the obituary for S. V. Shidlovskii (by his former students V. Levashev and N. Gusteran) which appeared in *Izvestiia imp. Voenno-Meditsinskoi Akademii* 25, no. 4 (1912): 779–794.

80. M. Ia. Kapustin, *Osnovnye voprosy zemskoi meditsiny* (St. Petersburg, 1889).

81. *Izvestiia imp. Voenno-Meditsinskoi Akademii* 25, no. 4 (1912): 783. For his contribution to the field of hygiene, see Z. G. Surovtsov, *Materialy dlia istorii Kafedry Gigieny v imperatorskoi Voenno-Meditsinskoi (byvshei Mediko-Khirurgicheskoi) Akademii* (St. Petersburg, Voennaia Tipografiia, 1898), 100–104.

82. The Medical Edict [*Vrachebnyi ustav*] may be found in *Svod zakonov Rossiiskoi imperii* 13 (St. Petersburg: Gosudarstvennaia Tipografiia, 1905).

83. Unlicensed practitioners were exempt from prosecution provided no money changed hands: article 226 of the Medical Edict sanctioned the activity of those who "from philanthropic motives and without compensation" offered advice and simple, harmless remedies to the sick.

84. *Zapiski vracha* by V. Veresaev [V. V. Smidovich] originally appeared in serial form in *Mir Bozhii* during 1901 and was subsequently published in several Russian editions and many translations. An English version appeared in 1916, Vikenty Veresayev, *The Memoirs of a Physician*, trans. Simeon Linden, with an introduction and notes by Henry Pleasants, Jr., M.D. (New York: Alfred A. Knopf, 1916).

85. Ibid., 287.

86. Frieden 1981, 271–275.

87. Valerianov, *Prava i obiazannosti vrachei*, 12–13.

88. Salary levels, static from 1859 until 1902, when they were increased substantially, were raised again between 1905 and 1914. In 1912, beginners earned 1,170 to 1,320 rubles; after five years, 1,400 to 2,080; senior regimental physicians and senior hospital physicians, 2,400 to 3,000. There were other benefits, including half-pay after twenty-five years, special disability pensions, and pensions for the widows and families of those killed on active service. Valerianov, *Prava i obiazannosti vrachei*, 23–25; also *Stoletie Voennogo Ministerstva*, 314.

89. Valerianov, *Prava i obiazannosti vrachei*, passim; Freiberg, *Vrachebno-Sanitarnoe Zakonodatel'stvo*, 33–70, 124–40.

90. Valerianov, *Prava i obiazannosti vrachei*, 15.

91. "A few of my comrades were fortunate enough to obtain hospital appointments elsewhere, others entered the service of the 'Zemstvos': but those who remained—including myself—failed to secure any such positions, and the only thing left us was to try and gain our bread by private practice," lamented Veresayev, *Memoirs*, 58.

2: PHYSICIANS, POLITICS, AND THE 1905 REVOLUTION

1. D. N. Zhbankov, "Proshloe i budushchee pirogovskogo obshchestva," *Zhurnal ORVP*, no. 5 (1906): 437–438.

2. On the involvement of physicians with the alcohol problem, see John F. Hutchinson, "Medicine, Morality and Social Policy in Imperial Russia: The Early Years of the Alcoholism Commission," *Histoire Sociale/Social History* 7 (1974): 202–236, and "Science, Politics, and the Alcohol Problem in Post-1905 Russia," *Slavonic and East European Review* 58 (1980): 232–254.

3. On the medical profession, prostitution, and venereal disease, see Bernstein, "Sonia's Daughters" and Laura Engelstein, "Morality and the Wooden Spoon: Russian Physicians View Syphilis, Social Class, and Sexual Behaviour, 1890–1905," *Representations* 14 (1986): 169–208.

4. This was one of the main themes in E. A. Osipov, I. V. Popov, and P. I. Kurkin, *Russkaia zemskaia meditsina* (Moscow, Obshchestvo Russkikh Vrachei, 1899).

5. For a brief examination of municipal public health issues in St. Petersburg, see James H. Bater, "Modernization and Public Health in St. Petersburg, 1890–1914," *Forschungen zur Osteuropäishchen Geschichte* 37 (1985): 357–372. Only in one civic hospital were residents and interns consulted about administrative decisions; see *Trudy obshchestva bol'nichnykh vrachei v S.-Peterburge za 1901 g.*, (St. Petersburg, 1903), 240 (hereafter cited as *Trudy OBV Spb*).

6. *Trudy OBV Spb*, 242.

7. Ibid., 3.

8. Ibid., 63.

9. See the lengthy report by S. S. Virsaladze in *Trudy OVB Spb*, 38–59, especially 56–59.

10. On the belief in science as a source of positive knowledge about society, see Alexander Vucinich, "Politics, Universities, and Science" in *Russia under the Last Tsar*, ed. T. G. Stavrou (Minneapolis: University of Minnesota Press, 1969), 177–178.

11. *Trudy OBV Spb*, 38.

12. Ibid., 233.

13. Ibid., 25.

14. *Trudy OBV Spb za 1903 g.*, 191–194.

15. Ibid., 20.

16. Ibid., 21.

17. *Russkii Meditsinskii Vestnik* 8 (1905): 30; on the banquet campaign itself, see Terence Emmons, "Russia's Banquet Campaign," *California Slavic Studies* 10 (1977): 43–86.

18. See the list of founding members in *Trudy OBV Spb za 1901*, 251–254, and the list of participants in *Pirogovskii S"ezd po Bor'be s Kholeroi, Moskva, 21–24 marta 1905 goda* (Moscow: S. P. Iakovlev, 1905), II: 252–275, (hereafter cited as *Pirogovskii S"ezd 1905 goda*).

19. Something of this tradition is apparent in Skorokhodov, *Materialy po istorii meditsinskoi mikrobiologii v dorevoliutsionnoi Rossii* (Moscow: Medgiz, 1948).

20. On Koch's position in Berlin, see Pauline M. H. Mazumdar, "Karl Landsteiner, and the Problem of Species, 1838–1868." Ph.D. diss., The Johns Hopkins University, 1976, 155.

21. Biographical and autobiographical fragments concerning some of the leading figures may be found in *Bor'ba za nauku v tsarskoi Rossii*. (Moscow-Leningrad, Gosudarstvennoe Sotsial'no-Ekonomicheskoe Izdatel'stvo, 1931).

22. For an analysis of a similar phenomenon in England, see Lloyd G. Stevenson, "Science down the Drain," *Bulletin of the History of Medicine* 29 (1955): 1–26.

23. For a fuller discussion of this confrontation, see John F. Hutchinson, "Tsarist Russia and the Bacteriological Revolution," *Journal of the History of Medicine and Allied Sciences*, 40 (1985): 428–429.

24. Frieden 1981, 241.

25. Hutchinson, "Tsarist Russia," 431–433.

26. The membership and powers of the Antiplague Commission are described by Dembo, *Vrachebnoe Pravo*, 52–53.

27. Hutchinson, "Tsarist Russia," 434–436.

28. For the reaction of physicians, see Frieden 1981, 291–295.

29. Ibid., 238–242.

30. Many of these criticisms, from a variety of sources, are cited in *Zhurnal ORVP*, no. 3–4 (1905): 318–322.

31. Dembo, *Vrachebnoe Pravo*, 54.

32. These developments are described in detail in Frieden 1981, 105–131, 201–228.

33. O. V. Petersen, "K istorii voznikoveniia Spb-ogo vrachebnogo obshchestva vzaimnoi pomoshchi," *Vestnik Spb-ogo vrachebnogo obshchestva vzaimnoi pomoshchi* 18 (1909): 15–18 (hereafter cited as *Vestnik SVOVP*).

34. Ibid., 17–18.

35. "Otchet Kaznacheia . . . 18-go marta 1900 g.," ibid., 38–42.

36. "Otchet Sekretaria . . . o deiatel'nosti obshchestva za 1900g.," ibid., 42–50.

37. M. N. Nizhegorodtsev, "Sanktpeterburgskoe vrachebnoe obshchestvo vzaimnoi pomoshchi i russkoe vrachebnoe soslovie," ibid., 4.

38. Ibid., 10–12.

39. For a full discussion, see O. Winkelmann, "Die Sitzungberichte der Ärztekammer Berlin-Brandenburg: Beitrag zur Geschichte der ärztlichen Strandespresse," *Zeitschrift für Ärztl. Fortbildung (Westberlin)* 53 (1964): 768–778.

40. On the role of the German government, see Kurt Glaser, *Vom Reichsgesundheitsrat zum Bundesgesundheitsrat: Ein Beitrag zur Geschichte des deutschen Gesundheitswesens* (Stuttgart, Thieme 1960).

41. Nizhegorodtsev, "Sanktpeterburgskoe vrachebnoe obshchestvo," 4.

42. See the entry on Councils of Barristers in *Entsiklopedicheskii slovar'* (St. Petersburg: Brokgauz-Efron, 1898) 25: 261.

43. For a full discussion, see M. N. Gernet, *Soslovnaia organizatsiia advokatury, 1864–1914. [Istoriia russkoi advokatury, tom 2.]* (Moscow: Izd. Sovetov Prisiazhnykh Poverennykh, 1916).

44. See Brian Levin-Stankevich, "Legal Professionals" in *Professionals and Professionalization in Tsarist Russia*, ed. Harley E. Balzer (Ithaca: Cornell University Press), forthcoming.

45. Nizhegorodtsev, "Sanktpeterburgskoe vrachebnoe Obshchestvo," 13.

46. His precise words enjoined them to "be steadfast, determined, holding on to those rights which we possess, seeking by legal means to achieve new and more equitable rights, and, while not exceeding the sphere of our competence, to work and work, guided by lessons of experience and sense, and relying on the dictates of our hearts." Ibid.

47. As an example of how "responsibly" Nizhegorodtsev and his colleagues were prepared to behave, one may cite their actions on behalf of the widow of a physician who was fatally beaten by the police: eschewing all publicity and criticism, they lobbied quietly behind the scenes, and the widow received 200 rubles from the office of His Imperial Majesty's Own Chancellery; for more information on such efforts, see *Vestnik SVOVP* 1 (1902): 38–42.

48. See, for example, A. Visloukh, "K kharakteristike fabrichno-zavodskoi meditsiny i eia predstavitelei," *Zhurnal ORVP*, no. 4 (1904): 303–319, and I. Voronov, "Obshche-stvennye usloviia zdorovia," *Meditsinskaia beseda* (Voronezh), no. 3–4 (1905): 65–77, no. 5–6: 114–130; see also R. B. Kaganovich, *Iz istorii bor'by s Tuberkulezom v Dorevoliutsionnoi Rossii* (Moscow, Izdatel'stvo Akademii Meditsinskikh Nauk SSSR, 1952).

49. Frieden 1981, 231–262.

50. According to E. I. Rodionova, *Ocherki istorii professional'nogo Dvizheniia Meditsinkikh Rabotnikov* (Moscow, Medgiz, 1962), 60, this council was to be composed of eleven physicians, two pharmacists, one feldsher, two nursing sisters, five interns, and an unspecified number of representatives of the city government.

51. On these events see Julie V. Brown, "The Professionalization of Russian Psychiatry: 1857–1911." Ph.D. diss., University of Pennsylvania, 1981, 352–357.

52. S. I. Mitskevich, *Zapiski vracha-obshchestvennika, 1888–1918 gg* (Moscow-Leningrad, Medgiz 1940), 134.

53. L. K. Erman, *Intelligentsiia v pervoi russkoi revoliutsii* (Moscow, Nauka, 1966), 83.

54. Mitskevich, *Zapiski vracha-obshchestvennika*, 134.

55. The work of the congress was divided into five sections: (1) history and epidemiology of cholera; (2) pathology and treatment; (3) bacteriology, vaccination, and disinfection; (4) general preventive measures; (5) specific organizational measures to combat an epidemic.

56. For the political background to these events, see S. Galai, *The Liberation Movement in Russia, 1900–1905* (Cambridge: Cambridge University Press, 1973) and T. Riha, *A Russian European: Paul Miliukov in Russian Politics* (Notre Dame: University of Notre Dame Press, 1969).

57. *Pirogovskii S"ezd 1905 goda*, II: vi–viii.

58. Frieden 1981, 297–305.

59. *Pirogovskii S"ezd 1905 goda*, I: 24.

60. Ibid., 22.

61. Ibid., 26.

62. All quotations in this paragraph are from the text of this resolution, which may be found in *Pirogovskii S"ezd 1905 goda*, II: 209–210.

63. These included demands for civil rights; equality before the law; equal rights for nationalities, languages, and religions; free compulsory education; separation of church and state; broad local autonomy; a progressive income tax; the abolition of redemption payments; a series of land reforms; the eight-hour day; a minimum wage; workers' insurance; and laws to protect occupational health and safety. Ibid., 210.

64. Ibid., 211.

65. This resolution was passed before the congress was declared closed, and the union's first meeting was held after a short break—a maneuver, as Frieden rightly observes, designed to protect the Pirogov Society from legal responsibility for the actions of the union. Frieden 1981, 305.

66. Mitskevich, *Zapiski vracha-obshchestvennika*, 138.

67. The text appears in *Pirogovskii S"ezd 1905 goda*, II: 211.

68. Rodionova, *Ocherki istorii professional'nogo dvizheniia*, 61. Sources are too sketchy to permit a breakdown of these figures; nevertheless, if the figure of 25,000 is even close to being accurate, then the union must have gained some adherents among medical personnel who were neither radical zemstvo nor hospital physicians.

69. Erman, *Intelligentsiia*, 100.

70. Rodionova, *Ocherki istorii professional'nogo dvizheniia*, 61–62.

71. Ibid.

72. Mitskevich, *Zapiski vracha-obshchestvennika*, 139. Militant radicalism among community physicians breathed its last in Moscow where, during the December general strike, some members of the local branch of the union organized an unofficial Red Cross committee to provide assistance to wounded strikers and other victims among the general populace. Ibid., 140; for a somewhat different version, see Rodionova, *Ocherki istorii professional'nogo dvizheniia*, 62.

73. G. I. Dembo's attempt to rally his conservative colleagues to support a revised version of a professional union of physicians was a dismal failure, as he later admitted in *Vestnik SVOVP* 23–24 (1912): 15.

3: COMMUNITY MEDICINE IN DISARRAY, 1907–1913

1. G. A. Berdichevskii, "K otsenke polozheniia," *Zhurnal ORVP*, no. 1 (1908): 5–27.

2. For a stimulating discussion of this problem in its American context, see Russell C. Maulitz, "'Physician versus Bacteriologist': The Ideology of Science in Clinical Medicine" in *The Therapeutic Revolution: Essays in the Social History of American Medicine*, eds. Morris J. Vogel and Charles E. Rosenberg (Philadelphia: University of Pennsylvania Press, 1979), 91–107.

3. The role of specialization in the development of modern medicine has been critically analyzed by Rosemary Stevens in separate works on England and the United States.

See her *Medical Practice in Modern England: The Impact of Specialization and State Medicine* (New Haven: Yale University Press, 1966) and *American Medicine and the Public Interest* (New Haven: Yale University Press, 1971).

4. On developments in Germany, see George Rosen, *From Medical Police to Social Medicine: Essays on the History of Health Care* (New York: Science History Publications, 1974), and Gertrud Kroeger, *The Concept of Social Medicine as Presented by Physicians and Other Writers in Germany, 1779–1932* (Chicago: Julius Rosenwald Fund, 1937).

5. The best account of Stolypin's reform plans and their fate is to be found in Weissman, *Reform in Tsarist Russia*, 124–175.

6. G. I. Dembo, "Voprosy vrachebnogo byta na X Pirogovskom S"ezde," *Vestnik SVOVP*, no. 15–16 (1907): 28.

7. "To achieve its goals the branch shall occupy itself with the elaboration of questions concerning public health by studying the medical-sanitary conditions of its own region, the occupational conditions of life and labour of the population, the organization of medical-sanitary affairs, of medical education, and of medical expertise of all kinds; [and] it shall establish mutual relations between medical institutions and societies in conformity with the basic tasks of the branch." Ibid., 28.

8. Its proceedings were published; see *Desiatyi s"ezd russkikh vrachei v pamiat' N. I. Pirogova*, pod. red. G. I. Dembo.

9. Dembo, "Voprosy Vrachebnogo byta," 29.

10. Ibid.

11. Ibid.

12. Ibid.

13. On this subject see Weissman, *Reform in Tsarist Russia*, 153–175; V. S. Diakin, "Stolypin i dvorianstvo (proval mestnoi reformy)" in *Problemy krest'ianskogo zemlevladeniia i vnutrennoi politiki Rossii* (Leningrad: Nauka, 1972), 231–274; A. Ia. Avrekh, *Stolypin i Tret'ia Duma* (Moscow: Nauka, 1968); Geoffrey A. Hosking, *The Russian Constitutional Experiment: Government and Duma, 1907–1914* (Cambridge: Cambridge University Press, 1973); Roberta Thompson Manning, "Zemstvo and Revolution: The Onset of the Gentry Reaction, 1905–1907" in *The Politics of Rural Russia 1905–1914*, ed. Leopold H. Haimson (Bloomington: Indiana University Press, 1979).

14. G. A. Berdichevskii, "K otsenke polozheniia," *Zhurnal ORVP*, no. 1 (1908): 5–27.

15. Ibid., especially 12 ff.

16. S. N. Igumnov, "K voprosu o krizise v zemskoi meditsine," *Zhurnal ORVP*, no. 3 (1908): 283–295.

17. Ibid., 289.

18. Ibid., 290.

19. Ibid., 294–295.

20. For recent treatments of the *Vekhi* controversy, see Christopher Read, *Religion, Revolution and the Russian Intelligentsia, 1900–1912* (London: The Macmillan Press Ltd., 1979), and Richard Pipes, *Struve: Liberal on the Right, 1905–1944* (Cambridge: Harvard University Press, 1980), 66–114.

21. N. A. Vigdorchik, "Voprosy narodnogo zdorov'ia i vrachebnogo byta. 1908-i god," *Obshchestvennyi Vrach*, no. 1 (1909): 13.

22. Ibid., 14.

23. *VOG*, part IV (1911): 1377. (See note 12, chapter 1.)

24. Ibid., 1062–1063.

25. Ibid., 1377.

26. See the report of a discussion of this problem by the sanitary council of Kostroma *guberniia* in 1910: *VOG*, part IV (1910): 874–875. On the eve of the war, the situation remained extremely difficult for northern provinces and towns in Siberia; see the advertisements for vacant positions in *VOG*, part IV (1914): 322–323.

27. *VOG*, part IV (1913): 1035.

28. Ibid.

29. *Obshchestvennyi Vrach*, no. 2 (1911): 43.

30. "O chastnoi praktike zemskikh vrachei," *Obshchestvennyi Vrach*, no. 2 (1911): 43–49. Slavskii had previously worked in the provinces of Tambov, Voronezh, Kaluga, and Nizhnii Novgorod.

31. Ibid., 45.

32. Despite the prevalence of stationary facilities such as hospitals and dispensaries in zemstvo provinces, physicians were liable to prosecution if they failed to go immediately to the assistance of a sick person who had summoned them.

33. Ibid., 48–49.

34. Ibid., 49.

35. D. N. Zhbankov, "Zemskaia meditsina i chastnaia praktika," *Obshchestvennyi Vrach*, no. 8 (1911): 14–28; other contributions were by R. E. Gorvits, "Po voprosu o chastnoi praktike zemskikh vrachei," ibid., no. 4 (1911): 63–66, and R. Matrasovich, "Po voprosu o chastnoi praktike zemskikh vrachei," ibid., no. 5 (1911): 32–35.

36. Zhbankov, "Zemskaia meditsina," 24.

37. His point about the burden of zemstvo taxation has been corroborated by modern research. See Dorothy Atkinson, "The Zemstvo and the Peasantry" in Emmons and Vucinich, *Zemstvo in Russia*, 101–105.

38. Zhbankov, "Zemskaia meditsina," 28. His hostility towards medical entrepreneurship must have been fortified by an incident that occurred in 1912 in Saratov *guberniia*. The sanitary council, informed that something was amiss at the zemstvo hospital in Petrovsk, discovered that the hospital physicians were holding surgery at home in the mornings; needless to say, such behavior was forbidden. *VOG*, part IV (1914): 137–138.

39. I. I. Molleson himself founded the sanitary bureau in Saratov, while the *narodnik* publicist M. S. Uvarov ran the bureau in Kherson. On Molleson's recommendation, Uvarov trained N. I. Teziakov, who went on to establish a sanitary bureau in Voronezh and then to succeed Molleson in Saratov. Kh. I. Idel'chik, *N. I. Teziakov i ego rol' v razvitii zemskoi meditsiny i stroitel'stve sovetskogo zdravo okhraneniia* (Moscow: Medgiz, 1960), 29–33.

40. For the text of this proposal, see *VOG*, no. 4 (1908): 1963–1966.

41. Vigdorchik, "Voprosy narodnogo," 14–15.

42. Ibid., 11.

43. Ibid., 15–16.

44. M. M. Gran', "Sposobny-li vrachi k ob"edineniiu?" *Vrachebnaia Gazeta*, no. 6 (1909): 178–184; no. 7: 208–215.

45. See A. V. Amsterdamskii's telling report on the 1910 Congress in *VOG*, part IV (1910): 1396–1415, especially 1406.

46. The proposed "Pirogov House" was designed to house the society's official, editorial, and committee activities and to provide a lecture theater and various amenities for members. Insufficient funds were collected to begin construction before war broke out in 1914, and the plan was shelved until the conclusion of hostilities. See Zhbankov's review of the proposal at the 1917 Congress: *Trudy chrezvychainogo s"ezda*, 55–56.

47. On this hostility, see the dissertation by Brown, "Professionalization," 166–195, 303–323.

48. G. I. Dembo, "Voprosy vrachebnogo byta na X Pirogovskom S"ezde," *Vestnik SVOVP*, no. 15–16 (1907): 22.

49. Ibid.

50. Its transactions were published in full; see *Trudy pervogo vserossiiskogo s"ezda fabrichnykh vrachei*, 2 vols. (Moscow, 1910).

51. Ibid., vol. II, 83–170.

52. *Trudy XI Pirogovskogo S"ezda* (St. Petersburg, 1913), vol. 3, 149–169.

53. A. Amsterdamskii, "XI Pirogovskii S"ezd 21–28 apr. 1910 g. v Peterburge," *VOG*, part IV (1910): 1400.

54. For its proceedings, see *Trudy soveshchaniia po bakteriologii, epidemiologii i prokaze* (St. Petersburg: A. E. Vineke, 1912).

55. *VOG*, part IV (1910): 1399.

56. *Trudy XI Pirogovskogo S"ezda* (St. Petersburg, 1911), vol. 1, 359–372.

57. *VOG*, part IV (1910): 1399.

58. Entitled "Novye puti v zemskoi meditsine," Brok's article appeared in *Vrachebno-Sanitarnyi Khronik Khersonskoi gubernii 1910, vypusk IV*; see also the summary in *VOG*, part IV (1911): 728–730.

59. Ibid., 729.

60. *VOG*, part IV (1910): 1681–1683. Sysin's article first appeared in *Svedeniia san. biuro Nizheg. zemstva*, no. 7 (1910).

61. Ibid., 1682.

62. S. N. Igumnov, "Osnovnoe napravlenie deiatel'nosti zemskikh sanitarnykh vrachei i ikh podgotovka," *Trudy XI Pirogovskogo S"ezda* (St. Petersburg, 1911), vol. 1, 352–355.

63. A. Amsterdamskii, "XI Pirogovskii S"ezd 21–28 apr. 1910 g. v. Peterburge," *VOG*, part IV (1910): 1397.

64. I. D. Strashun, *Russkaia obshchestvennaia meditsina v period mezhdu dvumia revoliutsiami, 1907–1917* (Moscow: Meditsina 1964), 84 ff. Igumnov's concerns about the role of bacteriology were shared outside Russia and well into the twentieth century. For an extraordinarily similar statement of the view that bacteriology is a deflection, if not an outright defection from the "organically sound development" of the public health movement, see Iago Galdston, "Humanism and Public Health," *Bulletin of the History of Medicine* 8 (1940): 1032–1039. A quite different objection to bacteriology, namely that it failed to distinguish between the separate settings of clinic and laboratory, was advanced by the German physician Ottomar Rosenbach; see his *Physician versus Bacteriologist*, trans. Achilles Rose (New York, 1904); for comment, see Maulitz's essay in Vogel and Rosenberg, *Therapeutic Revolution*, 97–98.

65. A. Amsterdamskii, "XI Pirogovskii S"ezd 21–28 apr. 1910 v. Peterburge," *VOG*, part IV (1910): 1398.

66. E. I. Iakovenko, "Zemskaia sanitarnaia gigieno-bakteriologicheskaia laboratoriia, eia zadachi i ustroistvo," *Trudy soveshchaniia po bakteriologii*, 104–109.

67. Ibid., 109–110.

68. Strashun, *Russkaia obshchestvennaia meditsina*, 91–92. The proceedings of both conferences have been published: *Trudy vtorogo soveshchaniia po voprosam bakteriologii i epidemiologii* (Moscow, 1912) and *Trudy soveshchaniia po sanitarnym i sanitarno-statisticheskim voprosam* (Moscow: Obshchestvennyi Vrach, 1912).

69. Strashun, *Russkaia obshchestvennaia meditsina*, 92.

70. For a sketch of Sysin's career, see I.D. Strashun, "A. N. Sysin kak obshchestvennyi deiatel'," *Gigiena i Sanitariia*, no. 6 (1957): 52–55; idem, *Russkaia obshchestvennaia meditsina*, 92.

71. See, for example, N. A. Kost', *Obschchestvennyi Vrach*, no. 1 (1913): 1–17.

72. For the origins and work of the commission, see Frieden 1981, 181–185.

73. Baldwin Latham's sanitary improvements in Croydon, England, seem to have been particularly influential; for an appreciation of his work by a Russian sanitary physician, see I. V. Poliak, "K voprosu ob ekonomicheskom znachenii narodnogo zdraviia," *Gigiena i Sanitariia*, no. 15–16 (1912): 137–140. For a full exposition of Latham's ideas and work, see Baldwin Latham, *Sanitary Engineering*, 2d ed. (London: E. & F. N. Spon, 1878).

74. E. [G.] M.[unblit], "Spetsializatsiia i obshchestvennost' v zemskoi meditsine," *Obshchestvennyi Vrach*, no. 6 (1912): 747.

75. Ibid., 750–751.

76. S. Igumnov, "Kharakter i obshchie zadachi zemskoi sanitarii v eia proshlom i nastoiashchem," *Obshchestvennyi Vrach*, no. 3 (1912): 307–319. Not all sanitary physicians of his generation were as resistant to change as Igumnov. N. I. Teziakov, who headed successively the sanitary bureaus of Perm, Kherson, Voronezh, and Saratov *gubernii*, strove to keep abreast of the latest scientific and technical information in hygiene and sanitation, while maintaining close connections with his *uchastok* physicians and organizing hygiene education for the people. For an appreciation of his career, see Idel'chik, *N. I. Teziakov*, passim.

77. On this point see Munblit, "Spetsializatsiia," 745, and Kost', *Obshchestvennyi Vrach*, no. 1 (1913): 17.

78. Munblit, "Spetsializatsiia," 752.

79. Kost', *Obschchestvennyi Vrach*, no. 1 (1913): 17.

80. Richard Charques, *Twilight of Imperial Russia* (Oxford: Oxford University Press, 1958), 140.

81. For an outstanding example of one Russian's ability to view the rest of the world through the prism of zemstvo medicine, see G. I. Dembo's four-part article, "V za-

koldovannom krugu. (K proektu o ministerstve narodnogo zdraviia)," *Vrachebnaia Gazeta*, no. 43 (1910): 1251–1255; no. 44: 1295–1301; no. 45: 1338–1443; no. 46: 1384–1391.

82. The English experience is thoroughly explored in R. A. Lewis, *Edwin Chadwick and the Public Health Movement, 1832–1854* (London: Longmans, 1952); S. E. Finer, *The Life and Times of Sir Edwin Chadwick* (London: Methuen, 1952); and R. J. Lambert, *Sir John Simon* (London: MacGibbon and Kee, 1964).

83. See A.-L. Shapiro, "Private rights, public interest, and professional jurisdiction: The French public health law of 1902," *Bulletin of the History of Medicine* 54 (1980): 4–22.

84. On this radical trend, see Louis Chevalier, *Labouring Classes and Dangerous Classes* (London: Routledge and Kegan Paul, 1973), 125–146; Erwin H. Ackerknecht, "Hygiene in France," *Bulletin of the History of Medicine* 22 (1948): 117–155; and William L. Coleman, *Death Is a Social Disease: Public Health and Political Economy in Nineteenth-Century France* (Madison: University of Wisconsin Press, 1982).

85. A. Amsterdamskii, "XI Pirogovskii S"ezd 21–28 apr. 1910 g. v Peterburge," *VOG*, part IV (1910): 1399–1400.

86. The pamphlet, entitled *K voprosu o Ministerstve Narodnogo Zdraviia*, was published as no. 5 in the *Biblioteka Zhurnala "Gigiena i Sanitariia"* (St. Petersburg, 1910); the original (untitled) version was the editorial in *Gigiena i Sanitariia* 2, no. 20–21: 398–428.

87. Gamaleia, *K voprosu*, 16–18.

88. Ibid., 29.

89. Ibid., 31.

90. Ibid., 32.

91. The editorial board for 1911 included K. V. Karaffa-Korbutt, a leading forensic physician; D. P. Nikol'skii, a specialist in industrial hygiene and social diseases; N. I. Teziakov, head of the sanitary bureau in Saratov *guberniia*; Z. G. Frenkel', physician and prominent member of the Constitutional Democratic Party; M. S. Uvarov, editor of the Ministry of the Interior's *Vestnik Obshchestvennoi Gigieny, Sudebnoi i Prakticheskoi Meditsiny;* and N. G. Freiberg, author of the authoritative compendium of Russian medical and sanitary law. With the exception of Karaffa-Korbutt, all of these individuals were active members of the Pirogov Society.

92. I. V. Poliak, "O roli pravitel'stvennykh i obshchestvennykh organov narodnogo zdraviia," *Gigiena i Sanitariia* II, no. 14 (1910): 55–75.

93. Ia. Iu. Kats, "O ministerstve narodnogo zdraviia," *Obshchestvennyi Vrach*, no. 1 (1911): 38–50. For earlier, negative opinions from zemstvo physicians on the need for a ministry of public health, see K. Turovskii, "Nuzhno-li Ministerstvo narodnogo zdraviia? (Mnenie zemskogo vracha)," *Russkii Vrach*, no. 1 (1911): 19–21, and V. Podel'skii, "Po povodu Ministerstva narodnogo zdraviia," ibid., no. 3 (1911): 91–92.

94. Kats, "O ministerstve," 46.

95. Ibid., 47.

96. Ibid., 50.

97. *Dvenadtsatyi Pirogovskii S"ezd, Peterburg, 29 maia–5 iiunia 1913 g. Vypusk II* (St. Petersburg, 1913), 150–152, 232–239.

4: THE GOVERNMENT AND MEDICAL REFORM

1. Riots during epidemics have a long history in Russia. The ugly incidents that occurred during the greatest outbreak of plague in the eighteenth century are described in John T. Alexander, *Bubonic Plague in Early Modern Russia: Public Health and Urban Disaster* (Baltimore: Johns Hopkins University Press, 1980), 177–201.

2. The zemstvo physicians' campaign against the Hospital Statute is described in detail in Frieden 1981, 166–173.

3. The best discussion of this problem from the point of view of the bureaucrats in St. Petersburg is Weissman, *Reform in Tsarist Russia*, 15–17.

4. For a discussion of public health organization in the major European states, see Albert Palmberg, *A Treatise on Public Health and Its Application in Different European Countries*, trans. Arthur Newsholme (London, Sonnenschein, 1895).

5. On the origins of this attitude, see George Rosen, "Cameralism and the Concept of Medical Police," *Bulletin of the History of Medicine* 27 (1953): 21–42; idem, "The Fate of

the Concept of Medical Police," *Centaurus* 5 (1957): 97–113; Marc Raeff, *The Well-Ordered Police State: Social and Institutional Change through Law in the Germanies and Russia, 1600–1800* (New Haven: Yale University Press, 1983), 130 ff.

6. See Orlovsky, *Limits of Reform,* passim.

7. On the origins of the Medical Council, see John T. Alexander, "Medical Chancery" in *The Modern Encyclopedia of Russian and Soviet History,* ed. Joseph L. Wieczynski (Gulf Breeze, Fla.: Academic International Press, 1981), 21: 167–173.

8. Its transactions were fully published: *Trudy Komissii uchrezdennoi pri meditsinskom sovete pod pred. S. P. Botkina po voprosu ob uluchenii sanitarnykh uslovii i umensheniia smert'nosti v Rossii* (St. Petersburg, Tipografiia Ministerstva Vnutrennikh Del', 1888). They also appeared in *Mezhdunarodnaia Klinika* 5 (1886) and 6 (1887). The commission is discussed in E. A. Osipov, I. V. Popov, and P. I. Kurkin, *Russkaia zemskaia meditsina* (Moscow, 1889), 35–36; see also Frieden 1981, 137–138.

9. See Frieden 1981, 135–178.

10. On the ministry's preference for "able men" (*sposobnye liudi*) rather than experts or specialists, see Orlovsky, *Limits of Reform,* 112.

11. The most detailed account of these changes is by V. Gubert, "Zapiska o preobrazovanii tsentral'nogo upravleniia grazhdanskoi meditsinskoi chast'iu . . . ," *Zhurnal ROONZ* 21, no. 2 (1911): 72–78; no. 3: 72–74; no. 4: 72–75. For contemporary medical reaction, see *Zhurnal ORVP,* no. 4 (1902): 255–259; no. 1–2 (1904): 113–115, no. 3 (1904): 243–249. For a recent account, see Frieden 1981, 288–290.

12. In 1905 von Anrep received a salary of 10,000 rubles, while that of his rival S. N. Gerbel was 12,000 rubles. Figures from *Spisok vysshikh chinov tsentral'nykh i mestnykh ustanovlenii Ministerstva Vnutrennikh Del' Chast' I* (St. Petersburg: Tipografiia Ministerstva Vnutrennikh Del', 1905), 74, 95.

13. It is regrettable that von Anrep, whose career spanned medical education and administration, government service, and politics—he was an Octobrist deputy in the Third Duma—left no memoirs; this account is based on the version given by G. E. Rein, *Iz perezhitogo 1907–1918* (Berlin, Parabola, n.d.), I: 70–71.

14. On the already difficult position of the provincial governors, see George L. Yaney, *The Systematization of Russian Government: Social Evolution in the Domestic Administration of Imperial Russia, 1711–1905* (Urbana: University of Illinois Press, 1973), 330–337, and Richard G. Robbins, Jr., *The Tsar's Viceroys: Russian Provincial Governors in the Last Years of the Empire* (Ithaca: Cornell University Press, 1987), 63–90.

15. On Stolypin's plans for local government, see Weissman, *Reform in Tsarist Russia,* 136–142.

16. On Stolypin's attempts to work with the Duma, see especially Hosking, *Russian Constitutional Experiment.*

17. Rein, *Iz perezhitogo,* I: 30. For reactions in the medical press to the proceedings of the Malinovskii Commission, see *Prakticheskii Vrach,* no. 12 (1907): 227–228; no. 22: 415–416; no. 39: 704–705; no. 43: 787–789.

18. Rein claims that Nicholas II's Imperial Rescript of 11 August 1908 was the first radical step in the reform of public health in Russia. It certainly was a significant departure from the established pattern of appointing special commissions to deal with epidemics only after they had assumed threatening proportions. Rein, *Iz perezhitogo,* I: ii.

19. The presidency had fallen vacant because of the retirement of L. F. Ragozin, who had been moved into the position in 1902 to curb his opposition to Plehve's reorganization of the MVD; see Frieden 1981, 287–289.

20. For Rein's account of his interview with Stolypin, see Rein, *Iz perezhitogo,* I: 5–6.

21. These biographical details were gleaned primarily from his memoirs. Rein, *Iz perezhitogo,* I: 7–14.

22. Rein, *Iz perezhitogo,* I: 72.

23. Ibid., 59.

24. For a thorough analysis of working conditions in the Donbass, see Theodore H. Friedgut, "Labor Violence and Regime Brutality in Tsarist Russia: The Iuzovka Cholera Riots of 1892," *Slavic Review* 46 (1987): 245–265.

25. *Russkoe Slovo,* no. 162 (16 July 1900): 4; no. 163 (17 July 1910): 4. Virtually every issue

of *Russkoe Slovo* for late July 1910 carries reports of riots or other incidents provoked by the cholera. In Kherson, physicians and feldshers working under police protection to bury the dead were threatened by a mob armed with rocks: ibid., no. 166 (21 July 1910): 3. In Voronezh, a feldsher was bombarded with rocks: ibid., no. 170 (25 July 1910): 4. The Governor of Samara *guberniia* arrested the president of the local branch of the right-wing Union of the Russian People for spreading (doubtlessly antisemitic) rumors about the cholera: ibid., no. 175 (31 July 1910): 3. In September, a doctor in the rural areas of Minsk *guberniia* was set upon by peasants who chanted, "drive out the doctor"; the peasants then went to a local "witch" to try to induce the cholera to move to another village: ibid., no. 218 (23 September 1910): 6.

26. The costs of special medical assistance, the council decided, were to be borne by the local zemstvo and municipal institutions (which could petition the Antiplague Commission for extra funds) and by the mineowners themselves. *Russkoe Slovo*, no. 167 (22 July 1910): 3. Significantly, S. N. Gerbel', a senior MVD official, publicly blamed the recurrence of cholera in South Russia on the appalling living conditions of the workers, especially those employed in mining. *Russkoe Slovo*, no. 171 (27 July 1910): 2.

27. Rein, *Iz perezhitogo*, I: 61–62; *Russkoe Slovo*, no. 171 (27 July 1910): 4.

28. Rein, *Iz perezhitogo*, I: 62.

29. *Russkoe Slovo*, no. 174 (30 July 1910): 3.

30. Rein, *Iz perezhitogo*, I: 62–64.

31. *Russkoe Slovo*, no. 176 (1 August 1910): 4.

32. Rein, *Iz perezhitogo*, I: 63.

33. Ibid.; *Russkoe Slovo*, no. 182 (10 August 1910): 3. While Rein was touring the stricken Don area, Chief Medical Inspector L. N. Malinovskii paid a visit to the city of Odessa to inspect its sanitary arrangements. There he aroused the ire of the *gradonachal'nik*, General Tolmachev, for pointing out faults in the city's antiplague measures: *Russkoe Slovo*, no. 211 (14 September 1910): 4. Tolmachev had directed a purge of liberals and socialists in Odessa after the 1905 Revolution: his clash with Malinovskii suggests that he found St. Petersburg bureaucrats no more palatable than local radicals.

34. *Russkoe Slovo*, no. 184 (10 August 1910): 3; ibid., no. 215 (19 September 1910): 4.

35. Rein, *Iz perezhitogo*, I: 64.

36. Rein reprints the full text of his report to the tsar; see ibid., I: 67–74.

37. Ibid., 72.

38. Ibid.

39. *Russkoe Slovo*, no. 236 (14 October 1910): 4.

40. Rein, *Iz perezhitogo*, I: 65.

41. Ibid., 66.

42. The Special Conference was set up on 22 October 1910, and its first meeting was held on 4 November.

43. L. B. Bertenson, V. N. Sirotinin, and V. G. Khlopin were elected by the Medical Council. Other members were S. N. Gerbel', *nachal'nik* of the Main Administration for Affairs of Local Economy, and his deputies N. N. Antsiferov and G. G. Vitte; Chief Medical Inspector L. N. Malinovskii and his assistants P. N. Bulatov and N. Ia. Shmidt. Rein, *Iz perezhitogo*, I: 91. Malinovskii, Bulatov, Antsiferov, and Vitte had already served on the earlier commission headed by von Anrep, as had Bertenson and Khlopin.

44. The text of the resolution appears in Rein, *Iz perezhitogo*, I: 75–88. Most of the eighty-three signatories were Octobrists, Nationalists, or Rightists. Several months earlier, the State Council had called upon the government to create a unified agency within the MVD to take charge of public health. See Rein, *Iz perezhigoto*, I: 74.

45. Ibid., 84.

46. Ibid., 84.

47. A full summary of the deliberations of the Krizhanovskii Conference is provided in Rein, *Iz perezhigoto*, I: 93–101.

48. The text of his report is reprinted in Rein, *Iz perezhigoto*, I: 104–123.

49. Ibid., 113.

50. Ibid., 105–108.

51. Ibid., 109.

52. Ibid., 96.
53. Ibid., 97.
54. Ibid., 98–99.
55. Ibid., 102.
56. Ibid., 156–157.
57. Ibid., 161–162.
58. N. G. Freiberg, *Vrachebno-sanitarnoe zakonodatel'stvo v Rossii*, 2nd ed. (St. Petersburg: V. Bezobrazov, 1908).
59. Soon after the formation of the Krizhanovskii Conference, Gamaleia, an admitted disciple of Havelock Ellis, had floated the idea of establishing an Institute of Public Health, which would draft sanitary legislation, train sanitary personnel to pass state examinations, and direct sanitary improvements at the local level. See his contribution to *Russkoe Slovo*, no. 270 (23 November 1910): 3. In all probability he saw himself as the first director of the institute; he continued to lobby for its establishment by means of his editorials in *Gigiena i Sanitariia*.
60. The names and positions of all those who served on the commission may be found in Rein, *Iz perezhigoto*, I: 175–179.
61. See, for example, the comments of A. S. Durnovo, "Sovremennaia zhizn' i narodnoe zdravie II," *Obshchestvennyi Vrach*, no. 10 (1912): 1218–1224.
62. Ibid., 1220.
63. See the complaints of an anonymous writer in *Promyshlennost' i Torgovlia*, no. 21 (1913): 402–403.
64. The draft statute, entitled "Osnovnye polozheniia glavnogo Upravleniia Gosudarstvennogo Zdravookhraneniia," may be found in Rein, *Iz perezhigoto*, I: 227–237. It was given final approval at the commission's meeting of 27 May 1913; see *Obshchii zhurnal*, 50–60, of the incomplete collection of papers of the Rein Commission in the possession of the National Library of Medicine, catalogued as *Russia. Mezhduvedomstvennaia Kommissiia po peresmotru vrachebno-sanitarnogo zakonodatel'stva. Sbornik* (hereafter cited as *Sbornik*).
65. On the role of *jurisconsults* in the MVD, see Orlovsky, *Limits of Reform*, 80–84.
66. On the intrusion of the central bureaucracy into the Russian countryside, see Yaney, *Systematization*, 230–248, 319–379.
67. For a summary, see Rein, *Iz perezhigoto*, I: 242–243.
68. The strengths of zemstvo medical and sanitary research lay in epidemic prevention, occupational mortality, and the sanitary condition of the laboring population. For a general survey, see P. E. Zabliudovskii, *Istoriia Otechestvennoi Meditsiny, Chast' I. Period do 1917 goda*, (Moscow: Tsentral'nyi Institut Usovershenstvovaniia Vrachei, 1960).
69. On the involvement of zemstvo physicians in the collection of medical statistics and the promotion of hygiene education, see Frieden 1981, especially 96–104, 179–199.
70. The details of the proposal may be found in K. P. Sulima, "Ob organizatsii vrachei v soslovie s pravami iurisdiktsii," *Obshchestvennyi Vrach*, no. 7 (1913): 814–825.
71. Ibid., 825.
72. For details, see Rein, *Iz perezhigoto*, I: 244.
73. Durnovo, "Sovremennaia zhizn'," *Obshchestvennyi Vrach*, no. 10 (1912): 1219, 1221.
74. *Russkoe Slovo*, no. 122 (29 May 1913): 2.
75. For a more detailed treatment of these events, see John F. Hutchinson, "Society, Corporation or Union? Russian Physicians and the Struggle for Professional Unity (1890–1913)," *Jahrbücher für Geschichte Osteuropas* 30 H.1 (1982): 50–51.
76. See the debate on this issue in the subcommittee on medical assistance: Rein Commission *Sbornik*, no. 7, *Obshchii zhurnal* II, 12–21.

5: WORLD WAR I AND THE CONTROL OF PUBLIC HEALTH
1. W. E. Gleason, "The All-Russian Union of Towns and the All-Russian Union of Zemstvos in World War I, 1914–1917." Ph.D. diss., Indiana University, 1972, 49 (hereafter cited as Gleason 1972).
2. M. V. Rodzianko, *The Reign of Rasputin: An Empire's Collapse*, trans. Catherine Zvegintsev (London: A. M. Philpot, 1927), 112.

3. For a description of the reform, see *Stoletie Voennogo Ministerstva 1802–1902*, tom VII, chast' IV, 338–344.

4. G. Gol'shukh, "K voprosu o sluzhebnom polozhenii tiuremnogo vracha," *Tiuremnyi Vestnik*, no. 4 (1910): 571.

5. The full list of serving personnel in the Main Military-Sanitary Administration may be found in *Stoletie*, tom VII, chast' IV, 349–351. Twenty-three of the fifty-five senior positions in the administration were held by physicians; of these, the majority were *doktory meditsiny* rather than *vrachi* and were graduates of the Military Medical Academy.

6. On the relative strength of the German and Russian armies in 1914, see Norman Stone, *The Eastern Front, 1914–1917* (London: Hodder and Stoughton, 1975), 37–43.

7. As late as December 1914, Evdokimov told a meeting of the medical committee of the Main Military-Sanitary Administration that the 100 beds available to his department at the Military Hospital in St. Petersburg, with 80 in reserve in Khar'kov, would suffice to deal with soldiers who became mentally ill during the war and that there was consequently no need for the Red Cross to become involved. His definition of war-related mental illness was so narrow that it failed to convince Russian psychiatrists, who believed that events had already proven him wrong. See *Psikhiatricheskaia Gazeta*, no. 24 (1914): 404, quoting a report in *Pravitel'stvennyi Vestnik*, 5 December 1914.

8. The full text of the *Polozhenie o Verkhovnom Nachal'nike sanitarnoi i evakuatsionnoi chasti* is reprinted in *Izvestiia po delam zemskogo i gorodskogo khoziaistva*, no. 10 (1914): 9–11.

9. The orders to Ol'denburg were drafted by the war minister and signed by Nicholas II. Suhkomlinov was thus implicated in exempting Ol'denburg's office from ministerial control. Although the last tsar is not known for driving shrewd political bargains, one wonders whether this was the price Suhkomlinov had to pay to protect Evdokimov and his deputies from imperial displeasure.

10. The origins of these two voluntary organizations are discussed in detail in Gleason 1972, 7–16.

11. According to the official report of the chief medical inspector, there were just over 24,000 civilian physicians in the empire at the end of 1913, 21,709 of them men and 2,322 women; the total number of beds available for civilian use was 227,868, of which 177,001 were in somatic hospitals, 43,324 in psychiatric hospitals, and 7,543 in maternity hospitals. Figures from *Otchet o sostoianii narodnogo zdraviia i organizatsiei vrachebnoi pomoshchi v Rossii za 1913 god* (St. Petersburg: Tipografiia Ministerstva Vnutrennikh Del', 1916). It was not official practice to record zemstvo medical services separately. One may reasonably estimate, however, that at least 25 percent of the physicians and 60 to 70 percent of the beds were controlled by the zemstvos and municipalities.

12. Gleason points out that Ol'denburg's line disregarded the fact that fifteen provincial zemstvos west of it had already joined the Union of Zemstvos. "The All-Russian Union of Zemstvos and World War I" in *Zemstvo in Russia*, Emmons and Vucinich, 366–367 (hereafter cited as Gleason 1982).

13. The use of line officers is reported by E. I. Lotova, "Sanitarno-epidemicheskoe sostoianie strany v gody pervoi mirovoi voiny (1914–1917)," *Sovetskoe zdravookhranenie*, no. 7 (1964): 77. For a unique account of the experiences of an American physician who worked with the Russian Army during the war, see Malcolm C. Grow, *Surgeon Grow: An American in the Russian Fighting* (New York: Stokes, 1918). I am indebted for this reference to Dr. Robert J. T. Joy.

14. Rein's recollections of the war period are in *Iz perezhitogo*, II, 49–133, 190–221. See also his testimony before the Investigating Commission of the Provisional Government in P. E. Shchegolev, ed., *Padenie Tsarskogo Rezhima* (Moscow-Leningrad: Gosizdat, 1926), vol. V, 1–31.

15. Z. P. Solov'ev, "Itogi vrachebno-sanitarnoi deiatel'nosti Zemskogo Soiuza i eia dal'neishie shagi," *Obshchestvennyi Vrach*, no. 7 (1916): 364.

16. The role, significance, funding, and staffing of the hospital trains are discussed in detail in Gleason 1972, 38–47. This section draws heavily on his account.

17. N. F. Nikolaevskii, "Obzor organizatsii i deiatel'nosti Sanitarnogo Otdela Glavnogo Komiteta Soiuza Gorodov," *Vrachebno-Sanitarnyi Vestnik*, no. 1–2 (1917): 74. On the general

state of urban sanitation on the eve of the war, see Lotova, "Sanitarno-epidemicheskoe sostoianie," 76–78. D. N. Zhbankov's survey of Russian towns was published by the Pirogov Society; see *Sbornik po gorodskomu delu.*

18. Lotova, "Sanitarno-epidemicheskoe-sostoianie," 78.

19. This incident is related in Teziakov's memoirs, the manuscript of which is in the Archive of the Semashko Institute in Moscow. Quoted by Lotova, "Sanitarno-epidemicheskoe sostoianie," 78.

20. Gleason 1972, 50, note 33.

21. Gleason, quoting *Izvestiia Vserossiiskogo Soiuza Gorodov,* no. 29 (15 December 1915): 19, reports a ratio of 1:16.4 in villages, compared with 1:20.8 in district towns and 1:43.5 in provincial towns. Gleason 1972, 50.

22. What follows summarizes his report, "Zemskaia meditsina v godinu voiny 1914–1915 gg.," published in *Obshchestvennyi Vrach,* no. 9–10 (1915): 537–562.

23. He made no estimate of the drop in local population owing to conscription, but it is highly unlikely that this reached 10 percent in one year in any one *uezd.*

24. Kurkin, "Zemskaia meditsina," 543.

25. Ibid., 542.

26. This account of the epidemiological consequences of the movement of refugees draws on Lotova, "Sanitarno-epidemicheskoe sostoianie," 79–80.

27. P. N. Diatroptov, "L. A. Tarasevich" in *Bor'ba za nauku,* 44.

28. Olga Metchnikoff, *Life of Elie Metchnikoff* (London: Constable, 1921), 210–218.

29. Ibid., 219.

30. The political sympathies of several *pirogovtsy* were first pointed out by P. Krug, "Russian Public Physicians and Revolution: The Pirogov Society, 1917–1920." Ph.D. diss., University of Wisconsin-Madison, 1979, 87–92. However, Krug classifies both Tarasevich and Diatroptov as "non-party medical scientists," a designation that obscures both the former's increasing radicalism and the latter's earlier arrest and exile for political reasons. Krug's attempt to divide the *pirogovtsy* into "professionals" and "politicals" is unfortunate; not only does it distort the position of individuals such as Tarasevich, but it also confers a nonexistent homogeneity of opinion upon the members of both groups. For example, although he classifies both D. N. Zhbankov and Z. P Solov'ev as "politicals," the abyss that separated the old-line *narodnik* from the Bolshevik *engagé* was enormous, probably greater than the distance that separated either of them from *pirogovtsy* who were neither Socialist Revolutionaries nor Social Democrats.

31. On Diatroptov's career see L. Ia. Skorokhodov, *Materialy po istorii meditsinskoi mikrobiologii v dorevoliutsionnoi Rossii* (Moscow: Medgiz, 1948), 292.

32. A useful summary of Solov'ev's prerevolutionary career is B. D. Petrov, "Zinovii Petrovich Solov'ev kak sanitarnyi vrach," *Gigiena i sanitariia,* no. 12 (1936): 8–16.

33. On Rusakov see B. D. Petrov, *Vrachi-Bolsheviki: Stroiteli Sovestkogo Zdravookhraneniia* (Moscow, Meditsina, 1973).

34. Sysin's remarkable career has been sympathetically reviewed by I. D. Strashun, "A. N. Sysin kak obshchestvennyi deiatel'," *Gigiena i sanitariia,* no. 6 (1957): 52–55.

35. Ibid., 53.

36. In 1907, he had published a damning attack on capitalist development and its effects on public health: L. B. Granovskii, "Obshchestvennoe zdravookhranenie i kapitalizm," *Zhurnal ORVP,* no. 5 (1907): 371–404; no. 6: 539–564.

37. On this see Gleason, "The All-Russian Union of Towns and the Politics of Urban Reform in Tsarist Russia," *Russian Review* 35, no. 3 (1976): 290–302 (hereafter cited as Gleason 1976); Gleason 1982, 365–382.

38. The extent to which the same individuals, wearing their two hats, dominated both the Pirogov Society and the medical staffs of the unions has not been fully appreciated. Thus Gleason 1972, 109–110, treats the wartime Pirogov conferences as if they were altogether separate organizations attended by representatives from the unions.

39. On the wartime activities of the Pirogov Society, see I. D. Strashun, *Russkaia obshchestvennaia meditsina v period mezhdu dvumia revoliutsiami 1907–1917* (Moscow, 1964), 177–83.

40. The best discussion of the wartime medical work of the unions is in Gleason 1972,

especially chapter 3, "Medical Operations on the Homefront," 33–55 and chapter 6, "The Health Crises," 107–137. See also T. I. Polner, *Russian Local Government during the War and the Union of Zemstvos* (New Haven, Yale University Press, 1930), and P. Gronsky and N. Astrov, *The War and the Russian Government* (New Haven: Yale University Press, 1929).

41. Its transactions were published by the Pirogov Society; see *Pirogovskoe soveshchanie bakteriologov i predstavitelei vrachebno-sanitarnykh organizatsii po bor'be s zaraznymi boleczniami v sviazi s voennym vremenem, Moskva, 28–30 dekabria 1914g.*; they were also printed in *Obshchestvennyi Vrach*, no. 2 (1915): 1–130.

42. Skorokhodov, *Materialy po istorii meditsinskoi mikrobiologii*, 316–317.

43. For a summary of the proceedings of the congress, see Strashun, *Russkaia obshchestvennaia meditsina*, 177–179; on the attitudes of physicians to the drink problem in the prewar period, see John F. Hutchinson, "Science, Politics and the Alcohol Problem in Post-1905 Russia," *Slavonic and East European Review* 58, no. 2 (April 1980): 232–254.

44. In this paragraph and those that follow, I have drawn heavily on Gleason's reconstruction of the unions' efforts to secure funds for antiepidemic work in the spring and summer of 1915; Gleason 1972, 109–122, especially 111–112.

45. Ibid., 112–115.

46. Ibid., 118–121.

47. The Special Council for Defense was created in August 1915 and brought together members of the State Duma, State Council, the two unions, the Central War-Industries Committee, and high military and civil bureaucrats. For varying assessments of its role see Bernard Pares, *The Fall of the Russian Monarchy* (New York: Knopf, 1939); Raymond Pearson, *Russian Moderates and the Crisis of Tsarism* (London: Macmillan, 1977); and George Katkov, *Russia 1917: The February Revolution* (London: Longmans Green, 1967).

48. Gleason 1972, 125–127. To be sure, vaccination programs and sanitary arrangements did not make the unions' medical personnel popular with the ordinary soldiers, sergeants, and junior officers, who liked to call them "Zemstvo hussars" [*zemgussari*] and taunt them with suggestions of cowardice. One does not expect common soldiers to have appreciated—as did their corps commanders—the army's medical requirements or the shortcomings of the Military-Sanitary Administration. The epidemiological problems involved were complex enough to tax physicians of many years' experience. It is, however, surprising to find the prejudices of contemporaries manifested again in the recent work of an American historian of the Russian army. Professor Allan Wildman repeats with unconcealed relish all the soldiers' gossip about *zemgussari* "stumbling over one another in the busy work [sic] of medical and delousing facilities, refugee evacuation centres, and backup supply services" and then barely manages to concede that "this dodge" did not always shelter "chronic shirkers from the grim side of war" by citing one memoir account of surgery in a field hospital. While it is undoubtedly true that there were some incompetents among union personnel at the front and in the rear, it is preposterous to suggest that all these activities were run by and for the benefit of privileged shirkers who, in Wildman's words, "nested in the swollen public organizations"; Allan K. Wildman, *The End of the Russian Imperial Army: The Old Army and the Soldiers' Revolt (March–April 1917)* (Princeton: Princeton University Press, 1980), 102–103.

49. Gleason 1972, 122, based on M. M. Kenigsberg's study for July–December 1915, published in *Izvestiia Vserossiiskogo Soiuza Gorodov*, nos. 31–32 (May 1916): 210–222.

50. For Lotova's assessment, see "Sanitarno-epidemicheskoe sostoianie," 80.

51. Z. P. Solov'ev, "Itogi vrachebno-sanitarnoi deiatel'nosti Zemskogo Soiuza i eia dal'neishie shagi," *Obshchestvennyi Vrach*, no. 7 (1916): 369.

52. S. Sukhanov, "O bol'nichnom prizrenii dushevno-bol'nykh v Rossii," *Psikhiatricheskaia Gazeta*, no. 24 (1914): 401.

53. Brown, "Professionalization of Russian Psychiatry," 341–376.

54. Ibid., 389. On the preference of local government for *patronazh* care in peasant families instead of institutionalization under professional psychiatrists, see her chapter 6, 301–335.

55. *Psikhiatricheskaia Gazeta*, no. 24 (1914): 404.

56. Ibid.

57. See the devastating critique of Evdokimov and the Russian Red Cross by L. B.

Blumenau, "Ob organizatsii vrachebnoi pomoshchi nervo-bol'nym voinam," *Psikhiatricheskaia Gazeta*, no. 1 (1915): 5–6.

58. No official statement to this effect was made, but see V. I. Iakovenko's speech to the meeting of city psychiatric hospital representatives in Moscow, reported in *Psikhiatricheskaia Gazeta*, no. 5 (1915): 83, and in *Russkie Vedomosti*, 16 February 1915.

59. On Bekhterev's role in the development of Russian psychiatry, see Brown, "Professionalization of Russian Psychiatry," 209–218; 230–231; 398, note 9.

60. The report is summarized in *Psikhiatricheskaia Gazeta*, no. 3 (1915): 51.

61. For the controversy over Diatroptov's action, see *Psikhiatricheskaia Gazeta*, no. 2 (1917): 43; no. 3: 77–79; no. 4: 106.

62. This seems a fair conclusion to draw from N. F. Nikolaevskii's description of the work of his bureau: "Obzor organizatsii i deiatel'nosti Sanitarnogo Otdela Glavnogo Komiteta Soiuza Gorodov," *Vrachebno-Sanitarnyi Vestnik*, no. 1–2 (1917): 73–87.

63. The physicians' deliberations on the problems expected to accompany demobilization may be followed in detail in the proceedings of the Medical-Sanitary Council of the Central Committee of the Union of Towns, beginning in late November 1916, printed in *Vrachebno-Sanitarnyi Vestnik*, no. 1–2 (1917): 105–153.

64. On this issue of urban reform, see Gleason 1976, 290–302.

65. Nikolaevskii blames the leadership of the Union of Towns for the delay in establishing a separate Sanitary Bureau; he also claims that "the peculiar constitution of the Central Committee" meant that little was done to improve sanitary conditions in cities along the front, evidently a euphemism for the committee's unwillingness to challenge the restrictions imposed by Prince Ol'denburg and the Russian Red Cross. N. F. Nikolaevskii, "Obzor organizatsii i deiatel'nosti Sanitarnogo Otdela Glavnogo Komiteta Soiuza Gorodov," *Vrachebno-Sanitarnyi Vestnik*, no. 1–2 (1917): 75–76, 84. For criticism of the union leadership for mishandling relations with the government over the anti-epidemic campaign, see *Vrachebno-Sanitarnyi Vestnik*, no. 1–2 (1917): 122.

66. Z. P. Solov'ev, "Itogi vrachebno-sanitarnoi deiatel'nosti Zemskogo Soiuza i eia dal'neishie shagi," *Obshchestvennyi Vrach*, no. 7 (1916): 363–373. A summary of its contents appears in the congress proceedings: *Pirogovskii s"ezd vrachei i predstavitelei vrachebno-sanitarnykh organizatsii 1916*, 4–6.

67. Solov'ev, "Itogi," 372. Although a new law establishing *volost'* zemstvo institutions was before the Fourth Duma, its property qualifications were regarded as a deliberate attempt by the government to restrict the role of the "village intelligentsia" in local affairs. For a discussion of the issues involved, see G. A. Kovalenko, "Volostnoe zemstvo i sel'skaia intelligentsia," *Volost' Zemstvo*, no. 2 (1917): 56–58.

68. Solov'ev, "Itogi," 372.

69. I. D. Strashun, "A. N. Sysin kak obshchestvennyi deiatel'," *Gigiena i Sanitariia*, no. 6 (1957): 53–54.

70. *Pirogovskii S"ezd Vrachei 1916*, 80–81.

71. Ibid., 78.

72. N. F. Nikolaevskii, "Obzor organizatsii i deiatel'nosti Sanitarnogo Otdela Glavnogo Komiteta Soiuza Gorodov," *Vrachebno-Sanitarnyi Vestnik*, no. 1–2 (1917): 85. All of the factual information in this paragraph comes from Nikolaevskii's report, 82–85.

73. Ibid., 86.

74. See "'Soveshchanie chlenov Sanitarno-Tekhnicheskikh Biuro Soiuza Gorodov (12–15 noiabriia 1916g.)," *Izvestiia Vserossiskogo Soiuza Gorodov*, no. 38 (April 1916): 115–151.

75. "Ot redaktsii," *Vrachebno-Sanitarnyi Vestnik*, no. 1–2 (1917): 1–2.

76. For an extraordinary example of this vision, in which Russian towns were to be turned into a sanitary reformer's paradise of cleanliness, discipline, hygiene education, and harmless amusements, see M. M. Kenigsberg, "Zadachi sanitarnykh popechitel'stv i organizatsiia obshchestvennogo prizreniia v obnovlennoi Rossii," *Vrachebno-Sanitarnyi Vestnik*, no. 1–2 (1917): 42–51.

77. "Municipal medicine has for too long followed in the footsteps of zemstvo medicine," said Granovskii at the meeting of 28 November 1916, in what was clearly an attempt to undermine the candidacy of L. A. Tarasevich and promote the election of A. N. Sysin

as President of the Council. When on 7 February 1917, it was proposed that the two unions cooperate in planning the conversion of their operations to a peacetime footing, Sysin spoke sharply of the "huge differences between city and country" which made such an alliance impossible, and Nikolaevskii and A. N. Merkulov agreed with him. Sysin proposed instead that the plan should be worked out by the newly created Central Bureau for Municipal Affairs of the Union of Towns. See *Vrachebno-Sanitarnyi Vestnik*, no. 1–2 (1917): 105–106, 137.

78. Rein described his maneuvering in some detail before the Extraordinary Investigating Commission in 1917; see P. E. Shchegolev, ed., *Padenie Tsarskogo Rezhima* (Moscow-Leningrad: Gosizdat, 1924), vol. V, 4–16.

79. Rein, *Iz perezhitogo*, II: 88; Shchegolev, *Padenie*, V: 16–17. Rein's old rival, L. N. Malinovskii, had been relieved of his post as Chief Medical Inspector in May 1916 and was simultaneously appointed to the Senate. His successor, A. N. Molodovskii, was a relative unknown in MVD circles. *Izvestiia po delam zemskogo i gorodskogo khozaistva*, no. 6–7 (1916): 16.

80. Rein, *Iz perezhitogo*, II: 132.

81. The frustration of the Council of Ministers over the increasing importance of the two unions is amply documented in M. Cherniavsky, *Prologue to Revolution: Notes of A. N. Iakhontov on the Secret Meetings of the Council of Ministers, 1915* (Englewood Cliffs, N.J., 1967).

82. This summary of his views is based on his own testimony: Shchegolev, *Padenie*, V: 8–9.

83. Ibid., 6.

84. See Zhbankov's report to the 1917 Pirogov Congress, *Trudy chrezvychainogo pirogovskogo s"ezda (Moskva. 4–8 Aprelia 1917 g.)*, 55–56 (hereafter cited as *Trudy 1917 g.*).

6: THE CLEANSING HURRICANE: MEDICAL POLITICS IN THE 1917 REVOLUTION

1. *Trudy 1917 g*, 56.

2. *Vestnik Vremmenogo Pravitel'stva*, no. 2/47 (7/20 March 1917): 2 (hereafter cited as *VVP*).

3. *VVP*, no. 3/49 (8/21 March 1917): 1; the appointment, initially *pro tem*, was confirmed four days later. Guchkov's precipitate actions earned him a stern but ineffectual rebuke from the Military-Sanitary Learned Committee, the members of which endeavored to carry on as if the regime had not collapsed: see *VVP*, no. 5/51 (10/23 March 1917): 3. Burdenko speedily replaced some of his section heads with experienced sanitary physicians; among the latter was N. I. Teziakov, appointed *nachal'nik* of the Sanitary Section of the Caucasian front. Idel'chik, *Teziakov*, 125–127.

4. The precise date and circumstances of the prince's dismissal are unclear, largely because his name was omitted from the published lists of tsarist officials relieved of their duties, but the news was certainly known by March 14, when the hastily reformed Red Cross executive held a meeting. See *VVP*, no. 10/56 (16/29 March 1917): 3.

5. *VVP*, no. 8/54 (14/27 March 1917): 3.

6. The full text of this resolution appears in *VVP*, no. 10/56 (16/29 March 1917): 3.

7. Zhbankov described this campaign in detail at the April 1917 Pirogov Congress. See *Trudy 1917 g*, 54–56.

8. For accounts of the trip to Petrograd by Tarasevich and Merkulov, see *Vrachebno-Sanitarnyi Vestnik*, no. 1–2 (March–April 1917): 101–102, 148–149. The version presented here draws on the report that Merkulov presented to a joint meeting of union, zemstvo, and municipal physicians in Moscow on 23 March 1917.

9. *Vrachebno-Sanitarnyi Vestnik*, no. 1–2 (March–April 1917): 101–102.

10. For a complete list of those attending and their institutional affiliations, see ibid., 101. Also in attendance were the Chief Medical Inspector of the City of Moscow and his assistant and I. V. Rusakov, official representative of the Pirogov Society executive.

11. Ibid., 102. The committee of eleven was to be composed of Commissar Almazov, plus one representative each from the Military-Sanitary Administration, the Fleet Sanitary Administration, the Office of the Chief Medical Inspector, the Red Cross, the Union of Zemstvos, the Union of Towns, and the Soviet of Workers' and Soldiers' Deputies and

three representatives of the Central Medical-Sanitary Council. One representative of the United Front Organizations was added to the proposal at the March 23 meeting. See *Vremennoe Polozhenie o tsentral'nykh vrachebno-sanitarnykh organov v Rossii,* ibid., 103–105.

12. Ibid., 102.

13. *Trudy 1917 g,* 57.

14. Indeed, at the meeting on 23 March 1917, K. G. Slavskii, a Moscow *uezd* physician, took the position that zemstvos and towns must be represented directly, not indirectly by the Union of Zemstvos or the Union of Towns. He was not alone in enunciating this viewpoint. See *Vrachebno-Sanitarnyi Vestnik,* no. 1–2 (March–April 1917): 102.

15. The published records of the 1917 Pirogov Congress are a historian's nightmare. Only the texts of the resolutions are reliable; both the debates and the reports depend entirely on versions supplied to the editor by the participants themselves. The minutes of the final session—at which the resolutions were adopted—are, unfortunately, especially cursory.

16. *Trudy 1917 g,* 53.

17. VVP, no. 23/69 (5/18 April 1917): 2. The funds, papers, and materials of the Rein Commission were transferred to the office of the Chief Medical Inspector "pending the holding of a congress to work out the bases for the administration of medical and sanitary affairs."

18. *Trudy 1917 g,* 57.

19. *Trudy 1917 g,* 58. Peter Krug's version of this speech suggests that Zhbankov was opposed only to a "bureaucratic" central agency, but not to one dominated by community physicians. Yet Zhbankov made no such qualification when issuing his blanket denunciation of central agencies, and he specifically called for the representation of citizens to ensure "the broadest and most active participation of the population in the creation of the new order." Ibid., 57. Zhbankov's naive populism assumed that scientists, physicians, and citizens would all instruct each other in an atmosphere of harmony; hence he saw no reason why community physicians should seek power for themselves. For Krug's treatment, see Krug, "Russian Public Physicians," 107.

20. For criticisms of Zhbankov's views, see *Trudy 1917 g,* 4, 6, 15.

21. *Trudy 1917 g,* 7.

22. Ibid.

23. *Trudy 1917 g,* 4–21, 59–61.

24. See, for example, Mark G. Field, "Medical Organization and the Medical Profession" in *The Transformation of Russian Society: Aspects of Social Change Since 1861,* ed. Cyril E. Black (Cambridge: Harvard University Press, 1960), 545–549. P. Krug's treatment correctly underlines continuing Pirogov suspicions about central bureaucratic agencies but misses the significance of the pressure exerted on Almazov by the union physicians from Moscow. See Krug, "Russian Public Physicians," 101–123.

25. Both the text of his proposal and his covering memorandum are printed in *Vrachebno-Sanitarnyi Vestnik,* no. 1–2 (March–April 1917): 98–100.

26. Ibid., 99.

27. For purposes of comparison, the composition of the council as in the Moscow proposal is given alongside that in Almazov's recommendation and that of his temporary advisory committee (see table, p. 225).

28. The text of this letter appears in *Vrachebno-Sanitarnyi Vestnik,* no. 1–2 (March–April 1917): 93–96.

29. Ibid., 94.

30. Ibid., 95.

31. The additional six included one representative each from the Ministry of Finance and the State Control, two elected by the Pirogov Congress, and two from the united hospital funds of Petrograd and Moscow. Ibid.

32. Ibid., 92.

33. *Vrachebnaia Zhizn',* no. 1 (15 August 1917): 10–11; VVP, no. 58/104 (19 May/1 June 1917): 2.

34. VVP, no. 64/110 (27 May/9 June 1917): 3.

COMPARISON OF COUNCIL COMPOSITION, 1917 (See Note 27)

	Composition of the Executive Committee, Moscow Proposal of 23 March 1917		Composition of the Central Medical Sanitary Council as Recommended by Almazov		Composition of Almazov's Temporary Advisory Committee
1	Commissioner	1		1	
1	Military Sanitary Administration	1		1	
1	Sanitary Administration of Fleet	1		1	
1	Office of Chief Medical Inspector	1	the same	1	the same
1	Red Cross	1		1	
1	Union of Zemstvos	1		1	
1	Union of Towns	1		1	
1	Soviet of Workers' & Soldiers' Deputies	1			
1	President of full Council	1	Central War Industries Committee		
1	United Front Organization	1	Ministry of Ways & Communications	1	Ministry of Ways & Communications
2	Representatives of Zemstvo members of Full Council	1	Main Administration of General Staff	1	(?) United Committee of the Military-Sanitary Organization of the Northern Front
1	Moscow municipal administration	1			
1	Moscow *guberniia* zemstvo	1		1	Petrograd City Committee, Union of Towns
1	Petrograd Municipal administration	1			
1	St. Petersburg *guberniia* zemstvo	1			
16		15		10	(?)

Source: *Vrachebno-Sanitarnyi Vestnik*, no. 1–2 (March–April 1917): 98–104.

35. According to a brief announcement in *VVP*, no. 58/104 (19 May/1 June 1917): 2, the agenda of the conference was (1) the organization of *oblast'* and *guberniia* medical/sanitary councils; (2) planning antiepidemic activity for the summer of 1917; (3) the organization of *oblast'* sanitary-technical bureaus; (4) the creation of new agencies to direct wartime psychiatric affairs.

36. *Vrachebnaia Zhizn'*, no. 1 (15 August 1917): 11.

37. Ibid.

38. Ibid.

39. Both his report on the reorganization of hospital administration and his proposed reorganization of public health within the MVD appear in *Vrachebnaia Zhizn'*, no. 5 (15 September 1917): 8–9.

40. Police and prison physicians were in practice exempt from the draft, as were, for security reasons, Jewish private practitioners.

41. This was a meeting of all physicians—military, Red Cross, and union—serving in

the regions of the XI and VII armies, which took place on 28–29 March. Its resolutions were reported in detail at the Pirogov Congress. See *Trudy 1917 g*, 42.

42. *Trudy 1917 g*, 77.

43. Ibid., 40.

44. Ibid., 36.

45. On the problems involved in organizing the exchange, see the report of G. N. Pinegin in *Vrachebnaia Zhizn'*, no. 5 (15 September 1917): 4–5.

46. See V. D. Markuzon's report to the Delegate Congress of Moscow Military *Okrug*, 8–11 May 1917, in *Vrachebnaia Zhizn'*, no. 2 (22 August 1917): 8–9.

47. *Vrachebnaia Zhizn'*, no. 5 (15 September 1917): 3.

48. The CMSC was not officially established until 16 July, and the decree that announced its formation was not published until 19 August, three days before the council's first plenary meeting. *VVP*, no. 134/180 (19 August/1 September 1917): 1.

49. *VVP*, no. 105/151 (15/28 July 1917): 1. See also *Vrachebnaia Zhizn'*, no. 1 (15 August 1917): 12–13. On the attempts of the Provisional Government to keep pace with the wave of revolutionary organizing in the army, see Wildman, *End of the Russian Imperial Army*, 246–290.

50. The vacancy was created by transferring the incumbent, N. A. Veliaminov, to the Sanitary Administration of Petrograd Military District. *VVP*, no. 101/147 (11/24 July 1917): 2. The fact that Veliaminov, who had been both a bastion of the prerevolutionary medical establishment and a close associate of G. E. Rein, retained his senior military position for more than four months after the February Revolution demonstrates again how easy it was for senior tsarist officials to survive under the Provisional Government.

51. War Ministry *prikaz* no. 412 to the Chief Military-Sanitary Inspector, 29 June 1917, printed in *VVP*, no. 105/151 (15/28 July 1917): 1. See also *Vrachebnaia Zhizn'*, no. 1 (15 August 1917): 13. Composition of the MMSC was as follows: the Chief Military-Sanitary Inspector and his deputy, representatives (unspecified) of front physicians, one representative from each interior military district, one representative (who must be a physician) from the Soviet of Workers' and Soldiers' Deputies, one representative from each existing medical organization [sic], representatives (the number to be fixed by mutual agreement) from the Red Cross, the Union of Zemstvos, and the Union of Towns. The CCF, headed by the Chief Field Sanitary Inspector, included representatives (numbers unspecified) of front sanitary councils, of the MMSC, the Red Cross, the Union of Zemstvos, and the Union of Towns.

52. *Vrachebnaia Gazeta*, no. 29 (1917), quoted in *Vrachebnaia Zhizn'*, no. 2 (22 August 1917): 16.

53. *Vrachebnaia Zhizn'*, no. 2 (22 August 1917): 14.

54. Ibid.

55. On the conflicts at the Golitsyn Hospital, see *Vrachebnaia Zhizn'*, no. 4 (7 September 1917): 9–10.

56. The count fired thirteen employees, including three physicians, who had organized a meeting to approve proposals for an elected hospital council. When the employees appealed to the city government to step into the dispute, the count announced that he would shut down the hospital rather than give in. The City Duma's committee on public health was evidently still discussing what to do about the situation when the Bolsheviks seized power in October. See *Vrachebnaia Zhizn'*, no. 4 (7 September 1917): 10.

57. This would involve closing the *guberniia* medical departments and replacing them and their agents, the *uezd* and *gorodovoi* physicians, with entirely new agencies run, presumably, by the zemstvos and municipalities, *Trudy 1917 g*, 75; *Vrachebnaia Zhizn'*, no. 1 (15 August 1917): 11.

58. *VVP* no. 91/137 (28 June/11 July 1917); quoted in *Vrachebnaia Zhizn'*, no. 1 (15 August 1917): 11–12.

59. On the opposition of community physicians to these institutions, established under the Rules of 24 August 1903, see Frieden 1981, 292–295, 301–307.

60. The text of the order, signed by Prince L'vov and by Pereverzev, Minister of Justice, appears in *VVP*, no. 134/180 (19 August/1 September 1917): 1.

61. *Vrachebnaia Zhizn'*, no. 6–7 (1917): 9.

62. Ibid., 9–10.

63. "Health-resort medicine" was the name given to specialist work in physiotherapy at special sanatoria; it was anticipated that the end of the war would bring enormous demand for programs to rehabilitate wounded and maimed soldiers.

64. For Mandel'berg's proposal, his defense of it, and an alternative proposal advanced by Kiriakov, see *Vrachebnaia Zhizn'*, no. 5 (15 September 1917): 6–9.

65. Ibid., 3.

66. *Vrachebnaia Zhizn'*, no. 3 (1 September 1917): 9.

67. William G. Rosenberg, "The Zemstvo in 1917 and under Bolshevik Rule" in Emmons and Vucinich, *Zemstvo in Russia*, 389–403.

68. For a thorough discussion of this theme, see Ferro, *October 1917*, 1–88.

69. Elected members of the Presidium of the CMSC at its plenary session on 22 August were: President—P. N. Diatroptov (Union of Zemstvos); Vice-Presidents—N. P. Vasilevskii (head of Petrograd *guberniia* zemstvo sanitary bureau) and Z. G. Frenkel' (Petrograd city sanitary physician and member of the Constitutional Democratic Party); Secretary—M. G. Rafes (head of Astrakhan *guberniia* zemstvo sanitary bureau). *Vrachebnaia Zhizn'*, no. 6–7 (22 September/1 October 1917): 16.

70. Both the Ministry of Labor and the Ministry of Public Welfare were forging ahead on their own with plans to reform (respectively) workers' medical care and medical charities.

71. Krug, "Russian Public Physicians," 115–116.

72. Ibid., 121.

73. *Vrachebnaia Zhizn'*, no. 2 (22 August 1917): 3.

74. *Vrachebnaia Zhizn'*, no. 3 (1 September 1917): 5.

75. *Vrachebnaia Zhizn'*, nos. 6–7 (22 September–1 October 1917): 3–6.

76. According to a report made to a congress of the CCF at Stavka in early August, about 900 physicians had been drafted into a new front reserve and about 500 more into a new rear reserve. (Drafted women physicians were assigned to service in the rear, whatever their capabilities.) Moreover, some 500 front physicians had been transferred to the rear, while another thousand were to be exchanged as soon as replacements arrived at the front. See the report on the proceedings of the CCF Congress of 5–7 August in *Vrachebnaia Zhizn'*, no. 6–7 (22 September/1 October 1917): 10–11.

77. *Vrachebnaia Zhizn'*, no. 5 (15 September 1917): 3–4.

78. Solov'ev attributed this proposal to Professor Iurevich, a colleague of Burdenko in the office of the Chief Military-Sanitary Inspector. Presumably the plan envisioned that private practitioners would be drafted in any case.

79. Ibid., 4.

80. Both Peter Krug and Mark Field have argued that the *pirogovtsy* defended the Provisional Government because it had given them so much influence over the direction of medical reform, an interpretation that seems to exaggerate the significance and achievement of the CMSC.

7: SOVIET MEDICINE: THE BOLSHEVIKS AND MEDICAL REFORM

1. On the formation of Red Guard medical units, see Rex A. Wade, *Red Guards and Workers' Militias in the Russian Revolution* (Stanford: Stanford University Press, 1984), 169–170.

2. M. I. Barsukov, *Velikaia Oktiabr'skaia sotsialisticheskaia revoliutsiia i organizatsiia sovetskogo zdravookhraneniia. X. 1917 g.–VII. 1918 g* (Moscow: Medgiz, 1951), 66.

3. A. I. Nesterenko, *Kak byl obrazovan Narodnyi Komissariat Zdravookhraneniia RSFSR: Iz istorii sovetskoqo zdravookhraneniia (oktiabr' 1917 g.-iul' 1918 g.)*, (Moscow: Meditsina, 1965), 13.

4. S. I. Mitskevich, *Zapiski vracha-obshchestvennika*, 133–134, 158–159.

5. Wade, *Red Guards*, 169; Barsukov, *Velikaia Oktiabr'skaia revoliutsiia*, 64–65, 72.

6. Barsukov, *Velikaia Oktiabr'skaia revoliutsiia*, 88.

7. Ibid., 73.

8. Nesterenko, *Kak byl obrazovan*, 13.

9. Barsukov, *Velikaia Oktiabr'skaia revoliutsiia*, 68; Nesterenko, *Kak byl obrazovan*, 15.

10. Barsukov, *Velikaia Oktiabr'skaia revoliutsiia*, 70–71.

11. Nesterenko, *Kak byl obrazovan*, 16–17.

12. Mitskevich, *Zapiski vracha-obshchestvennika*, 202–203. This strike did not affect the Military-Sanitary Administration.

13. Members of the colleges were as follows: Internal Affairs (NKVD)—A. N. Vinokurov, I. S. Veger, S. I. Mitskevich; State Welfare—A. E. Artemenko, A. L. Berkovich, D. I. Glezer; Ways and Communications—M. I. Barsukov, M. V. Golovsinkii, M. G. Vecheslov; Enlightenment—V. M. Bonch-Bruevich, M. I. Barsukov, and several others. Barsukov, *Velikaia Oktiabr'skaia revoliutsiia*, 103; Nesterenko, *Kak byl obrazovan*, 20.

14. Nesterenko, *Kak byl obrazovan*, 17; Mitskevich, *Zapiski vracha-obshchestvennika*, 181.

15. Nesterenko, *Kak byl obrazovan*, 18, note 2.

16. Nesterenko, *Kak byl obrazovan*, 14–15, 18; M. I. Barsukov, "Vospominaniia Glavnogo Komissara Vrachebno-Sanitarnogo otdela Voenno-revoliutsionnogo komiteta M. I. Barsukova" in *Doneseniia Komissarov Petrogradskogo Voenno-revolutsionnogo Komiteta* (Moscow: Gos. Izd-vo politicheskoi literatury, 1957), 247–248; A. N. Vinokurov, "V. I. Lenin i sotsial'noe obespechenie" in *Vospominaniia o Vladimire Il'iche Lenine*, II (Moscow: Gos. Izd-vo politicheskoi literatury, 1957), 289.

17. On the liquidation of the Military Revolutionary Committee, see T. H. Rigby, *Lenin's Government: Sovnarkom 1917–1922* (Cambridge: Cambridge University Press, 1979), 19–20.

18. *Obshchestvennyi Vrach*, no. 9–10 (1917): 79–80.

19. Dorf and Zhbankov were undoubtedly supporters of the Socialist Revolutionaries; Granovsky and Levitskii were probably sympathetic to the Mensheviks; Kanel', Shvaitsar, and Mol'kov were probably sympathetic to the Kamenev-Zinoviev wing of the Bolsheviks.

20. Krug, "Russian Public Physicians," 133.

21. *Obshchestvennyi Vrach*, no. 9–10 (1917): 408–410. For Krug's treatment, see Krug, "Russian Public Physicians," 134–135; see also Barsukov, *Velikaia Oktiabr'skaia revoliutsiia*, 91.

22. Barsukov, *Velikaia Oktiabr'skaia revoliutsiia*, 93.

23. *Obshchestvennyi Vrach*, no. 3–4 (1918): 30; Barsukov, *Velikaia Oktiabr'skaia revoliutsiia*, 54, 89; Krug, "Russian Public Physicians," 129.

24. Barsukov, *Velikaia Oktiabr'skaia revoliutsiia*, 120–123.

25. The appeal was published in *Sobranie ukazanii i rasporiazhenii rabochego i krest'ianskogo pravitel'stva*, no. 5, otdel pervyi, 16 dekabria, st. 81 (1917): 72–73.

26. Nesterenko, *Kak byl obrazovan*, 23–24.

27. Ibid., 25.

28. Ibid., 23.

29. Barsukov, *Velikaia Oktiabr'skaia revoliutsiia*, 117–118.

30. Details in Nesterenko, *Kak byl obrazovan*, 26–27.

31. Nesterenko, *Kak byl obrazovan*, 25–26.

32. Barsukov, *Velikaia Oktiabr'skaia revoliutsiia*, 137; Nesterenko, *Kak byl obrazovan*, 26.

33. Mitskevitch, *Zapiski vracha-obshchestrennika*, 186.

34. *Obshchestvennyi Vrach*, no. 9–10 (1917): 408–410; Krug, "Russian Public Physicians," 134–135; Barsukov, *Velikaia Oktiabr'skaia revoliutsiia*, 148–149. In November 1917, a full meeting of the CMSC had been called for 12–15 January 1918 in Petrograd, but it had to be abandoned for lack of a quorum.

35. For the text, see Nesterenko, *Kak byl obrazovan*, 32; also printed in *Dekrety Sovestkoi vlasti*, I (Moscow: Lenizdat, 1957), 478–480.

36. As quoted in Krug, "Russian Public Physicians," 142.

37. Barsukov, *Velikaia Oktiabr'skaia revoliutsiia*, 132, 150. The union—founded in 1917—was headed by A. A. Lozinskii and the old *pirogovets* G. I. Dembo; together they also edited *Vrachebnaia Gazeta*, which became a strongly anti-Bolshevik organ. See, for example, M. M. Gran's scathing attack on the new government in *Vrachebnaia Gazeta*, no. 78 (1918): 53–59.

38. Krug, "Russian Public Physicians," 143.

39. Ibid.

40. Ibid., 144. The translation is Krug's.

41. "Otkliki sovetskoi pechati na Pirogovskii s"ezd vrachei," *Izvestiia sovestkoi meditsiny*, no. 1 (1918): 12.

42. "Sovetskie meditsinskie rabotniki o "pirogovtsakh," ibid., 11–12.
43. Barsukov, *Velikaia Oktiabr'skaia revoliutsiia*, 179–181.
44. Ibid., 181.
45. M. A. Neviadomskii, as quoted in Krug, "Russian Public Physicians," 147.
46. N. Shvaitsar, as quoted in Barsukov, *Velikaia Oktiabr'skaia revoliutsiia*, 168.
47. Barsukov, *Velikaia Oktiabr'skaia, revoliutsiia*, 168–169.
48. "Soiuz meditsinskogo personala na platforme priznaniia vlasti sovetov," *Izvestiia sovestkoi meditsiny*, no. 1 (1918): 9.
49. Nesterenko, *Kak byl obrazovan*, 59–60.
50. Ibid., 37. V. A. Obukh was appointed head of the Medical Department of the Moscow Soviet.
51. Barsukov, *Velikaia Oktiabr'skaia revoliutsiia*, 75, 77; Nesterenko, *Kak byl obrazovan*, 37.
52. Barsukov, *Velikaia Oktiabr'skaia revoliutsiia*, 73.
53. Nesterenko, *Kak byl obrazovan*, 37, 43; Barsukov, *Velikaia Oktiabr'skaia revoliutsiia*, 177. Other members of the reorganized Administration of the Medical Sector in the NKVD were Rusakov, Veger, Golubkov, Semashko, Veisbrod, and Barsukov.
54. Nesterenko, *Kak byl obrazovan*, 44.
55. Barsukov, *Velikaia Oktiabr'skaia revoliutsiia*, 182.
56. Ibid.
57. E. I. Lotova and Kh. I. Idel'chik, *Bor'ba s infektsionnymi boleezniami v SSSR. 1917–1967 gg.* (Moscow: Meditsina, 1967), 101.
58. Ibid.; see also Nesterenko, *Kak byl obrazovan*, 46–47; Barsukov, *Velikaia Oktiabr'skaia revoliutsiia*, 188; Krug, "Russian Public Physicians," 191–192. Other members of the Pirogov Commission on Epidemics were Levitskii, Kats, Kurkin, and Mol'kov. These four, all of whom had signed the anti-Bolshevik declaration, did not go to the May 23 meeting. Diatroptov was the only signatory who did attend.
59. Nesterenko, *Kak byl obrazovan*, 46.
60. Barsukov, *Velikaia Oktiabr'skaia revoliutsiia*, 188.
61. Nesterenko, *Kak byl obrazovan*, 49.
62. *Obshchestvennyi Vrach*, no. 11–12 (1918): 107; Barsukov, *Velikaia Oktiabr'skaia revoliutsiia*, 190–191; Nesterenko, *Kak byl obrazovan*, 51. Proceedings of the meeting of the commission may be found in *Obshchestvennyi Vrach*, no. 11–12 (1918): 92–107.
63. Barsukov, *Velikaia Oktiabr'skaia revoliutsiia*, 162, 177.
64. Ibid., 201.
65. Among the scholars present at this meeting were Zabolotnyi, Tarasevich, Diatroptov, Martsinovskii, Kurkin, Levitskii, Kats, V. V. Ivanov, and A. V. Martynov. Krug, "Russian Public Physicians," 191; Barsukov, *Velikaia Oktiabr'skaia revoliutsiia*, 202.
66. Barsukov, *Velikaia Oktiabr'skaia revoliutsiia*, 202.
67. Ibid., 202–204.
68. Nesterenko, *Kak byl obrazovan*, 42, 44. T. H. Rigby, perhaps overly impressed by Barsukov's claims, ascribes to Semashko the role of major legislative draftsman; Rigby, *Lenin's Government*, 131–132.
69. Barsukov, *Velikaia Oktiabr'skaia revoliutsiia*, 255, 258.
70. The first issue of *Izvestiia sovetskoi meditsiny*, no. 1 (15 May 1918), included announcements regarding the organization of *SMK*, the abolition of the CMSC, Soviet medicine at the local level, the unionization of medical workers, comments about the *pirogovtsy* by "Soviet medical workers," coverage of the 1918 Pirogov Congress in the pro-Bolshevik press, and various other topics.
71. Ibid., 1.
72. Nesterenko, *Kak byl obrazovan*, 73.
73. *Izvestiia sovetskoi meditsiny*, no. 5–6 (1918): 13–18.
74. Nesterenko, *Kak byl obrazovan*, 71.
75. Ibid., 72.
76. Ibid.
77. Barsukov, *Velikaia Oktiabr'skaia revoliutsiia*, 252, 254. For example, under Pervukhin's plan, the administration of prison medicine, on being transferred from the

Commissariat of Justice to *NKZ*, would have continued as a separate *otdel* within *NKZ*, staffed by experts in the field.

78. Nesterenko, *Kak byl obrazovan*, 76; Barsukov, *Velikaia oktiabr'skaia revoliutsiia*, 275–276. There seems to have been a tug-of-war during June 1918 between *SMK* and the Commissariat for Military Affairs for control over military medicine. On 4 June, *SMK* transferred the entire evacuation and hospital administration from Army Headquarters to the Main Military Sanitary Administration (*GMSU*) and ordered *GMSU* to take over all Red Cross facilities on 7 June. Then on 15 June the Commissariat for Military Affairs announced that the *GMSU* would no longer be run by a collegial administration (i.e., by *SMK*) but by a single *nachal'nik* and appointed A. A. Tsvetaev to this position. An opponent of Solov'ev's plans for the unification of all medical affairs under *NKZ*, Tsvetaev quickly became a thorn in the side of Solov'ev and Barsukov. On this conflict see Barsukov, *Velikaia Oktiabr'skaia revoliutsiia*, 236–239.

79. Barsukov, *Velikaia Oktiabr'skaia revoliutsiia*, 276.

80. Others proposed for membership in the college were: M. F. Vladimirskii, V. M. Bonch-Bruevich, P. G. Dauge, M. G. Vecheslov, and I. S. Veger.

81. This account is based on Nesterenko, *Kak byl obrazovan*, 78–80; Barsukov, *Velikaia Oktiabr'skaia revoliutsiia*, 277–278; Mitskevich, *Zapiski vracha-obshchestvennika*, 189; N. A. Semashko, *Prozhitie i perezhitie* (Moscow, Gosudarstvennoe izdatel'stvo politicheskoi literatury, 1960), 70. See also Krug, "Russian Public Physicians," 187.

82. Nesterenko, *Kak byl obrazovan*, 80–82; the text of the letter from Sovnarkom to *SMK*, 12 July 1918, is printed in Barsukov, *Velikaia Oktiabr'skaia revoliutsiia*, 279.

83. The text of the *NKZ polozhenie* is printed in Nesterenko, *Kak byl obrazovan*, 85–87.

84. Nesterenko, *Kak byl obrazovan*, 82. Sovnarkom stipulated that 3 million rubles were to be sent to Tsaritsyn immediately, while *SMK* and the Petrograd *NKZ* were to agree on an appropriate sum for anticholera measures in that city.

85. Nesterenko, *Kak byl obrazovan*, 89.

86. Ibid., 87; the text of this announcement appeared in *Izvestiia VTsIK*, 23 July 1918.

87. Nesterenko, *Kak byl obrazovan*, 87.

88. Ibid., 89.

89. Barsukov, *Velikaia Oktiabr'skaia revoliutsiia*, 280; Nesterenko, *Kak byl obrazovan*, 88.

90. Nesterenko, *Kak byl obrazovan*, 89.

91. *Izvestiia sovetskoi meditsiny*, no. 4 (1918): 2–5.

92. By a decree of *SMK*, 14 May 1918, new enrollments in feldsher schools were stopped; those already trained at feldsher schools were encouraged to enroll in medical schools; untrained (*rotnye*) feldshers were ordered to attend the feldsher schools to upgrade their skills. Clearly the intention of *SMK* was to get rid of feldshers as soon as possible. Barsukov, *Velikaia Oktiabr'skaia revoliutsiia*, 297–298.

93. Dorf, as quoted in Krug, "Russian Public Physicians," 143.

94. For the full text of this resolution, see Barsukov, *Velikaia Oktiabr'skaia revoliutsiia*, appendix V, 303.

95. Barsukov, *Velikaia Oktiabr'skaia revoliutsiia*, 269.

96. On the pharmacists, see Jonathan Sanders, "Drugs and Revolution: Moscow Pharmacists in the First Russian Revolution," *The Russian Review*, 44, no. 4 (1985): 351–378.

SELECT BIBLIOGRAPHY

Unless otherwise indicated, the place of publication is Moscow (M), St. Petersburg (Spb), Petrograd (P), or Leningrad (L).

REFERENCE WORKS

Bulatov, P. N., Ed. *Kalendar' dlia vrachei vsekh vedomstv na 1916 god.* P: 1916.

Durdenevskii, V., and Bernitskii, S. *Opyt bibliografii obshchestvennykh nauk za revoliutsionnoe trekhletie (1918–1920).* M-L: 1925.

Ezhegodnik Russkoi Meditsinskoi Pechati. Obzor 1911g. M: 1912; *Obzor 1912g.* M: 1914.

Lotova, E. I. *Bibliografiia i obzor osnovnykh rabot po istorii gigieny i sanitarii (1917–1957).* M: 1959.

Margolin, D. *Spravochnik po vysshemu obrazovaniiu.* P-Kiev: 1915.

Matskina, R. Iu. *Istoriia razvitiia meditsiny i zdravookhraneniia v Rossii. Obzor dokumental'nykh materialov.* M-L: 1958.

Spisok grazhdanskim chinam voennogo vedomstva . . . sostavlen po 1-e ianvaria 1904 goda. Spb: 1904.

Spisok vysshikh chinov tsentral'nykh i mestnikh ustanovlenii ministerstva vnutrennikh del'. Spb: 1905.

Vsia administrativnaia Rossiia. Kiev: 1913.

Zhbankov, D. N. *Bibliograficheskii ukazatel' po zemskoi meditsinskoi literature.* M: 1890.

———. *Bibliograficheskii ukazatel' po obshchestvennoi meditsinskoi literature za 1890–1905 gg.* M: 1907.

DISSERTATIONS

Adams, Bruce F. "Criminology, Penology and Prison Administration in Russia, 1863–1917." Ph.D. diss., University of Maryland, 1981.

Brown, Julie Vail. "The Professionalization of Russian Psychiatry: 1857–1911." Ph.D. diss., University of Pennsylvania, 1981.

Gleason, William E. "The All-Russian Union of Towns and the All-Russian Union of Zemstvos in World War I: 1914–1917." Ph.D. diss., Indiana University, 1972.

Graf, Daniel William. "The Reign of the Generals: Military Government in Western Russia, 1914–1915." Ph.D. diss., University of Nebraska, 1972.

Hildreth, Martha L. "Doctors, Bureaucrats and Public Health in France, 1888–1902." Ph.D. diss., University of California, Riverside, 1983.

Krug, Peter F. "Russian Public Physicians and Revolution: The Pirogov Society, 1917–1920." Ph.D. diss., University of Wisconsin-Madison, 1979.

Lindenmeyr, Adele. "Public Poor Relief and Private Charity in Late Imperial Russia." Ph.D. diss., Princeton University, 1980.

Mazumdar, Pauline M. H. "Karl Landsteiner and the Problem of Species, 1838–1868." Ph.D. diss., Johns Hopkins University, 1976.

Zyrianov, P. N. "Krakh vnutrennoi politiki tret'eiun'skoi monarkhii v oblasti mestnogo upravleniia (1907–1914gg.)." Ph.D. abstract. University of Moscow, 1972.

PERIODICALS

Bol'nichnaia Gazeta Botkina.
Gigiena i Sanitariia.
Gigiena i Sanitarnoe Delo.
Izvestiia Narodnogo Komissariata Zdravookhraneniia.
Izvestiia Narodnogo Komissariata Zdravookhraneniia Soiuza Kommun Severnoi Oblasti.
Izvestiia Sovetskoi Meditsiny.
Meditsinskaia Beseda.
Meditsinskoe Obozrenie.
Ministerstvo Vnutrennikh Del'. Meditsinskii Department. *Vestnik Obshchestvennoi Gigieny, Sudebnoi i Prakticheskoi Meditsiny.*
Ministerstvo Vnutrennikh Del'. Sovet po delam mestnogo khozaistva. *Izvestiia po Delam Zemskogo i Gorodskogo Khozaistva.*
Ministerstvo Vnutrennikh Del'. Upravlenie Glavnogo Meditsinskogo Inspektora. *Rossiiskii Meditsinskii Spisok.*
Moskovskaia Gorodskaia Duma. *Izvestiia Moskovskoi Gorodskoi Dumy.*
Obshchestvennoe-sanitarnoe Obozrenie.
Obshchestvennyi Vrach.
Prakticheskaia Meditsina.
Prakticheskii Vrach.
Psikhiatricheskaia Gazeta.
Russkii Meditsinskii Vestnik.
Russkii Vrach.
Sovetskoe Zdravookhranenie.
Tretii Element.
Vestnik Sanktpeterburgskogo Vrachebnogo Obshchestva Vzaimnoi Pomoshchi.
Volostnoe Zemstvo.
Vrach.
Vrachebnaia Gazeta.
Vrachebnaia Zhizn'.
Vrachebnoe Delo.
Vrachebno-sanitarnyi Vestnik.
Vrachebnye Vedomosti.
Vrachebnyi Vestnik.
Vserossiiskii zemskii soiuz pomoshchi bol'nym i ranenym voinam. *Izvestiia Glavnogo Komiteta.*
Zemskaia Meditsina.
Zemskii Vrach.
Zemskoe Delo.
Zhurnal Obshchestva Russkikh Vrachei v pam. N.I. Pirogova.
Zhurnal Russkogo Obshchestva Okhraneniia Narodnogo Zdraviia.

MEMOIRS

Bertenson, V. B. *Za tridtsat' let (1875–1905).* Spb: 1914.
Gamaleia, N. F. *Vospominaniia.* M: 1947.
Gurko, V. I. *Features and Figures of the Past: Government and Opinion in the Reign of Nicholas II.* Stanford, 1939.
Kryzhanovskii, S. E. *Vospominaniia.* Petropolis: n.d. (1938).
Mitskevich, S. I. *Na grani dvukh epokh. Ot narodnichestva k marksizmu.* M: 1937.
———. *Zapiski vracha-obshchestvennika, 1888–1918.* M-L: 1940.
Rein, G. E. *Iz perezhitogo 1907–1918.* 2 vols. Berlin: n.d. (1935).
Rodzianko, M. V. *The Reign of Rasputin: An Empire's Collapse. Memoirs.* Translated by Catherine Zvegintzoff. London: 1927.
Rudinskii, N. *Zapiski zemskogo vracha.* 2d ed. Spb: 1910.
Sokolov, D. *25 let bor'by. Vospominaniia vracha, 1885–1910.* Spb: 1910.
Sukhomlinov, V. A. *Vospominaniia.* Berlin: 1924.
Teziakov, N. I. "Iz perezhitogo.—Vospominaniia." *Gigiena i epidemiologiia,* no. 11 (1927); no. 4 (1928).

Turovskii, K. G. "Iz istorii zemskoi meditsiny." *Vestnik sovremennoi meditsiny*, no. 15–16: (1927): 991–1002; no. 17: 1079–1090; no. 19: 1217–1228.

Zalenskii, E. Ia. *Iz zapisok zemskogo vracha.* Pskov: 1908.

DOCUMENTS AND OTHER PRIMARY SOURCES

Government Publications

Ministerstvo Vnutrennikh Del'. Glavnoe upravlenie po delam mestnogo khozaistva. *Vrachebno-Politseiskii Nadzor za Gorodskoi Prostitutsiei.* Spb: 1910.

———. Meditsinkii Department. *Otchety 1877–1899 gg.* Spb: 1878–1900.

———. Meditsinskii Department. *Kratkii ocherk sanitarnogo sostianiia gorodov Rossii v 1892 g.* Spb: 1895.

———. Meditsinskii Department. *Sanitarnoe sostoianie gorodov Rossiiskii Imperii v 1895 po dannim Med. Dep. MVD.* Spb: 1898.

———. Meditsinskii Sovet. *Trudy komissii uchrezdennoi pri meditsinskom sovete pod pred. S.P. Botkina po voprosu ob uluchenii sanitarnykh uslovii i umensheniia smertnosti v Rossii.* Spb: 1888.

———. *Spisok vysshikh chinov tsentral'nykh i mestnykh ustanovlenii Ministerstva Vnu-trennikh Del'. Chast' I.* Spb: 1905. *Chast' II.* Spb: 1910.

———. Upravlenie Glavnogo Meditsinskogo Inspektora. *Otchety o sostoianii narodnogo zdraviia i organizatsii vrachebnoi pomoshchi v Rossii, 1892–1916.* Spb., 1904–14, P., 1915–16.

———. Upravlenie Glavnogo Meditsinskogo Inspektora. *Sanitarnoe sostoianie gorodov Rossiiskoi Imperii v 1895 g.* Spb., 1898.

[Russia.] *Svod mnenii gubernatorov po voprosu o preobrazovanii gubernskogo upravleniia.* Spb., n.d.

[Russia.] *Vysochaishe uchrezdennaia mezhduvedomstvennaia komissia po peresmotru vrachebo-sanitarnogo zakonodatel'stva. Sbornik.* Spb., 1913.

[U.S.S.R.] Tsentral'noe staticheskoe upravlenie. Otdel voennoi statistiki. *Rossiia v mirovoi voine 1914–1918 goda. (v tsifrakh).* M., 1925.

Publications of the Pirogov Society of Russian Physicians

Desiatyi s"ezd russkikh vrachei v pamiat' N. I. Pirogova, pod. red. G. I. Dembo. M: 1907.

Dnevnik sed'mogo s"ezda russkikh vrachei, pod. red. Prof. A. V. Levashova. Kazan': 1899.

Dvenadtsatyi Pirgovskii S"ezd, Peterburg, 29 maia–5 iunia 1913 g. 2 vols. Spb: 1913.

Gran', M. M., Frenkel', Z. G., and Shingarev, A. I., eds. *Nikolai Ivanovich Pirogov i ego nasledie: Pirogovskie s"ezdy, iubileinoe izdanie.* Spb: 1911.

Pirogovskii S"ezd po bor'be s kholeroi. 2 vols. M: 1905.

Pirogovskii s"ezd vrachei i predstavitelei vrachebno-sanitarnykh organizatsii zemstv i gorodov po vrach-san. voprosam v sviazi s usloviami nastoiashchego vremeni. Petrograd, 13–18 apr. 1916 g. P: 1916.

"Pirogovskoe soveshchanie bakteriologov i predstavitelei vrachebno-sanitarnykh organizatsii po bor'be s zaraznymi boleziami v sviazi s voennym vremenem. Moskva, 28–30 dek. 1914 g.," *Obshchestvennyi Vrach*, no. 2 (1915): 1–130.

Shidlovskii, K. I. *Svod postanovlenii i rabot I–VI s"ezdov.* M: 1899.

Trudy chrezvychainogo pirogovskogo s"ezda (Moskva, 4–8 Aprelia 1917 g.) M: 1918.

Trudy IX Pirogovskogo S"ezda. 6 vol. Spb: 1904–1906.

Trudy odinnadtsatogo s"ezda russkikh vrachei, pod. red. Dr. P. N. Bulatova. 3 vols. Spb: 1910.

Trudy XII Pirogovskogo S"ezda. 3 vols. Spb: 1910–1913.

Vos'moi Pirogovskii S"ezd (Moskva, 3–10 ianvaria 1902). M: 1902.

Zhbankov, D. N. *Sbornik po gorodskomu vrachebno-sanitarnomu delu v Rossii.* M: 1915.

———, ed. *Sbornik po obshchestvenno-sanitarnym i vrachebno-bytovym voprosam.* M: 1909.

———, ed. *Zemsko-meditsinskii sbornik.* 7 vols. M: 1890–1893.

Other Primary Sources

Bazhenov, N. N. "Psikhologiia i politika." *Moskovskii Ezhenedel'nik*, no. 16 (1906): 15–26; no. 17: 19–28.

Blinov, I. *Gubernatory: Istoriko-Iuridicheskii Ocherk*. Spb: 1906.

Blumental', F. M. *Ocherki Gosudarstvennogo Zdravookhraneniia na Zapade*. Spb: 1914.

Cherniavsky, Michael. *Prologue to Revolution: Notes of A. N. Iakhontov on the Secret Meetings of the Council of Ministers, 1915*. Englewood Cliffs, N J., 1967.

Chertov, A. A. *Gorodskaia Meditsina v Evropeiskoi Rossii. Sbornik svedenii ob ustroistve vrachebno-sanitarnoi chasti v gorodakh*. M: 1903.

D., B. G. *Strakhovanie rabochikh po zakonam 23 iunia 1912g. Spb*: 1913.

Dagaev, Iu. V. *Narodnoe zdravie i nasushchnye voprosy meditsinskoi organizatsii*. Spb: 1906.

Dembo, L. I. *Vrachebnoe pravo: Vypusk 1-yi. Sanitarno-sotsial'noe zakonodatel'stvo*. 1914.

Freiberg, N. G. *Vrachebno-Sanitarnoe Zakonodatel'stvo v Rossii*. 2d ed. Spb: 1908.

Frenkel', Z. G. *Ocherki Zemskogo Vrachebno-sanitarnogo dela*. Spb: 1913.

God raboty Narodnogo komissariata zdravookhraneniia RSFSR, 1918–19. M: 1919.

Golovin, N. N. *The Russian Army in the World War*. New Haven, Conn.: 1931.

Gubert, V. O. *XXV let nauchno-prakiticheskoi deiatel'nosti russkogo obshchestva okhraneniia narodnogo zdraviia*. Spb: 1904.

Gvozdev, S. *Zapiski Fabrichnogo Inspektora*. M: 1911.

Imperatorskii Institut Eksperimental'noi Meditsiny (1890–1910). Spb: 1911.

Iur'ev, N. P. *K voprosu o material'nom polozhenii vrachei, sluziashchikh po vedomstvu M.V.D. v guberniiakh i oblastiakh Rossii*. Spb: 1904.

K., M. M. "Nuzhny-li nam sanitarye ili sanitarno-blagotvoritel'nye popechitel'stva?" *Prizrenie i Blagotvoritel'nost' v Rossii*, no. 8–10 (1914): 967–979.

Kanel', V. Ia. *Fabrichnaia meditsina i biurokratiia*. M: 1906.

Kapustin, M. Ia. *Obrazovanie i Zdorov'e. Kazan: 1904*.

———. *Osnovnye voprosy zemskoi meditsiny*. Spb: 1889.

———. "Zadachi gigieny v sel'skoi Rossii." *Russkaia Mysl'*, no. 5 (1902): 1–27.

Khar'kovskoe meditsinskoe obshchestvo, 1861–1911 gg. Khar'kov: 1913.

K-ov. A. "Ozdorovlenie Rossii i sredstva k tomu." *Vestnik Evropy*, no. 4 (1907): 729–753.

Koz'minykh-Lanin', I. M. *Vrachebnaia pomoshch' fabrichno-zavodskim rabochim v uezdakh Moskovskoi gubernii*. M: 1912.

Levitskii, M. "Sel'skaia meditsina v ne-zemskikh guberniakh." *Vestnik Evropy*, no. 8 (1895): 789–807.

Metchnikoff, Elie [I. I. Mechnikov]. *The New Hygiene: Three Lectures on the Prevention of Infectious Diseases*. Translated by E. Ray Lankester. London, 1906.

Ministerstvo Vnutrennikh Del'. Istoricheskii Ocherk. 3 vols. Spb: 1902.

Moiseev, A. I. *Meditsinskii Sovet M.V.D*. Spb: 1913.

Moskovskoe gorodskoe upravlenie. Sanit.-statist. biuro. *Kratkii ocherk razvitiia i sovremennogo sostoianiia gorodskoi vrachebnoi sanitarnoi organizatsii*. M: 1911.

Nikol'skii, D. P. "Gigiena v sviazi s sotsial'nymi usloviami." *Obrazovanie*, no. 7 (1906): 151–172.

Osipov, A. E., Popov, I. V., and Kurkin, P. I. *Russkaia zemskaia meditsina*. M: 1899.

Otchet o sostoianii i deiatel'nosti Spb. Zhenskogo Meditsinskogo Instituta za 1908–1912 gg. Spb: 1914.

Pirumova, N. M. *Zemskoe liberal'noe dvizhenie: Sotsial'nye korni i evoliutsiia do nachala XX veka*. M: 1977.

Seguel [initials?] "L'assistance publique en Russie." *Revue philanthropique* 20 (1906–7): 744–775.

Semashko, N. A. "Friedrich Erismann, the dawn of Russian public hygiene and public health." Translated by H. E. Sigerist. *Bulletin of the History of Medicine* 20 (1946): 1–9.

———. *Osnovy Sovetskoi meditsiny*. M: 1919.

Shchegolev, P. E., ed. *Padenie Tsarskogo Rezhima*. 7 vols. M.-L: 1924–7.

Shevchenko, I. F. *Smertnost' naseleniia S.-Peterburga po vozrastnym gruppam v zavisimosti ot roda zaniatii*. Spb: 1904.

Shingarev, A. I. "Obshchestvennaia meditsina v budushchem demokraticheskom stroe Rossii." *Russkaia Mysl'*, no. 6 (1907): 124–155.

———. *Vymiraiushchaia Derevnia*. Spb: 1907.

[Slobozhanin, M.] *Iz istorii i opyta zemskikh uchrezhdenii v Rossii. Ocherki M. Slobozhanina*. Spb: 1913.

Solov'ev, Z. P. *Izbrannye proizvedeniia, pod. red. B. D. Petrova*. M: 1956.

———. *Stroitel'stvo sovetskogo zdravookhraneniia*. M: 1932.

Soobshcheniia i protokoly zasedanii Spb-ogo meditsinskogo obshchestva [za 1900–1911]. Spb. 1901–1912.

Stoletie Voennogo Ministerstva, 1802–1902 gg. T.IX, Ch.II: Imperatorskaia Voenno-meditsinskaia akademiia do 1902 g. vkliuch. Spb: 1911.

Surovtsov, Z. G. *Materialy dlia istorii kafedry gigieny v Imperatorskoi Voenno-Meditsinskoi Akademii*. Spb: 1898.

Sysin, A. N. "Sanitarnoe sostoianie Rossii v nastoiashchem i proshlom." *Sotsial'naia gigiena, sbornik izd. Narkomzdrav RSFSR*. M: 1923.

[Tarasevich, L. A.] "Epidemics in Russia since 1914: Report to the Health Committee of the League of Nations by Professor L. Tarassevitch (Moscow)." *Epidemiological Intelligence*, no. 2 (1922): 2–33, no. 5: 2–55.

Tarasevich, L. A. "Rabota I. I. Mechnikova v oblasti meditsiny i mikrobiologii." *Priroda*, no. 5 (1915): 707–724.

Teziakov, N. I. *Besedy po gigieny v primenenii eia k narodnoi shkole*. P: 1915.

Trudy obshchestva bol'nychnykh vrachei v Spb. za 1901 [1902, 1903]. Spb: 1902–1905.

Trudy pervogo vserossiiskogo s"ezda fabrichnykh vrachei i predstavitelei fabrichno-promyshlennosti (pod red. D. I. Orlova). 2 vols. M: 1910.

Trudy pervogo vserossiiskogo s"ezda po bor'be s pianstvom. 3 vols. Spb: 1910.

Trudy soveshchaniia po bakteriologii, epidemiologii i prokaze (3–9 ian. 1911 g.). Spb: 1912.

Trudy soveshchaniia po sanitarnym i sanitarno-statisticheskim voprosam. Moskva, 31-go marta–3-e aprelia 1912 g. M: 1912.

Trudy soveshchaniia predstavitelei zemstv po voprosam osushchestvleniia zemstvami pomoshchi uvechnym voinam. 5–7 okt. 1916 g. M: 1916.

Trudy vserossiiskogo s"ezda prakticheskikh deiatelei po bor'be s alkogolizmom (Moskva, 6–12 avg. 1912 g.). 3 vols. P: 1914–16.

Trudy vtorogo vserossiiskogo s"ezda fabrichnykh vrachei i predstavitelei fabrichno-zavodskoi promyshlennosti (pod. red. I. D. Astrakhana). 2 vols. M: 1911.

Trutovskii, V. *Sovremennoe Zemstvo*, P: 1914.

Usilenie gubernatorskoi vlasti. Proekt von Pleve. Paris, 1904.

Valerianov, L. *Prava i obiazannosti vrachei*. Spb: 1913.

Verekundov, S. P. *Ministerstvo narodnogo zdraviia. K istorii voprosa*. Spb: 1899.

Veresaev, V. V. "Po povodu 'zapisok vracha' (Moim kritikam)." *Mir' bozhii, no. 10 (1902)*: 1–33.

———. *[V. V. Smidovich] Zapiski vracha*. Spb: 1902.

Veselovskii, B. *Istoriia zemstva za sorok let*. 4 vols. Spb. 1909–11.

Veselovskii, B. B., and Frenkel', Z. G. *Iubileinyi Zemskii Sbornik 1864–1914*. Spb: 1914.

Vigdorchik, N. A. *Sotsial'noe strakhovanie*. Spb: 1912.

von Pettenkofer, Max. "The Value of Health to a City, Two Lectures delivered in 1873." Translated by H. E. Sigerist. *Bulletin of the History of Medicine* 10 (1941): 473–503, 593–613.

Vserossiiskii s"ezd vrachei psikhiatrov i predstavitelei zemstv, gorodov i zainteresovannykh vedomstv po organizatsii prizreniia dushevno-bol'nykh voinov . . . v Petrograde, 24–27 noiabria, 1916 g. P: 1917.

Vserossiskii Zemskii Soiuz pomoshchi bol'nym i ranenym boitsam. Postanovleniia soveshchaniia po voprosam frontovykh vrachebno-sanitarnykh organizatsii Zemskogo Soiuza. Moskva, 25–27 Ianvaria 1916 g. M: 1916.

Witte, S. Iu. *Samoderzhavie i zemstvo*. Stuttgart: 1901.

Zdravookhranenie v Sovetskoi Rossii: Sbornik statei k s"ezdu sovetov. M: 1919.

Zhbankov, D. N. *O deiatel'nosti sanitarnykh biuro i obshchestvenno-sanitarnykh uchrezhdenii v zemskoi Rossii*. M: 1910.

———. "Vsesoslovnaia volost' i zemskaia meditsina." *Zemstvo, no. 25 (1882): 2–4.

SECONDARY SOURCES

Ackerknecht, Erwin. *Rudolf Virchow: Doctor, Statesman, Anthropologist.* Madison: 1953.
Alexander, John T. *Bubonic Plague in Early Modern Russia: Public Health and Urban Disaster.* Baltimore: 1980.
Alston, Patrick L. *Education and the State in Tsarist Russia.* Stanford: 1969.
Barsukov, M. I. *Velikaia Oktiabr'skaia sotsialisticheskaia revoliutsiia i organizatsiia sovetskogo zdravookhraneniia. (Okt. 1917g–Iul', 1918).* M: 1951.
————. "Voprosy organizatsii zdravookhraneniia v Rossii vo vremia fevral'skoi burzhuazno-demokraticheskoi revoliutsii." *Sovetskoe Zdravookhranenie (1947),* no. 4: 43–51.
————, ed. *Ocherki istorii zdravookhraneniia SSSR (1917–1956).* M: 1957.
Bater, J. H. "Modernization and Public Health in St. Petersburg, 1890–1914." *Forschungen zur osteuropäischen Geschichte* 37 (1985): 357–372.
————. *St. Petersburg: Industrialization and Change.* Montreal: 1976.
Beilikhis, G. A. *Iz istorii bor'by za sanitarnuiu okhranu truda v tsarskoi Rossii.* M: 1957.
Bor'ba za nauku v tsarskoi Rossii: Neizdannye pis'ma i stati. M-L: 1931.
Bradley, Joseph. *Muzhik and Muscovite: Urbanization in Late Imperial Russia.* Berkeley: 1985.
Brand, Jeanne L. *Doctors and the State: The British Medical Profession and Government Action in Public Health, 1870–1912.* Baltimore: 1965.
Burbank, Jane. *Intelligentsia and Revolution: Russian Views of Bolshevism, 1917–1922.* New York: 1986.
Chermenskii, E. D. *Burzhuazia i Tsarizm v Pervoi Russkoi Revoliutsii.* M: 1970.
————. *IV-aia Gosudarstvennaia Duma i sverzhenie tsarizma v Rossii.* M: 1976.
Diakin, V. S. *Russkaia burzhuazia i tsarizm v gody pervoi mirovoi voiny (1914–1917).* L: 1967.
————. *Samoderzhavie, burzhuazia i dvorianstvo v 1907–1911 gg.* L: 1978.
————. "Stolypin i dvorianstvo (proval mestnoi reformy)." In *Problemy krest'ianskogo zemlevladeniia i vnutrennoi politiki Rossii: Dooktiabr'skoi period.* L: 1972.
Emmons, Terence, and Vucinich, Wayne S., eds. *The Zemstvo in Russia: An Experiment in Local Self-Government.* Cambridge: 1982.
Engel, Barbara A. "Women Medical Students in Russia, 1872–1882: Reformers or Rebels?" *Journal of Social History* 12 (1979): 394–414.
Engelstein, Laura. *Moscow, 1905: Working-Class Organization and Political Conflict.* Stanford: 1982.
Erman, L. K. *Intelligentsia v Pervoi Russkoi Revoliutsii.* M: 1966.
Fallows, Thomas. "Politics and the War Effort in Russia: The Union of Zemstvos and the Organization of the Food Supply, 1914–1916." *Slavic Review* 37 (1978): 70–90.
Ferro, Marc. *October 1917: A Social History of the Russian Revolution.* London: 1980.
Field, Mark. *Doctor and Patient in Soviet Russia.* Cambridge, Mass.: 1957.
————. *Soviet Socialized Medicine: An Introduction.* New York: 1967.
50 let Pervogo Leningradskogo Meditsinskogo Instituta im. I. P. Pavlova. L: 1947.
Frenkel', Z. G. *Obshchestvennaia meditsina i sotsial'naia gigiena.* L: 1926.
Frieden, Nancy Mandelker. "Physicians in Pre-revolutionary Russia: Professionals or Servants of the State?" *Bulletin of the History of Medicine* 49 (1975): 20–29.
————. "The Russian Cholera Epidemic, 1892–93, and Medical Professionalization." *Journal of Social History* 10 (1977): 538–559.
————. *Russian Physicians in an Era of Reform and Revolution, 1856–1905.* Princeton: 1981.
Fuller, William C., Jr. *Civil-Military Conflict in Imperial Russia, 1881–1914.* Princeton: 1985.
Galai, Shmuel. *The Liberation Movement in Russia, 1900–1905.* Cambridge: 1973.
George, Mark. "Liberal Opposition in Wartime Russia: A Case Study of the Town and Zemstvo Unions, 1914–1917." *Slavonic and East European Review* 65 (1987): 371–390.
Geyer, Dietrich. *Russian Imperialism: The Interaction of Domestic and Foreign Policy, 1860–1914.* New Haven: 1987.
Gleason, William E. "The All-Russian Union of Towns and the Politics of Urban Reform in Tsarist Russia," *Russian Review* 35 (1976): 290–302.
Griaznov, I. *Nikolai Fedorovich Gamaleia.* M: 1949.

Gronsky, Paul P., and Astrov, Nicholas J. *The War and the Russian Government*. New Haven: 1929.

Haimson, Leopold H. "The Problem of Social Stability in Urban Russia, 1905–1917." *Slavic Review* 23 (1964): 619–642; 24 (1965): 1–22.

———, ed. *The Politics of Rural Russia, 1905–1914*. Bloomington: 1979.

Hasegawa, Tsuyoshi. *The February Revolution*. Seattle: 1981.

Hume, E. E. *Max von Pettenkofer*. New York: 1927.

Hutchinson, John F. "Society, Corporation or Union? Russian Physicians and the Struggle for Professional Unity (1890–1913)." *Jahrbücher für Geschichte Osteuropas* 30 (1982): 37–53.

———. "Tsarist Russia and the Bacteriological Revolution." *Journal of the History of Medicine and Allied Sciences* 40 (1985): 420–439.

Idel'chik, Kh. I. *N. I. Teziakov i ego rol' v razvitii zemskoi meditsiny i stroitel'stve Sovetskogo zdravookhraneniia*. M: 1960.

Igumnov, S. N. *Ocherk razvitiia zemskoi meditsiny*. Kiev: 1940.

Istoriia russkoi advokatury. 2 vols. M: 1914–16.

Kaganovich, R. B. *Iz istorii bor'by s tuberkulezom v dorevoliutsionnoi Rossii*. M: 1952.

Kal'iu, P. I., ed. *Ocherki istorii Russkoi obshchestvennoi meditsiny*. M: 1965.

Kanevskii, L. O., Lotova, E. I., and Idel'chik, Kh. I. *Osnovnye cherty razvitiia meditsiny v Rossii v period kapitalizma (1861–1917)*. M: 1956.

Karpov, L. N. *Zemskaia sanitarnaia organizatsiia v Rossii*. L: 1964.

Kovrigina, M., ed. *Sorok let Sovetskogo zdravookhraneniia (1917–1957)*. M: 1957.

Kroeger, Gertrud. *The Concept of Social Medicine as Presented by Physicians and Other Writers in Germany, 1779–1932*. Chicago: 1937.

Krug, Peter F. "The Debate over the Delivery of Health Care in Rural Russia." *Bulletin of the History of Medicine* 50 (1976): 226–241.

Laverychev, V. Ia. *Tsarizm i Rabochii Vopros v Rossii (1861–1917 gg.)*. M: 1972.

Leikina-Svirskaia, V. R. *Intelligentsia v Rossii vo vtoroi polovine XIX veka*. M: 1971.

———. *Russkaia intelligentsia v 1900–1917 godakh*. M: 1981.

Levin, Alfred. "Russian Bureaucratic Opinion in the Wake of the 1905 Revolution." *Jahrbücher für Geschichte Osteuropas* 11 (1963): 1–12.

Lieven, D. C. B. "Russian Senior Officialdom under Nicholas II: Careers and Mentalities." *Jahrbücher für Geschichte Osteuropas* 32 (1984): 199–223.

Lotova, E. I. *Russkaia Intelligentsia i Voprosy Obshchestvennoi Gigieny*. M: 1962.

Manning, Roberta T. *The Crisis of the Old Order in Russia: Gentry and Government*. Princeton: 1982.

McGrew, Roderick E. *Russia and the Cholera, 1823–1832*. Madison: 1965.

Mercier, P. "Les instituts Pasteur d'outre-mer: Leur objectifs et moyens d'action." *Bulletin de l'Academie nationale de Medicine* 165 (1981): 441–448.

Metchnikoff [Mechnikov], O. *Life of Elie Metchnikoff, 1845–1916*. London: 1921.

Milenushkin, Y. I. *N. F. Gamaleia: Ocherk zhizni i deiatel'nosti*. M: 1954.

Nesterenko, A. I. *Kak byl obrazovan Narodnyi komissariat zdravookhraneniia RSFSR: Iz istorii Sovetskogo zdravookhraneniia (oktiabr' 1917g.–iul' 1918g.)* M: 1965.

Orlovsky, Daniel T. *The Limits of Reform: The Ministry of Internal Affairs in Imperial Russia, 1802–1881*. Cambridge, Mass.: 1981.

Palmberg, Albert. *A Treatise on Public Health and Its Application in Different European Countries*. Translated by A. Newsholme. London: 1895.

Pearson, Raymond. *Russian Moderates and the Crisis of Tsarism, 1914–1917*. London: 1977.

Perkal', S. I. "Z. P. Solov'ev kak stroitel' sovetskogo zdravookhraneniia i sotsial'noi gigieny." *Sovetskii vrachebnyi zhurnal* (1938): 942–947.

Petrov, B. D. *Vrachi-Bolsheviki: Stroiteli Sovetskogo Zdravookhraneniia*. M: 1973.

———. *Z. P. Solov'ev*. M: 1967.

———, ed. *Istoriia razvitiia meditsiny i zdravookhraneniia v Rossii*. M-L: 1958.

Petrov, B. D., and Potulov, B. M. *Z. P. Solov'ev*. M: 1976.

Pilipenko, D. S. "O sanitarnykh poteriakh russkoi armii v pervuiu mirovuiu voinu." *Voenno-meditsinskii Zhurnal* 9 (1964): 86–89.

Pintner, W. M., and Rowney, D. K., eds. *Russian Officialdom: The Bureaucratization of Russian Society from the Seventeenth to the Twentieth Centuries*. Chapel Hill: 1980.

Ramer, Samuel. "Who Was the Russian Feldsher?" *Bulletin of the History of Medicine* 50 (1976): 213–225.

Read, Christopher. *Religion, Revolution and the Russian Intelligentsia, 1900–1912.* London: 1979.

Das Reichsgesundheitsamt 1876–1926: Festschrift herausgeben vom Reichsgesundheitsamt aus Anlass seines fünfzig-jahrigen Bestehens. Berlin: 1926.

Robbins, Richard G., Jr. *Famine in Russia, 1891–1892: The Imperial Government Responds to a Crisis.* New York: 1975.

Rodionova, E. I. *Ocherki istorii professional'nogo dvizheniia meditsinskikh rabotnikov.* M: 1962.

Rogger, Hans. *Russia in the Age of Modernisation and Revolution, 1881–1917.* London: 1983.

Rosen, George. *From Medical Police to Social Medicine: Essays on the History of Health Care.* New York: 1974.

Rosenberg, W. G. *Liberals in the Russian Revolution: The Constitutional Democratic Party, 1917–1921.* Princeton: 1974.

Rowney, Don Karl. "Higher Civil Servants in the Russian Ministry of Internal Affairs: Some Demographic and Career Characteristics, 1905–1916." *Slavic Review* 31 (1972): 101–110.

Shatsillo, K. F. *Rossiia pered pervoi mirovoi voiny.* M: 1974.

Sidorov, A. L., ed. *Pervaia mirovaia voina, 1914–1918.* M: 1968.

Sigerist, H. E. *Socialized Medicine in the Soviet Union.* New York: 1937.

Skorokhodov, L. Ia. *Materialy po Istorii Meditsinskoi Mikrobiologii v Dorevoliutsionnoi Rossii.* M: 1948.

Startsev, V. I. *Revoliutsiia i vlast': Petrogradskii sovet i vremennoe pravitel'stvo v marte-aprele 1917 g.* M: 1978.

————. *Vnutrenniaia politika vremennogo pravitel'stva pervogo sostava.* L: 1980.

Stavrou, T. G., ed. *Russia under the Last Tsar.* Minneapolis: 1969.

Stone, Norman. *The Eastern Front, 1914–1917.* London: 1975.

Strashun, I. D. *Russkaia obshchestvennaia meditsina v period mezhdu dvumia revoliutsiami 1907–1917 gg.* M: 1964.

————. "Z. P. Solov'ev kak professor sotsial'noi gigieny (1876–1928)." *Sotsial'naia gigiena,* no. 1 (1929): 3–13.

Suny, Ronald Grigor. "Toward a Social History of the October Revolution." *American Historical Review,* 88 (1983): 31–52.

Sysin, A. N. "Erisman kak predstavitel' russkoi gigienicheskoi shkoly XIX veka." In *Trudy nauchnoi konferentsii posviashchennoi pamiati F. F. Erismana,* edited by V. A. Riazanov. M: 1947.

Thurston, Robert W. *Liberal City, Conservative State: Moscow and Russia's Urban Crisis, 1906–1914.* New York: 1987.

Vucinich, Alexander. *Science in Russian Culture, 1861–1917.* Stanford: 1970.

Wagner, W. G. "Tsarist Legal Policies at the End of the Nineteenth Century: A Study in Inconsistencies." *Slavonic and East European Review* 54 (1976): 371–394.

Weissman, Neil B. *Reform in Tsarist Russia: The State Bureaucracy and Local Government, 1900–1914.* New Brunswick, N.J.: 1981.

Wildman, Allan K. *The End of the Russian Imperial Army: The Old Army and the Soldiers' Revolt, March–April 1917.* Princeton: 1979.

Wilkinson, A. "Disease in the Nineteenth-Century Urban Economy: The Medical Officer of Health and the Community." *Society for the Social History of Medicine Bulletin* 27 (1980): 24–26.

Yaney, George L. *The Systematization of Russian Government: Social Evolution in the Domestic Administration of Imperial Russia, 1711–1905.* Urbana: 1973.

Zabliudovskii, P. E. *Istoriia Otechestvennoi Meditsiny: Chast' I. Period do 1917 goda.* M: 1960.

Zabliudovskii, P. E., et al. *Istoriia meditsiny.* M: 1981.

Zaionchkovskii, P. A. *Rossiiskoe Samoderzhavie v Kontse XIX Stoletiia.* M: 1970.

Zhuk, A. P. *Razvitie obshchestvennoi-meditsinskoi mysli v Rossii v 60–70gg. XIX veka.* M: 1963.

Zinoviev, I. A. *K istorii vysshego meditsinskogo obrazovaniia v Rossii.* M: 1962.

INDEX

Alcohol, 129, 136
Alcoholism, 30
Alexander I *(tsar)*, xvii
Alexander II *(tsar)*, xvii–xviii
Alexander III *(tsar)*, 4
All-Russian Alliance of Professional Associations of Physicians (VSPOV), 182, 185
All-Russian Congress on the Health of Towns, 138
All-Russian Congress of Medical Personnel, proposed, 174
All-Russian League for Struggle with Tuberculosis, 122, 189
All-Russian Pirogov Society, 62–63. *See also* Pirogov Society of Russian Physicians
All-Russian Union of Medical Personnel: collapse of, 52; congress of, 1905, 47–48; formation of, 46; moderate reaction against, 52; political diversity in, 48; program of, 47–48, 80; and proposed strike, 48, 52; Rusakov in, 123
All-Russian Union of Towns, 187, 188, 189; Antiepidemic Bureau, 123; assets nationalized, 181, 187; and cadet rebellion, 174; Central Bureau for Municipal Affairs, 138; democratization of, 148–49, 153; established, 112; establishes hospitals, *113–14*, 116–17; and Joint Sanitary Organization for the Northern Region, 144; Medical Bureau, 145–46, 148–49, 157, 201; Medical Bureau transferred to Commissariat of Health Protection, 192–93; and Military-Sanitary Administration, 112, 127; Medical-Sanitary Council, 139, 159; obsolescence of, 148; political possibilities of, 124–27; postwar plans by, 132, 135–39, 147; provides military

medical services, 108–9, 116–17; Provisional Government's financing of, 165; relations with Pirogov Society, 127–28; Sanitary Bureau, 124, 128, 135, 138, 148–49; and sanitary medicine, 128, 136; sanitary physicians and engineers in, 138; Sanitary-Technical Consultation Department, 138; Sysin and, 165; tension with All-Russian Union of Zemstvos, 139; in the war, 108, 112–15, 128–30. *See also* Physicians, union; Voluntary organizations, wartime
All-Russian Union of Zemstvos, 136, 187, 188, 189; and cadet rebellion, 174; democratization of, 148–49, 153; Diatroptov in, 122, 135, 170; dissolved and assets nationalized, 181, 187; established, 112; establishes hospital trains, 116–18; establishes medical facilities and hospitals, 116–17; General Brusilov and, 115; and Joint Sanitary Organization for the Northern Region, 144; L'vov as president of, 142, 144; Medical Bureau, 135, 145–46, 148–49, 157; Medical Bureau transferred to Commissariat of Health Protection, 192–93; and Military-Sanitary Administration, 112, 127; obsolescence of, 148; opposes the October Revolution, 174; political possibilities of, 124–27; postwar plans by, 135–39, 147; Provisional Government's financing of, 165; relations with Pirogov Society, 127–28; Sanitary Bureau, 109, 122–23, 128, 148–49; Solov'ev in, 122–23; Tarasevich in, 122, 159; tension with All-Russian Union of Towns, 139; in the war, 108, 112–15, 128–30. *See also* Physicians, union; Voluntary organizations, wartime

Almazov, V. I.: appointed commissar of Sanitary and Evacuation Section, 145; and the Army, 146; asks cooperation of wartime voluntary organizations, 145–46; and Joint Sanitary Organization for the Northern Region, 145; and medical reform, 145, 150, 151; meets with Diatroptov, Tarasevich, and Merkulov, 145–46; and military medical coordination, 145–46; and Ministry of the Interior, 154–56; proposes Central Medical-Sanitary Council, 153–54, 156–57, 161; and Red Cross, 146; and Rein, 145; temporary advisory committee to, 156–57, 159, 162

American Medicine and the Public Interest (Stevens), xv–xvi

Amsterdamskii, A. V., 57–58

Antiepidemic campaign: Bolshevik government and, 186–88; congress (1918), 187–88; and preventive vaccination program as political issue, 187–88

Antiepidemic campaign, wartime: Army intervenes on behalf of, 131–32, 136; Council of Ministers denies funds for, 129–31; and disinfection program, 125–26, 128–29; and isolation facilities, 128–29, 131; Maklakov denies funds for, 129–31; Pirogov Society and, 128–29, 131; and preventive vaccination program, 128, 131, 135; Special Commission for Measures against Plague and, 130–32, 135; Special Council for Defense and, 131–32; success of, 131–32; Sysin and, 165, 202; union physicians and, 128–32

Antiplague Commission. *See* Special Commission for Measures against Plague

Antituberculosis League. *See* All-Russian League for Struggle with Tuberculosis

Antsiferov, N. N., 93–95

Army: Almazov and the, 146; democratization of, 161, 169; intervenes on behalf of wartime antiepidemic campaign, 131–32, 136; low status of physicians in, 25; Provisional Government and loyalty of, 162; Provisional Government and reform of, 144–45, 149; retreats, 119; tsar assumes command of the, 111, 120; wartime voluntary organizations provide medical services to, 108–9, 116–17, 158, 166, 200

Army medical corps: cooperates with Red Cross, 112, 117, 168; inadequacy of, 108, 110–11, 158, 171–72, 200; inspectors in, 4–5, 9, 110; and reform of, 159

"Authority of knowledge" vs. "authority of

office," 28, 29–30, 31, 36–37, 38, 80, 105–6

Avdakov, N. S., 89

Bacteriologists: and "Cholera" Congress of 1905, 44; cooperate with Bolshevik government, 187; criticize zemstvo medicine, 65; and formation of medical union, 38; political activism among, 35, 37–38; and public health policy, 30, 35–38, 65; in Revolution of 1905, 200; support central health administration, 148; and wartime epidemics, 121, 128

Bacteriology: community phyisicians and, 36, 51, 56, 65–66, 199; criticism of, 35–36, 51, 56; Erismann on, 35–36, 51; at Imperial Military-Medical Academy, 36; at Institute of Experimental Medicine, 36, 188; Mechnikov and, 35–36; as medical specialization, 63–69

Bacteriology and Epidemiology, Conference on: 1st (1911), 65, 67; 2nd (1912), 69, 123–24

Bacteriology Institute, 36

Barsukov, M. I.: and Bolshevik government's health policy, 189; calls for popular support of medical reform, 178–79; as Commissar of Military Revolutionary Committee Medical-Sanitary Section, 173, 186; as Council of Medical Boards member, 185; and democratic social medicine, 174; on Lenin, 176; Lenin blocks proposals of, 174, 178, 180–81; on Pirogov Congress (1918), 183–84; Pirogov Society opposes proposals of, 174, 176–77; plans Committee for the Protection of Public Health, 175–77; and sovietization of Red Cross, 181

Battleship Potemkin (film), 25

Bekhterev, V. M.: as head of St. Petersburg Psycho-Neurological Institute, 134; as leading physician, 20; in Revolution of 1905, 134

Berdichevskii, G. A., 54–56

Berestnev, N. M. 35

Bismarck, Otto von, 51

Bloody Sunday massacre, 43, 44

Bogutskii, V. M., 146, 168, 171

Bolshevik government: and antiepidemic campaign, 186–88; bacteriologists cooperate with, 187, 188; blamed for state of public health in Russia, 183, 202; cadet rebellion against, 174; civil service strike against, 175; Military-Sanitary Administration opposes, 174; non-Bolshevik physicians cooperate with, 187, 188, 194; physicians and support of, 184–85;

Pirogov Congress (1918) denounces, 182–85, 194; Pirogov Society denounces, 176–78, 180, 201; and public health education, 186–87; public health policy of, 176, 186, 189–92, 195, 201–3; Red Cross opposes, 174; transferred to Moscow, 177, 185. *See also* Central Executive Committee of the Soviet (VTsIK); Sovnarkom

Bolshevik Revolution. *See* October Revolution (1917)

Bolsheviks, 43–44, 122, 168–71

Bonch-Bruevich, V. M., 173, *190;* and Bolshevik government's health policy, 189–90; and Commissariat of Health Protection, 192; at Congress of Soviet Medical Departments, 191

Botkin Commission, 82, 84, 202

Botkin, S. P., 6, 82, 107

Botkin, S. S., 20

Brand, Jeanne, xv

Brok, T. M., 65–66

Brown, Julie, 133

Brusilov, A. A. *(general),* 115

Bulygin, I. A., 48

Burdenko, N. N.: appointed Chief Military-Sanitary Inspector, 144, 159; as director of field hospitals, 144; as head of Main Military-Sanitary Council, 161; and military medical coordination, 144; and military medical reform, 159, 161

Catherine the Great *(empress),* xvii

Central Council, 152–53

Central Council of Fronts, 161

Central Executive Committee of the Soviet (VTsIK), 180–82. *See also* Bolshevik government; Sovnarkom

Central Medical Sanitary Council (CMSC), 175, 181, 183, 188; Almazov proposes, 153–54, 156–57, 161; Chief Medical Inspector ordered to cooperate with, 157; and Council of Ministers, 168; and democratization of hospital management, 167; Diatroptov as president of, 170, 177, 181; dissolution of, 177, 179, 183; February Revolution and, 167–68; ineffectiveness of, 168, 194, 201; and local medical reform, 167–68, 169, 172; meets with Pirogov Society, 181–82; Ministry of the Interior and, 154–55; Petrograd Soviet and, 163; Pirogov Society and, 155, 159; plenary meeting (1917), 165, 166–68, 170, 172; proposed representation on, 154; and Provisional Government, 165, 168–69; Solov'ev attacks, 170–71, 186; Sovnarkom dissolves, 181–82; Standing Council, 165–66, 167;

Sysin and, 166; Tarasevich and, 160; union physicians and, 154, 201

Central War Industries Committee, 144, 154

Chadwick, Edwin, 74

Chambers of Physicians (Germany), 40

Chief Medical Inspector, Office of, 150, 151, 153, 155; opposes Military Revolutionary Committee Medical-Sanitary Section, 175; ordered to cooperate with Central Medical-Sanitary Council, 157

Clinical Institute of Grand Duchess Elena Pavlova, 19–20, 83

Commissariat for Internal Affairs (NKVD), 180, 186. *See also* Ministry of the Interior

Commissariat for Local Self-Government, 180

Commissariat of Health Protection (NKZ): and antiepidemic campaign, 193; authority of, 192–93; established, xvi, 191–94; jurisdiction over military medicine, 193–94; Solov'ev and, 166, 202

Commissariat of Labor, 195

Commissariat for Military Affairs, 174. *See also* Ministry of War

Commissariat of Popular Enlightenment, 175

Commissariat of State Welfare, 175

Commissariat of Ways and Communications, 175. *See also* Ministry of Ways and Communications

Commission to Reform Higher Educational Institutions, 87

Committee for the Protection of Public Health, 175–77

Community medicine. *See* Zemstvo medicine

Community Physician. See Obshchestvennyi Vrach (periodical)

Community physicians, xvii–xviii, 4, 25; and bacteriology, 36, 51, 56, 65–66, 199; collegial activities among, 33; conservative reaction among, 50–51, 136; dissatisfaction with union physicians, 158; dominate Pirogov Society, 28, 42, 109; expanded opportunities in the war, 108–9, 120–21, 128, 158, 200; as generalists, 61–62; Igumnov on traditional role of, 55–56, 72; and local Bolshevik disruption, 180; at May Congress (1905) of Union of Unions, 47; and medical professionalism, 109; and medical reform, 109, 163–64, 169, 198; and medical reform proposal, 146–47; Ministry of War conscripts, 118–19, 158, 167, 171; misunderstanding of sanitary reform outside Russia, 73–74; and mobiliza-

66, 89–90, 97; cholera (1918), 186,
187–88, 193; fear of, 37–38; government
ignores in wartime, 120; prisoners of
war and, 128; Red Cross and, 57, 89;
Sanitary-Executive Commissions' ineffectiveness against, 66, 90, 164–65; and
social disorder, 91; as threat to authority, 78; *Uezd* physicians ineffective
against, 66, 90, 99; zemstvo medicine's
ineffectiveness against, 66, 78, 90
Epidemics, wartime: bacteriologists and,
121; causes of, 117–20, 200; community
physicians and, 121–23; Ministry of the
Interior and, 130–32; refugees and,
119–20, 128, 131, 200; Rein on, 140; results of, 131–32
Epidemiology. *See* Bacteriology
Erismann, F. F., 22, 61, 199; on bacteriology, 35–36, 51; and public health
reform, 7–8
Evdokimov, A. Ia.: as Chief Military-
Medical Inspector, 19; as Chief Military-
Sanitary Inspector, 111, 117, 130–31, 144;
and definition of mental illness,
133–34; and mentally ill soldiers,
133–34; refuses to cooperate with Red
Cross, 111; resigns, 144

Factory medicine, 52; first All-Russian
congress (1909), 64; government and,
65; as medical specialization, 62–65,
199; relationship to zemstvo medicine,
64–65, 150, 199
Factory physicians, 62, 64
February Revolution (1917), 132, 138–39,
142, 152, 201; and Central Medical-
Sanitary Council, 167–68; failure of the,
168, 169; and medical reform, 160, 162,
167, 169; Ministry of the Interior and
the, 156–57; peasants and the, 167; Red
Cross supports the, 145; Zhbankov and
the, 143, 194
Fenomenov, N. N., 19
Ferro, Marc, 168
Fischer, Alfons, xv
Fleet Sanitary Administration, 153
Fortunatova, T. A., 174, 178
France: sanitary medicine in, 73–74
Freiberg, N. G., 96
Frenkel', Z. G., 171
Frieden, Nancy, 4, 25, 36, 42; on "Cholera"
Congress of 1905, 45; *Russian Physi-
cians in an Age of Reform and Revolu-
tion, 1856–1905*, xix–xx
Front physicians. *See* Physicians, army
Fundamental Laws (Article 18), 139–40,
141

Gabrichevskii, G. N., 35; at "Cholera" Con-
gress of 1905, 44; establishes Bacteri-
ology Institute, 36
Gamaleia, N. F.: serves on the Rein Com-
mission, 96, 199; supports centralized
public health administration, 74–76,
96, 199
Germany: sanitary reform in, 75, 94,
199–200; social medicine in, 51
*Geschichte des Deutsches Gesundheits-
wesens* (Fischer), xv
Gigiena i Sanitariia (periodical), 74, 76, 96
Gleason, William, 108
Golitsyn Hospital (Moscow), 163
Golovinskii, M. V., 185, 195
Golubkov, A. P., 186, 192
Gorodovoi physicians: functions of,
16–18; proposed disbanding of, 157;
working conditions of, 18
Government, local, 135–39
Government, prerevolutionary. *See*
Tsarist government
Gran', M. M., 63, 174
Granovskii, L. B., 138–39; background of,
124; and medical reform proposal, 152;
in Revolution of 1905, 124; and role of
technology in public health reform,
124; supports Bolsheviks, 171
Great Britain: medical practices in, 74;
sanitary reform in, 73–74, 75, 94,
199–200
Gubert, V. O., 20
Guchkov, A. I., 144

Health. *See* Public Health
Healthification *(ozdorovlenie)*, xv–xvi, 28,
45, 48, 50, 105, 171, 201
Hoppe-Seyler, Felix, 21
Hospital Insurance Law, 150
Hospital management: Congress of Soviet
Medical Departments on, 195; democ-
ratization of, 167; hostility toward re-
form of, 32–33; Rubel' on reform of, 33;
Society of Hospital Physicians of St.
Petersburg attempts to reform, 31–35,
43
Hospitals: authoritarian management of,
in St. Petersburg, 30–35; collegial man-
agement of, in St. Petersburg, 30–31; in-
effective supervision of, 15; Military-
Sanitary Administration of, 117; in St.
Petersburg, 19, 20, 30–35; wartime
shortage of, 128–29; workers' control
of, 150, 152
Hospital Statute of 1894, 73, 76, 78
Hospital trains, 116–18
Hygiene. *See* Public health; Sanitary
reform

Main Medical Administration: Botkin Commission recommends, 82, 84, 202; proposed in Ministry of the Interior, 9–10, 82–83; Von Anrep supports, 84, 202

Main Military-Sanitary Council, 161

Makarov, A. A., 95–96

Maklakov, N. A.: denies funds for wartime antiepidemic campaign, 129–31; dismissed from office, 132; as Minister of the Interior, 115

Malaria, 36

Malinovskii, L. N.: ambitions of, 95; as Chief Medical Inspector, 81, 85, 93, 94–95; and the Kryzhanovskii Conference, 93, 94–95, 151; serves on the Rein Commission, 96

Mandel'berg, Dr. 167, 171

Manifesto of 17 October 1905, 48–49, 84

Markuzon, F. D., 169

Martsinovskii, E. I., 187

May Conference of Commissar Almazov (1917), 156–57, 160, 164, 165

Mechnikov, I. I., 35–36, 122

Mechnikova, Olga, 122

Medical collegiality, 31, 143, 198

Medical coordination, military: Almazov and, 145–46; Burdenko and, 144; Pirogov Society and, 144, 146; Von Anrep and, 145–46

Medical Council, 20, 21, 24, 75, 84, 134; dissolved, 188; ignores wartime epidemics, 120; ineffectiveness of, 5–6, 10, 82–83; and Kryzhanovskii Conference, 92; Main Administration for State Health Protection and 98–99; and medical reform, 84–85, 93; as political threat to Ministry of the Interior, 82–83; proposed reform of, 9–11; Ragozin as president of, 11, Ragozin and reorganization of, 11–13; Rein appointed president of, 85, 88; Rein as member of, 87; Sirotinin proposes reorganization of, 152; Zhbankov demands elimination of, 150

Medical Department. *See* Ministry of the Interior (MVD)

Medical Edict, 24–25

Medical education, 151; Main Administration for State Health Protection and, 99–100, 105–6

Medical inspectors, provincial, 16–17, 165

Medical Life (periodical), 168–72

Medical private practice. *See* Physicians: in private practice

Medical professionalism, 151, 183–84; government and problem of, 80–82, 101; Gran' on problem of, 63; Main Admin-

istration for State Health Protection and problem of, 101–3, 106; physicians and problem of, 62–63, 106; Pirogov Society and problem of, 62–63; and proposed central health administration, 8–9; Rein and, 101, 141

Medical reform: Almazov and, 145, 150, 151; Central Medical-Sanitary Council and, 167–68, 169, 172; community physicians and, 109, 163–64, 169, 198; Duma and, 96; February Revolution and, 160, 162, 167, 169; government and, 78–82, 84–85, 88–89, 99–100, 128; Kiriakov and, 164, 165–66, 167; Lenin on, 176; Medical Council and, 84–85, 93; Ministry of the Interior and, 79–80, 151, 164, 169; Moscow Soviet and, 163, 187; Petrograd Soviet and, 162–63; Pirogov Congress (1917) proposes, 146, 149–53, 159–60; Pirogov Society and, 163–64; Pirogov Society as obstacle to, 148; Provisional Government and, 143–46, 149, 151–52, 159, 160, 169, 201; Sanitary-Executive Commissions and, 80; Stolypin and, 84–85, 88, 91–93, 151, 198; Von Anrep on, 83–85, 91; zemstvo medicine as obstacle to, 79, 91, 93, 151–52, 194, 197. *See also* Public health reform

Medical reform, military: Army physicians and, 158–59, 169; Burdenko and, 159, 161; Ministry of War and, 161; Tarasevich and, 161; union physicians and, 161, 169

Medical research: criticism of, 56; Igumnov on, 67; Main Administration for State Health Protection and, 100; Ministry of the Interior Medical Department and, 79; and public health policy, 30; sanitary physicians and, 66–67; tsarist government supports, 29–30; *Uchastok* physicians and, 66–67

Medical-Sanitary Bureau (Soviet), 170, 171

Medical societies, 38, 62–63, 105

Medical specialization: bacteriology as, 63–69; Ministry of the Interior's hostility toward, 85; Munblit attacks, 71–72; Pirogov Society's hostility toward, 51–52, 63–64, 70–71, 199; psychiatry as, 133; sanitary engineering as, 70–71

Medical students, 119

Medical unions, 28–29, 38, 44–48, 52–53, 62, 102, 105, 181–82, 198

Medicine, 73–77, 78–79, 99–100

Medicine, industrial. *See* Factory medicine; Occupational medicine

Medicine, social. *See* Social medicine

Medicine, zemstvo. *See* Zemstvo medicine

Mensheviks, 44, 173, 177, 191

Mentally ill soldiers, 128; Council of Ministers and, 133, 135; Council of Ministers refuses funding for, 134–35; Evdokimov and, 133–34; Military-Sanitary Administration and, 132; Ol'denburg and, 134; psychiatrists and, 132–33; Red Cross and, 132–35; Sisters of Mercy and, 133–34; union physicians and, 132–35

Merkulov, A. N., 146

Military-Medical Administration, 25, 110

Military Revolutionary Committee (MRC), 173–75, 176

Military-Sanitary Administration, 90, 153; ignores wartime epidemics, 120; ineffectiveness of hospitals, 117; ineffectiveness of management, 158; and Joint Sanitary Organization for the Northern Region, 144; and mentally ill soldiers, 132; opposes the Bolshevik government, 174; relations with wartime voluntary organizations, 112, 127; reorganization of, 110, 160–61; transferred to Commissariat of Health Protection, 193–94; transferred to Council of Medical Boards, 180

Ministry of Education, 157

Ministry of Finance, 99, 157

Ministry of the Imperial Court, 98

Ministry of the Interior (MVD), 121, 150, 160, 165, 199, 201; Almazov and, 154–56; and Central Medical-Sanitary Council, 154–55; and "Cholera" Congress of 1905, 44; Economic Department, 10–11; established, xvii; and the February Revolution, 156–57; hostility toward medical specialization, 85; ignores wartime epidemics, 120; innovation in, 82; inspectors in, 112; Main Administration for Local Economic Affairs, 12, 35, 83–84, 92, 93–94, 141; and Main Administration for State Health Protection, 98–99, 102; Medical Council as political threat to, 82–83; Medical Department, 5, 9–10, 79; and medical reform, 79–80, 151, 164, 169; and medical research, 79; Plehve reorganizes, 11, 79, 83, 180; proposed Main Medical Administration in, 9–10, 82–83; and public health policy, 1–2, 37–38, 74–75, 197–98; reorganization of, 79; St. Petersburg Physicians' Mutual Assistance Society as rival to, 40–41; Uvarov in, 150–51; Veterinary Committee, 98–99; and wartime epidem-

ics, 130–32; and zemstvo medicine, 151. *See also* Commissariat for Internal Affairs

Ministry of Labor, 157, 170

Ministry of Public Health: proposed establishment of, 74–76, 79, 82; Rein recommends establishment of, 90–91, 93–94, 115–16, 120–21, 154

Ministry of Public Instruction, 21

Ministry of War, 37, 90, 98; Army physicians and, 161; conscript community and sanitary physicians, 118–19, 167, 171; and military medical reform, 161; Solov'ev attacks, 171; and transportation of "unreliables," 117–18, 128, 200. *See also* Commissariat for Military Affairs

Ministry of Ways and Communications, 157. *See also* Commissariat of Ways and Communications

Ministry of Welfare, 157

Mitskevich, S. I.: at "Cholera" Congress of 1905, 46; in Commissariat for Internal Affairs, 180; on fall of Provisional Government, 175; at May Congress (1905), 47; radical politics of, 43–44, 173; in Revolution of 1905, 43, 173

Molleson, I. I., 199

Moscow: Bolshevik government transferred to, 177, 185; Hospital Commission, 32; medical establishment in, 24; municipal Duma of, 32, 163; public health administration in, 16, 17; radical medical activities in, 43

Moscow Commissariat of Public Health, 185

Moscow Higher Women's Courses, 122

Moscow Psychiatric Commission, 135

Moscow–St. Petersburg Medical Society. *See* Pirogov Society of Russian Physicians

Moscow Sanitary Bureau, 123–24

Moscow Society of Factory Physicians, 43

Moscow Soviet, 163, 187

Moscow Stock Exchange, 97

Moscow Union of Medical Workers, 183

Moscow University, 36, 39, 121

Moscow Zemstvo Union, 187

Munblit, E. G., 71–72

Municipal physicians. *See* Community physicians

Municipal Statute (1892), 4, 94, 127

Nesterenko, A. I., 187, 191, 193

Neznamov, E. A., 96

Nicholas II (*tsar*), 7, 8, 29, 75, 88, 90, 109; abdication of, 142, 143, 167; approves establishment of Rein Commission, 96;

Physicians, union (*continued*)
with, 158; and Council of Ministers, 140;
demand postwar political reforms, 136,
141, 201; exempt from conscription, 158;
frustration of, 132; future plans by,
135–39; hostility to Bolsheviks, 172;
hostility to Red Cross, 132–33, 134; and
lack of funding for mentally ill soldiers,
135; and medical reform proposal, 148;
and mentally ill soldiers, 132–35; and
military medical reform, 161; and mobilization of physicians, 159; perform
preventive vaccinations, 131; postwar
plans of, 147; and public health financing, 165; radical politics among, 132;
and reform of Army medical corps, 159;
Rein and, 140–41; and the Soviets, 163;
support central health administration,
148; and tuberculosis, 136; and venereal
disease, 135–36; and wartime antiepidemic campaign, 128–32
Pirogov Commission on Epidemics, 188,
193; Sysin as head of, 186–87, 189
Pirogov Congresses, 8, 9, 23, 42, 123; 2nd
(1881), 7, 35; 3rd (1889), 38; 6th (1896),
7–8; 9th (1904), 44; 10th (1907), 52–53,
56, 62, 64; 11th (1910), 63, 64–65, 72, 74;
12th (1913), 69, 72, 77; antiepidemic conferences (1914–15), 128–29; call for mobilization of physicians (1917), 159–60,
171; call for political reforms (1916), 137,
141; of 1917, 143, 146, 158; "Cholera" Congress of 1905, 35, 38, 44–47, 49, 52, 80,
137, 198; criticized (1918), 183–84, 189;
denounce the Bolshevik government
(1918), 182–85, 189, 194; Extraordinary
(1916), 127, 132, 136–37; and formation
of medical union, 28–29; and the mentally ill, 133; of 1918, 186; propose medical reform (1917), 146, 152–53, 154, 155,
159–60, 195; and zemstvo medicine
(1918), 183
Pirogov Society of Russian Physicians,
xvii, 4, 157, 168, 172, 195, 201; anti-
Bolshevik declaration of, 176–78, 180,
201; association with Tarasevich, Diatroptov, and Solov'ev, 123, 170; and
Central Medical Sanitary Council, 155,
159; Central Medical Sanitary Council
meets with, 181–82; Commission for
the Diffusion of Popular Hygiene Education, 70–71; community physicians
dominate, 28, 42, 109; and compilation
of medical statistics, 100; conservative
reaction to, 50–51; criticizes bacteriology, 51; criticizes Special Commission for Measures against Plague, 130;
decline in membership of, 62; defends

zemstvo medicine, 104–5; denounces
Rein Commission proposals, 104,
149–51; Eberman and formation of, 38;
establishment of, xviii, 38; excluded
from the Rein Commission, 97, 101;
government interferes with, 62–63;
government's reaction against, 52; hostility toward medical specialization,
51–52, 63–64, 70–71, 199; increased
militancy in, 42–43, 87, 109; journal
(see *Obshchestvennyi Vrach*); Lenin's
relations with, 175–77, 178; and local
medical reform, 163–64; Malaria Commission, 36–37; and medical collegiality, 31, 143; and medical reform
proposal, 147; and military medical
coordination, 144, 146; as obstacle to
medical reform, 148; opposes Barsukov's proposals, 174, 176–77; opposes
central health administration, 8–9, 11,
82–83, 176; opposes state involvement
in public health, 77; Petrograd Soviet
and, 163; and problem of medical professionalism, 62–63; and proposed
new union, 52–54; and public health
education, 70–71, 101; and public
health reform, 7–8, 28, 198; rejects Sulima's proposals, 104; relations with
wartime voluntary organizations,
127–28; Rusakov and, 123; Rusakov and
Solov'ev resign from, 177, 186; and St.
Petersburg Physicians' Mutual Assistance Society, 42; survey of public
health (1913), 116; Veger and, 177; and
wartime antiepidemic campaign,
128–29; wartime increase in power of,
127–28; Zhbankov as administrator of,
60, 143, 145. *See also* All-Russian Pirogov Society
Plague Fort (Kronstadt), 120
Plehve, V. K.: assassinated, 11, 13; as Minister of the Interior, 11, 33, 79, 83; reorganizes Ministry of the Interior, 11, 79, 83,
180
Pliushchevskii-Pliushchik, Ia. A., 96
Poliak, I. V., 76
Police, 15–16
Police physicians. *See Gorodovoi*
physicians
Political activism: among bacteriologists,
35, 37–38; among community physi-
cians, 4, 33–35, 36
Political reform, 137
Prisoners of war, 128
Proletarian Red Cross, 174–75, 178. *See
also* Red Cross
Provisional Government, xx, 175; and
Army reform, 144–45, 149; Central

Medical Sanitary Council and, 168–69; Constitutional Democratic Party and, 143; established, 142; establishes Central Medical Sanitary Council, 165; fall of, 172, 177; Kornilov's attempted coup against, 168; and loyalty of the Army, 162; L'vov as head of, 142, 144; and medical reform, 143–46, 149, 151–52, 159, 160, 169, 201; Mitskevitch on fall of, 175; and proposed Central Medical Sanitary Council, 153–54, 156–57; and public health financing, 165–66; Red Cross and, 144–45; Solov'ev attacks, 171, 186

Psychiatrists, 63, 132–33

Public health: community physicians' populist position on, 72–73, 76–77, 78, 97, 202; Gamaleia supports centralized administration of, 74–76, 96; ineffective local administration of, 12, 13–18, 75–76, 90; Kats opposes centralized administration of, 76–77; local government and, 135–36; Main Administration for State Health Protection and education in, 101; Pirogov Society and education in, 70–71, 101; Pirogov Society opposes state involvement in, 77; as political issue, xv–xvii, 1, 88–89, 92–93, 167–70; Provisional Government and financing of, 165–66; Solov'ev on reform of, 170; Soviets and, 183; state of, in Europe, 1–2; state of, in Russia, 1–2, 78, 116, 138, 183, 197–98. *See also* Health; Sanitary physicians; Sanitary reform

Public health policy: bacteriologists and, 30, 35–38, 65; of Bolshevik government, 176, 186, 189–92, 195, 201–3; enforced by police, 15–16; medical research and, 30; Ministry of the Interior and, 1–2, 37–38, 74–75, 197–98; venereal disease and, 30

Public health reform: Botkin and, 6; in Germany, 51; and lack of centralized organization, 4–7; Orthodox Church and, 80; Pirogov Society and, 7–8, 28, 198; resolution in Duma for, 92–93; Revolution of 1905 and, 28–29, 47, 78–79; role of technology in, 124; Sipiagin opposes, 11; Veliaminov on, 1–3, 4–5, 9–11, 17. *See also* Medical reform

Ragozin, L. F., 11–13
Red Army, 194
Red Cross. *See* Proletarian Red Cross; Russian Red Cross
Red Guards, 172, 174, 180, 194

Refugees, wartime, 119–20, 128, 131, 200

Rein, G. E., *103*, 152, 179, 192, 195; Almazov and, 145; appointed Main Administrator for State Health Protection, 140, 142; appointed President of the Medical Council, 85, 88; arrested by Provisional Government, 142, 143, 168; background of, 86; and cholera epidemic of 1909, 88; and cholera epidemic of 1910, 89–90, 97; elected to the Duma, 86, 87–88; and government medical reform, 82, 115–16; as landowner, 87; and medical professionalism, 141; as member of the Medical Council, 87; monarchist politics of, 85–89, 105–6, 141; and problem of medical professionalism, 101; as proponent of antisepsis, 86, 88; recommends establishment of central health administration, 90–91, 93–94, 115–16, 120–21, 139–41, 154, 194, 199, 202; on Sanitary-Executive Commissions, 90; and sanitary reform, 105; serves on Kryzhanovskii Conference, 92–94; supports tsarist government, 85–86; and union physicians, 140–41; and the war, 106–7, 108, 115–16, 120, 128, 130, 139, 200; on wartime epidemics, 140; and zemstvo medicine, 86–87, 93–94, 139–41

Rein Commission, 140–41; activities of, 96–98, 199; broad membership of, 96–97; Diatroptov denounces, 104; disbanded, 149–50; Durnovo denounces, 104; Makarov supports establishment of, 95–96; nonpolitical approach of, 97; Pirogov Society denounces proposals of, 104, 149–51; Pirogov Society excluded from, 97, 101; proposes Councils of Physicians, 102–3; proposes establishment of Main Administration for State Health Protection (GUGZ), 19, 98–99, 105–6, 108–9, 115–16; Tsar and Council of Ministers approve establishment of, 96; zemstvo medicine and proposals of, 104–6, 108–9

Revolution of 1905, xx, 23, *39*, 85, 87, 109; bacteriologists in, 200; Bekhterev in, 134; community physicians in, 28–29, 30, 43, 80, 84, 109; failure of, 29, 48–49, 50, 73, 136, 198, 200; Granovskii in, 124; Mitskevich in, 43, 173; and public health reform, 28–29, 47, 78–79; Tarasevich and, 121

Rodzianko, M. V., 110
Rosenberg, William, 167
Rozanov, P. P., 45
Rubel', A. N., 33, 35

Rusakov, I. V., 185; in All-Russian Union of Medical Personnel, 123; background of, 123; and Commissariat of Health Protection, 192; and Congress of Medical Workers, 182; at Congress of Soviet Medical Departments, 190–91; on Pirogov Congress (1918), 183; and Pirogov Society, 123; radical politics of, 43, 123; resigns from Pirogov Society, 177; supports Bolsheviks, 169, 177; on zemstvo medicine, 171–72

Russia: effects of medical advances in, 51–52; political divisions, *xxii;* public health survey in (1913), 116; state of public health in, 1–2, 78, 116, 138, 183, 197–98

Russian Physicians in an Age of Reform and Revolution, 1856–1905 (Frieden), xix–xx

Russian Red Cross, 24, 25, 140, 161, 189; Almazov and, 146; Army medical corps cooperates with, 112, 117, 168; asks for supreme wartime medical authority, 145; Barsukov and sovietization of, 181; and cadet rebellion, 174; and epidemics, 57, 89; Evdokimov refuses to cooperate with, 111; Guchkov and, 144; hostility toward union physicians, 132–33, 134; and Joint Sanitary Organizations for the Northern Region, 144; and mentally ill soldiers, 132–35; nursing school, 19, 20; Ol'denburg as head of, 111; opposes Bolshevik government, 174–75; physicians exempt from conscription, 158; Pirogov Congress (1916) attacks, 137; and Provisional Government, 144–45, 165; and reform of Army medical corps, 159; and the Rein Commission, 97; relations with wartime voluntary organizations, 112, 115, 127; reorganized and assets nationalized, 181; sovietization of, 178; supports the February Revolution, 145; Von Anrep on executive board of, 112. *See also* Proletarian Red Cross

Russian Society for the Protection of Public Health, 20, 21, 22, 30

Russian Union of Psychiatrists, 133

St. Petersburg: City Duma, 89; hospitals in 19, 20, 30–35; medical establishment in, 18–24, 28, 43, 197; medical establishment's political position, 49, 80; municipal Duma of, 31; public health administration in, 16, 17; threatened by the Germans, 172. *See also* Petrograd

St. Petersburg Obstetrics and Gynecology Society, 87

St. Petersburg Physicians' Mutual Assistance Society (SPMAS), 22, *33,* 53; activities of, 42, 101–2; Eberman as first president of, 38; formation of, 38–40; Nizhegorodtsev and purpose of, 40–41, 42, 47; and Pirogov Society, 42; as rival to Ministry of the Interior Medical Department, 40–41

St. Petersburg Psycho-Neurological Institute, 134

Sanitary and Evacuation Section: Almazov appointed commissar of, 145; discontinued, 144–45, 160; Ol'denburg appointed Supreme Head of, 111–12, 200; proposal to disband, 153

Sanitary engineering: in All-Russian union of Towns, 138; and cholera epidemic of 1910, 90; community physicians and, 69–71; Igumnov on, 72; introduction of, 69; Kost' promotes, 69, 72; as medical specialization, 70–71; Nikolaevskii promotes, 138; outside Russia, 71; sanitary physicians and, 70; Sysin promotes, 69; as threat to zemstvo medicine, 69–72, 199; Tsvetaev promotes, 69

Sanitary-Executive Commissions (SECs), 28, 73; community physicians oppose, 37–38, 80; disbanded, 165–66; establishment of, 36; function of, 61; ineffectiveness against epidemics, 66, 90, 164–65; and medical reform, 80; operations of, 37–38; physicians boycott, 45–46; as political issue, 45–46; Rein on, 90; *uchastok* physicians and, 71, 72

Sanitary physicians, 123; in All-Russian Union of Towns, 138; Conference of (1912), 69, 76; ineffectiveness of, 72, 90; and medical research, 66–67; Ministry of War conscripts, 118; and proposed Ministry of Public Health, 75; qualifications of, 63; and sanitary engineering, 70; Sysin's ideal of, 70; *uchastok* physicians as, 61, 72; wartime shortage of, 128–29; and zemstvo medicine, 105

Sanitary reform: All-Russian Union of Towns and, 128, 136; in France, 73–74; in Germany, 75, 94; in Great Britain, 73–74, 75, 94; Iakovenko on, 67–69; in Japan, 75; in Military-Medical Administration, 110; Rein and, 105; Sysin and, 123–24; in the United States, 75. *See also* Public health

Science, physicians' faith in, 32, 37

Semashko, N. A., *190;* and Bolshevik government's health policy, 189–90, 195; in Commissariat for Internal Affairs medical college, 186; as Commissar of

Health Protection, 190, 192–93; at Congress of Soviet Medical Departments, 190; as member of Council of Medical Boards, 185; in the October Revolution (1917), 185; and reorganization of All-Russian Union of Towns, 181

Shcherbatov, Prince, 132

Sheremet'ev, Count S. D., 163

Sheremet'ev Hospital (Moscow), 163

Shidlovskii, K. I., 8–9, 149

Shidlovskii, S. V., 23

Shingarev, A. I.: and centralized public health administration, 77; criticizes zemstvo medicine, 65, 74; as Minister of Agriculture, 143

Shvaitsar, S. M., 43

Sinandino, P. V., 92

Sipiagin, D. S., 9–10, 11

Sirotinin, V. N., 20, 152

Sisters of Mercy, 133–34

Slavskii, K. G., 59–60, 61

Social Democratic Party, 122–24

Socialist Revolutionary Party, 44, 173, 177, 191

Social medicine. See Democratic social medicine

Society of Hospital Physicians of St. Petersburg, 31–35, 43

Society of Physicians of Petrograd, 152

Solov'ev, Z. P., *166*; in All-Russian Union of Zemstvos, 122–23, 136, 189; association with Pirogov Society, 123, 170, 190, 201; attacks Central Medical-Sanitary Council, 170–71, 186; attacks conscription of physicians, 171–72; attacks ineffective local government, 136–37; attacks Ministry of War, 171; attacks Provisional Government, 171, 186; background of, 122–23, 189; and Bolshevik government's health policy, 186, 189–91, 195; and Commissariat of Health Protection, 166, 202; in Commissariat for Internal Affairs medical college, 186; and Congress of Soviet Medical Departments, 187, 189–90; on Council of Ministers, 132; demands democratic political reforms, 137; as Deputy Commissar of Health Protection, 192; in February Revolution, 160; and guidelines for learned advisory bodies, 188; as head of Commissariat for Internal Affairs Administration of the Medical Sector, 186; and medical reform proposal, 146, 168; and the October Revolution, 174, 201; as president of Commissariat for Internal Affairs, 186; on public health reform, 170; radical politics of, 122–23, 136–37, 189; resigns

from Pirogov Society, 177, 186; supports Bolsheviks, 166, 168–71, 177; supports centralized health administration, 189–92; supports Lenin, 186; and tuberculosis, 136, 189; wartime activities of, 121–23, 189; and wartime antiepidemic campaign, 128, 132

Soviets: demands by the, 163, 167, 169; evaluation of, 184; and public health, 183

Soviet Union. See Russia

Sovnarkom, 188, 192, 193; dissolves Central Medical Sanitary Council, 181–82. *See also* Bolshevik government; Central Executive Committee of the Soviet (VTsIK)

Special Commission for Measures against Plague, 6–7, 28, 29, 36–37, 73, 80, 188, 200; community physicians oppose, 83, 165; disbanding of, 167; Duma and Pirogov Society criticize, 130; ignores wartime epidemics, 120, 130–31; independent establishment of, 83; as political issue, 7, 45; and wartime antiepidemic campaign, 130–32, 135

Special Council for Defense, 131–32

Specialists, medical. See Medical specialization

State: medicine's proper relationship to the, 73–77, 78–79, 99–100. *See also* Tsarist government

State Control, Office of, 157

Stevens, Rosemary, *American Medicine and the Public Interest*, xv–xvi

Stolypin, P. A.: abandons proposed reforms, 50, 53, 65, 198; alters electoral law, 50, 53–54; assassinated, 95–96, 199; establishes Kryzhanovskii Conference, 92; and medical reform, 84–85, 88, 91–93, 151, 199; ordered by the tsar to eliminate epidemics, 85, 91; as premier, 50, 73; reaction to Revolution of 1905, 50, 52; and zemstvo medicine, 54, 91

Sukhomlinov, V. A., 111

Sulima, K. P., 101–3, 104

Sysin, A. N., 72, 138–39; and All-Russian Union of Towns, 165; background of, 123; and Bolshevik government's health policy, 186; and Central Medical Sanitary Council, 166; as community physician, 123; at Congress of Soviet Medical Departments, 190; cooperates with Bolshevik government, 186–87, 194; criticizes zemstvo medicine, 66; demands democratic political reforms, 137; and democratization of wartime voluntary organizations, 148–49, 160; in February

Sysin, A. N. (*continued*)
Revolution, 160; as head of Moscow
Sanitary Bureau, 69, 123–24; as head of
Pirogov Commission on Epidemics,
186–87, 189; on medical reform,
146–47; and medical reform proposal,
146, 168; on the October Revolution,
194; at Pirogov Congress (1918), 186; in
Pirogov Society, 186; promotes sanitary
engineering, 69; radical politics of, 71,
123, 137; and reorganization of All-
Russian Union of Towns, 181; and role
of technology in public health reform,
124; and sanitary medicine, 123–24;
supports Bolsheviks, 169, 171; wartime
activities of, 123–24; and wartime antiepidemic campaign, 128, 165, 194, 202

Tarasevich, L. A., 35, *68*, 72, 85, 172, 187; in
All-Russian Union of Zemstvos, 122,
159; appointed Chief Field Sanitary inspector, 161; association with Pirogov
Society, 123; attends May Conference,
156; background of, 121–23; calls for
mobilization of physicians, 159–60;
and Central Medical Sanitary Council,
160; as head of Central Council of
Fronts, 161; as head of Learned Medical Committee, 193; meets with Almazov, 145–46; and military medical
reform, 161; radical politics of, 122; and
Revolution of 1905, 121; teaches at
Moscow Higher Women's Courses, 122;
wartime activities of, 121–22; and wartime antiepidemic campaign, 128
Tatiana Committee, 140
Teziakov, N. I., *70*, 117
Timashev, S. I., 89
Treaty of Brest-Litovsk (1918), 185
Tsarist government: and factory medicine, 65; ineffectiveness of, in the war,
108–9, 120, 183; interferes with Pirogov
Society, 62–63; and medical reform,
78–82, 84–85, 88–89, 99–100, 128; nature of, 29–30; poor relations with the
Duma, 141; and problem of medical
professionalism, 80–82, 101; reaction
against Pirogov Society, 52; reaction to
Revolution of 1905, 50–51; Rein and
medical reform under, 82, 115–16; Rein
supports, 85–86; supports medical research, 29–30. *See also* State
Tsvetaev, A. A.: and Commissariat of
Health Protection, 192; and Military-
Sanitary Administration, 193–94; promotes sanitary engineering, 69; and
radical politics, 71

Tuberculosis, Solov'ev and, 136, 189
Tutyshkin, P. P., 149–52

Uchastok physicians, 59, 119, 123; as generalists, 61–62; idealization of, 61; and
medical research, 66–67; and Sanitary-
Executive Commissions, 71, 72; as sani-
tary physicians, 61, 72; working condi-
tions of, 64
Uezd physicians: functions of, 16–18, 26;
indifference toward zemstvo medicine,
58; ineffective against epidemics, 66,
90, 99; proposed disbanding of, 157;
working conditions of, 18, 57–58, 62, 67
Union of Liberation, 44
Union of Medical Workers Acknowledg-
ing Soviet Power, 185
Union of Michael the Archangel, 57
Union of Physicians of the Army and the
Fleet, 157, 160, 183
Union of the Russian People, 57
Union of 17 October 1905, 23, 49
Union of Unions, 47
United States, public health in, 75
Uvarov, M. S., *81;* and medical reform pro-
posal, 149–51; in Ministry of the Inte-
rior, 150–51

Vasilevskii, N. P., 170
Vecheslov, M. G., 173; and Commissariat
of Health Protection, 192; as member of
Council of Medical Boards, 185; and
public health education, 186–87
Veger, I. S.: and Commissariat of Health
Protection, 192; in Commissariat for In-
ternal Affairs, 180; and guidelines for
learned advisory bodies, 188; and Piro-
gov Society, 177; radical politics of, 173,
175–77
Veisbrod, B. S., 186
Veliaminov, N. A., *14;* as Chief Physician of
the Imperial Household and Court
Medical Inspector, 1, 9–10, 19, 96; personal ambitions of, 9–11; on public
health reform, 1–3, 4–5, 9–11, 17;
serves on Rein Commission, 96, 199
Venereal disease, 30, 135–36
Veresaev, V., *Notes of a Physician,* 25
Vigdorchik, N. A., 56–57
Vinokurov, A. N., 173, 175, 182; and Commissariat of Health Protection, 192; in
Commissariat for Internal Affairs, 180;
as Commissar of Social Welfare, 193;
and guidelines for learned advisory
bodies, 188; on Lenin, 176; as president
of Council of Medical Boards, 180
Vitte, G. G., 93–95

Voluntary organizations, wartime: Almazov asks cooperation of, 145–46; and medical reform proposal, 146–49; Ol'denburg cooperates with, 112–14, 129, 139; proposed democratization of, 148–49, 160; provide military medical services, 108–9, 116–17, 158, 168, 200; relations with Red Cross, 112, 115, 127. *See also* All-Russian Union of Towns; All-Russian Union of Zemstvos

Von Anrep, V. K., *81*, 107; background of, 83; as Chief Medical Inspector, 83, 146; as Deputy Head of Sanitary and Evacuation Section, 112; as Director of the Medical Department, 11, 83; elected to the Duma, 85, 92, 112; on medical reform, 83–85, 91; and military medical coordination, 145–46; on Red Cross executive board, 112; supports central health administration, 83, 84, 91, 92, 199, 202; on zemstvo medicine, 84

Vrachebnaia Gazeta (periodical), 183

Vrachebnaia Zhizn'. See Medical Life (periodical)

Vrachebno-Sanitarnyi Vestnik (periodical), 138

Vyskovich, V. K., 35

Warsaw, public health administration in, 16

Witte, S. Iu, 8, 106

Women's Medical Institute (Petrograd), 19, 24, 83, 187

Workers' Hospital Funds, 150, 152, 167, 170, 193, 199

World War I, xx, 19; activities of municipal dumas in, 109; cause of epidemics in, 117–20; community physicians' expanded opportunities in, 108–9, 120–21, 128, 158; disease among Russian soldiers in, 117; failure of medical leadership in, 120, 183; government's ineffectiveness in, 108–9, 120, 183; mental illness in, 128, 132–35; Rein and, 106–7, 108, 115–16, 120, 128, 130, 139, 200; Russian casualty rate in, 112–15; wartime voluntary organizations in, 108, 112–15, 158; zemstvo medicine depleted in, 118–19, 183

Zabolotnyi, D. K., 35, *68*, 85, 187–88; and cholera epidemic of 1910, 89; serves on the Rein Commission, 97

Zemstvo assemblies, xvii–xviii

Zemstvo medicine, xviiii–xix, 8, 11, 15, 24, 44, 169; achievements of, 72, 197; advantages of, 26; Amsterdamskii on, 57–58; bacteriologists criticize, 65; Berdichevskii on future of, 54–56; Brok attacks, 65–66; compared to democratic social medicine, 163; conservative reaction in, 49, 50–51, 52, 60, 121, 136, 198–99; depleted in the war, 118–19, 183; factory medicine's relationship to, 64–65, 150, 199; ideology of, 51, 56–57, 60–61, 63, 73, 147, 152, 199; Igumnov on traditional role of, 55–56, 61, 67; ineffectiveness of, against epidemics, 66, 78, 90; internal crisis in, 50–51, 55–61, 109, 198–99; Kurkin and effect of the war on, 118–19; Ministry of the Interior and, 151; as obstacle to medical reform, 79, 91, 93, 151–52, 194, 197; Pirogov Congress (1918) and, 183; Pirogov Society defends, 104–5; and proposals of the Rein Commission, 104–6, 108–9; and proposed Ministry of Public Health, 75; quality of, 59–60; Rein and, 86–87, 93–94, 139–41; Rusakov on, 171–72; sanitary engineering as threat to, 69–72, 199; sanitary physicians and, 105; Shingarev criticizes, 65, 74; Slavskii criticizes, 59–60, 61; state origins of, 73; Stolypin and, 54, 91; Sysin criticizes, 66; as threat to authority, 78; Von Anrep on, 84; Zhbankov on, 60, 72

Zemstvo physicians. *See* Community physicians

Zemstvo Statute (1890), 4, 94, 127, 137

Zhbankov, D. N., *57*; as administrator of Pirogov Society, 60, 143, 145; arrested, 62–63; criticizes private practice, 60–61, 195; demands elimination of the Medical Council, 150; and the February Revolution, 143, 194; and medical reform proposal, 149–50; opposes central health administration, 147–48; supports formation of Pirogov Society, 63; survey of public health (1913), 116; on zemstvo medicine, 60–61, 72

Zinoviev, G. E. 177

POLITICS AND PUBLIC HEALTH IN REVOLUTIONARY RUSSIA,
1890–1918

Designed by Christopher Harris/Summer Hill Books
Composed by G&S Typesetters, Inc., in Zapf Book Light and Demibold, and
   Zapf International Heavy
Printed by the Maple Press Company, Inc., on Glatfelter 50-lb Eggshell Cream
   offset paper